MEDITERRANEAN DIET
SPECIAL EDITION

4 Books in 1: A Simple Guide to Start the Mediterranean Diet suitable for Vegetarian and Athlete with more 400+ Recipes! 4-Week Keto Meal Plan Included! Start to be Healthy and Fit!

A collaboration between

Alexander Sandler

Elizabeth Roberts

Kristen Potter

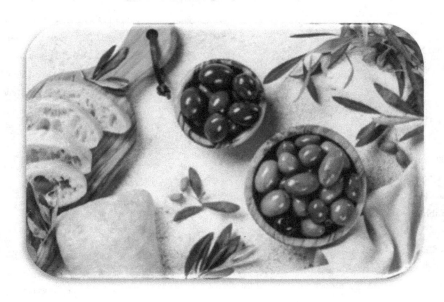

TABLE OF CONTENT

PART I: INTRODUCTION

Today, many people, especially teenagers, fill their plates with pizza, white bread, refined sugar, and processed food with lots of preservatives.

But analysis and research on processed foods such as frozen food, white bread, and carbonated beverages have led to surprising facts. Habitual consumption of these foods can tax the body. Excessive consumption can lead to high insulin production. This can cause diabetes, obesity, and coronary artery malfunction.

The reality of animal fats is not much different. Saturated fats in these foods can hurt our bodies. It causes the accumulation of extra fat in our body and disturbs our body mass index. Saturated fat in animal products like milk and butter increases lousy cholesterol or LDL. In short, it can damage the health of the coronary arteries.

In this technologically advanced society, when we can accomplish our tasks with little effort, physical activities are negligible. Poor health conveniently comes into play. It becomes essential to switch to a healthier diet that meets our body's nutritional needs while keeping us full.

The Mediterranean diet can do this. It is an eating pattern that overflows with whole grains, a plant-based diet in which olive oil is a fat source. This diet has no room for processed foods loaded with sugar or artificial sweeteners. The low amount of fat keeps your heart healthy and provides both essential nutrients and agility. Give it a try, and you won't look back. You will leap into a healthy future.

I wish you all the best in healthy eating.

START TO GET FAMILIAR WITH THE MEDITERRANEAN DIET

When you read the word "Mediterranean," you tend to think of the sea. This brings to mind seafood. The diet has its roots in the Mediterranean basin, a land that has historically been called a powerhouse of societal evolution. This area of the Nile Valley was good land for the peoples of the East and West. The frequent interaction of people from different regions and cultures had a significant effect on customs, languages, religion, and outlook and positively impacted lifestyles. This integration and cultural clash further influenced eating habits.

Looking at the Mediterranean diet's food content, one can see the reflection of different cultures and classes. Bread, wine, and oil reflect agriculture; lettuce, mushrooms, and mallow further complement this. There is a slight preference for meat but much preference for fish and seafood. This shows the greedy nature of the people of Rome. Here we also have the Germanic flavor of pork with garden vegetables. Beer was made from grains.

The food culture of bread, wine, and oil went beyond the Germanic and Christian Roman culture and entered the borders of the Arabs. The reason was their existence on the southern shore of the Mediterranean. Their food culture was unique because of the variety of leafy vegetables they grew. They had eggplant, spinach, sugarcane, and fruits such as oranges, citrus, lemon, and pomegranate. This influenced the cooking style of the Latinos and influenced their recipes.

The great geographical event that is the discovery of America by Europeans has a great additional impact on the Mediterranean diet. This event added several new foods such as beans, potatoes, tomatoes, chili peppers, and peppers. The tomato, the red plant, was first ornamental and then considered edible. It then became an essential part of the Mediterranean diet.

Historical analysis of the Mediterranean diet shows how the Egyptians' diet at the discovery of America gave us the Mediterranean diet of today. The Mediterranean diet's nutritional model is intimately linked to the Mediterranean people, lifestyle, and history.

Some established health and cultural platforms, such as UNESCO, define the Mediterranean diet, explaining the meaning of the word "diet," which comes from the word "data," meaning lifestyle or way of life. It focuses on food from landscape to table, covering cooking, harvesting, processing, preparation, fishing, cooking, and a specific form of consumption.

There is a variation in the Mediterranean diet in different countries due to ethnic and cultural differences, other religions, and economic disparity. According to the description and recommendation of dieticians and food experts, the Mediterranean diet has the proportion of the following food. In grains, there are whole grains and legumes. For fats, olive oil is the primary source. Onion, garlic, tomatoes, leafy greens, and peppers are the main vegetables. Fresh fruit is the main one in snacks and desserts. Eggs, milk, yogurt, and other dairy products are taken moderately. Foods such as red meat, processed foods, and refined sugar are handled as little as possible.

This diet has a fat ratio of 25% to 35% in calories, and saturated fat never exceeds 8%. As for oil, alternatives are depending on the region. In central and northern Italy, butter and lard are commonly used in cooking. Olive is used primarily for snacks and salad dressing.

This diet reflects Crete's dietary pattern, the rest of Greece, and much of Italy in the early 1960s. It gained widespread recognition in the 1990s. There is an irony to the Mediterranean diet. Although people who live in this region tend to consume a high amount of fat, they enjoy much better cardiovascular health than people in America who consume an equal amount of fat.

The Mediterranean diet tradition offers a cuisine rich in color, taste, flavor, and aroma. Above all, it keeps us closer to nature. It may be simple in appearance, but rich in health and has much to offer that is in no way inferior to any other healthy diet. Some Americans describe the Mediterranean diet as homemade pasta with parmesan sauce and enriched with a few pieces of meat. It includes lots of fresh vegetables with just olive oil drizzled on top. Desserts in this diet include fresh fruit.

An excellent Mediterranean diet does not include soy, canola, or any other refined oil. There is no room for processed meat, refined sugar, white bread, refined grains, white pasta, or pizza dough containing white flour.

This diet features a balanced use of foods with high amounts of fiber, unsaturated fat s, and antioxidants. Besides, there is an approach that prioritizes health by cutting unhealthy animal fats and meat consumption. This way, a balance is achieved between the amount of energy intake and its consumption. This magical diet is not only a preferred approach to health, with a wide range of magical recipes but also a channel between the most diverse cultures. The inhabitants of this region are children of the earth, and so is their food from the land and soil. It can ensure if consumed rationally, the effectiveness of various bodily functions.

Some well-known health organizations worldwide have designed food pyramids to clarify the most common forms of the Mediterranean region. It has become popular among health activists because people from this region have high life expectancy despite less access to healthcare facilities. It has been stated by the American Heart Association and the American Diabetes Association that the Mediterranean diet lowers the risk of cardiovascular disease and type 2 diabetes. If a Mediterranean diet plan is followed, it can have a lasting effect on health and help reduce and maintain a healthy weight.

THE BENEFITS OF THE MEDITERRANEAN DIET

The Mediterranean diet has gained popularity in medical fields because of its documented benefits for heart health. But, much research has shown that the Mediterranean diet may have a much longer list of health benefits that go beyond the heart. This will review just a few of the many improvements you can experience with your health when you start following the Mediterranean diet.

REDUCES AGE-RELATED MUSCLE AND BONE WEAKNESS

Eating a well-balanced diet that provides a wide range of vitamins and minerals is essential for reducing muscle weakness and bone degradation. This is especially important as you age. Accident-related injuries, such as tripping, falling, or slipping while walking, can cause serious injuries. As you age, this becomes even more concerning because some simple falls can be fatal. Many accidents occur because of weakening muscle mass and loss of bone density. Women, especially those entering the menopausal stage of their lives, are more at risk of severe injuries from accidental falls because estrogen levels decrease significantly during this time—this decrease in estrogen results in a loss of bone muscle mass. Reduced estrogen can also cause bone thinning, which over time develops into osteoporosis.

Maintaining healthy bone mass and muscle agility as you age can be a challenge. When you don't get the proper nutrients to promote healthy bones and muscles, you increase your risk of developing osteoporosis. The Mediterranean diet offers an easy way to meet the dietary needs necessary to improve bone and muscle function.

Antioxidants, vitamins C and K, carotenoids, magnesium, potassium, and phytoestrogens are essential minerals and nutrients for optimal musculoskeletal health. Plant-based foods, unsaturated fats, and whole grains help provide the necessary balance of nutrients that keep bones and muscles healthy. Following a Mediterranean diet can improve and reduce bone loss as you age.

The Mediterranean diet consists of many foods that increase the risk of Alzheimer's, such as processed meats, refined grains like white bread and pasta, and added sugar. Foods that contain dactyl, which is a chemical commonly used in the refining process, increase the buildup of beta-amyloid plaques in the brain. Microwave popcorn, margarine, and butter are some of the most frequently consumed foods that contain this harmful chemical. It's no wonder that Alzheimer's is becoming one of the leading causes of death among Americans.

On the other hand, the Mediterranean diet includes a wide range of foods that have been shown to boost memory and slow cognitive decline. Dark leafy vegetables, fresh berries, extra virgin olive oil, and fresh fish contain vitamins and minerals that can improve brain health. The Mediterranean diet can help you make necessary diet and lifestyle changes that can significantly decrease your risk of Alzheimer's.

The Mediterranean diet encourages improvement in both diet and physical activity. Thanks to these two components are the most important factors that will help you manage the symptoms of diabetes and reduce your risk of developing the condition.

HEART HEALTH AND STROKE RISK REDUCTION

Heart health is strongly influenced by diet. Maintaining healthy cholesterol levels, blood pressure, blood sugar, and staying within a beneficial weight results in optimal heart health. Your diet directly affects each of these components. Those at increased risk are often advised to start on a low-fat diet. A low-fat diet eliminates all fats, including those from oils, nuts, and red meat. Studies have shown that the Mediterranean diet, which includes healthy fats, is more effective at lowering cardiovascular risks than a standard low-fat diet: (that's processed red meat, 2019). This is because the unsaturated fats consumed in the Mediterranean diet lower bad cholesterol levels and increase good cholesterol levels.

The Mediterranean diet emphasizes the importance of daily activity and stress reduction by enjoying quality time with friends and family. Each of these elements, along with eating more plant-based foods, significantly improves heart health and reduces the risk of many heart-related conditions. By increasing your intake of fresh fruits and vegetables and adding regular daily activities, you improve not only your heart health but your overall health.

ADDITIONAL BENEFITS

Aside from the significant benefits to your heart and brain, the Mediterranean diet can significantly improve many other key factors in your life. Since the Mediterranean diet focuses on eating healthy, exercising, and connecting with others, you can see improvements to your mental health, physical health and often feel like you're living a more fulfilling life.

PROTECTS AGAINST CANCER

Many plant-based foods, especially those in the yellow and orange color groups, contain cancer-fighting agents. Increasing the antioxidants consumed by eating fresh fruits and vegetables, and whole grains can protect the body's cells from developing cancer cells. Drinking a glass of red wine also provides cancer-protective compounds.

ENERGY

Following a Mediterranean diet focuses on fueling your body. Other diets focus only on filling your body, and this is often done through empty calories. When your body gets the nutrients it needs, it can function properly, which results in feeling more energized throughout the day. You won't need to rely on sugary drinks, excess caffeine, or sugar-filled energy bars to get you going and keep you moving. You'll feel less weighed down after eating, and that translates into a greater capacity for output.

GET BETTER SLEEP

Sugar and caffeine can cause significant sleep disturbances. Besides, other foods, such as processed foods, can make it harder to get the right amount of sleep. When you eat the right foods, you can see a change in your sleep patterns. Your body will want to rest to recover and properly absorb the vitamins and minerals consumed during the day. Your brain will switch into sleep mode with ease because it has received the vitamins it needs to function correctly. When you get the right amount of sleep, you will, in turn, have more energy the next day, and this can also significantly improve your mood. The Mediterranean diet increases nutrient-dense food consumption and avoids excess sugar and processed foods known to cause sleep problems.

Besides, the Mediterranean diet allows you to maintain a healthy weight, reducing the risk of developing sleep disorders such as sleep apnea. Sleep apnea is common in individuals who are overweight and obese. It causes the airway to become blocked, making it difficult to breathe. This results in not getting enough oxygen when you sleep, which can cause sudden and frequent awakenings during the night.

LONGEVITY

The Mediterranean diet, indeed, helps reduce the risk of many health problems. Its heart, brain, and mood health benefits translate into a longer, more enjoyable life. When you eliminate the risk of developing certain conditions such as cardiovascular disease, diabetes, and dementia, you increase your lifespan. But eliminating these health risks is not the only cause of increased longevity with the Mediterranean diet. Increased physical activity and deep social connection also play a significant role in living a longer life.

CLEAR SKIN

Healthy skin starts on the inside. When you provide your body with healthy foods, it radiates through your skin. The antioxidants in extra virgin olive oil alone are enough to keep your skin young and healthy. But the Mediterranean diet includes many fresh fruits and vegetables that are full of antioxidants. These antioxidants help repair damaged cells in the body and promote the growth of healthy cells. Eating a variety of healthy fats also keeps your skin supple and can protect it from premature aging.

MAINTAINING A HEALTHY WEIGHT

With the Mediterranean diet, you eat mostly whole, fresh foods. Eating more foods rich in vitamins, minerals, and nutrients is essential to maintaining a healthy weight. The diet is easy to stick to, and there are no calorie restrictions to follow strictly. This makes it a highly sustainable plan for those who want to lose weight or maintain a healthy weight. Keep in mind; this is not an option to lose weight fast. This is a lifestyle that will allow you to maintain optimal health for years, not just a few months.

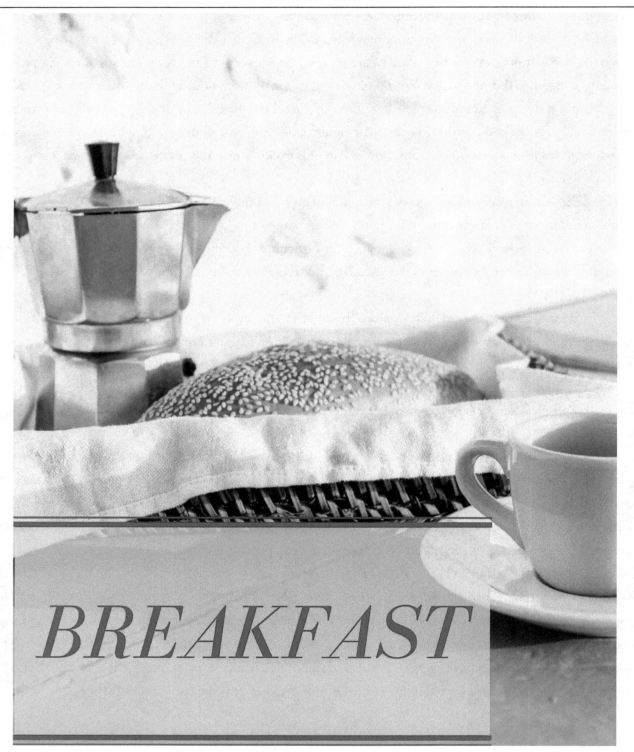

BREAKFAST

1) CAULIFLOWER FRITTERS AND HUMMUS

Cooking Time: 15 Minutes   **Servings:** 4

Ingredients:

- ✓ 2 (15 oz) cans chickpeas, divided
- ✓ 2 1/2 tbsp olive oil, divided, plus more for frying
- ✓ 1 cup onion, chopped, about 1/2 a small onion
- ✓ 2 tbsp garlic, minced
- ✓ 2 cups cauliflower, cut into small pieces, about 1/2 a large head
- ✓ 1/2 tsp salt
- ✓ black pepper
- ✓ Topping:
- ✓ Hummus, of choice
- ✓ Green onion, diced

Directions:

- ❖ Preheat oven to 400°F
- ❖ Rinse and drain 1 can of the chickpeas, place them on a paper towel to dry off well
- ❖ Then place the chickpeas into a large bowl, removing the loose skins that come off, and toss with 1 tbsp of olive oil, spread the chickpeas onto a large pan (being careful not to over-crowd them) and sprinkle with salt and pepper
- ❖ Bake for 20 minutes, then stir, and then bake an additional 5-10 minutes until very crispy
- ❖ Once the chickpeas are roasted, transfer them to a large food processor and process until broken down and crumble - Don't over process them and turn it into flour, as you need to have some texture. Place the mixture into a small bowl, set aside
- ❖ In a large pan over medium-high heat, add the remaining 1 1/2 tbsp of olive oil
- ❖ Once heated, add in the onion and garlic, cook until lightly golden brown, about 2 minutes. Then add in the chopped cauliflower, cook for an additional 2 minutes, until the cauliflower is golden
- ❖ Turn the heat down to low and cover the pan, cook until the cauliflower is fork tender and the onions are golden brown and caramelized, stirring often, about 3-5 minutes
- ❖ Transfer the cauliflower mixture to the food processor, drain and rinse the remaining can of chickpeas and add them into the food processor, along with the salt and a pinch of pepper. Blend until smooth, and the mixture starts to ball, stop to scrape down the sides as needed
- ❖ Transfer the cauliflower mixture into a large bowl and add in 1/2 cup of the roasted chickpea crumbs (you won't use all of the crumbs, but it is easier to break them down when you have a larger amount.), stir until well combined
- ❖ In a large bowl over medium heat, add in enough oil to lightly cover the bottom of a large pan
- ❖ Working in batches, cook the patties until golden brown, about 2-3 minutes, flip and cook again
- ❖ Distribute among the container, placing parchment paper in between the fritters. Store in the fridge for 2-3 days
- ❖ To Serve: Heat through in the oven at 350F for 5-8 minutes. Top with hummus, green onion and enjoy!
- ❖ Recipe Notes: Don't add too much oil while frying the fritter or they will end up soggy. Use only enough to cover the pan. Use a fork while frying and resist the urge to flip them every minute to see if they are golden

Nutrition: Calories:333;Total Carbohydrates: 45g;Total Fat: 13g;Protein: 14g

2) ITALIAN BREAKFAST SAUSAGE AND BABY POTATOES WITH VEGETABLES

Cooking Time: 30 Minutes   **Servings: 4**

Ingredients:

- ✓ 1 cup baby carrots
- ✓ 2 tbsp olive oil
- ✓ 1/2 tsp garlic powder
- ✓ 1/2 tsp Italian seasoning
- ✓ 1 tsp salt
- ✓ 1/2 tsp pepper

- ✓ 1 lbs sweet Italian sausage links, sliced on the bias (diagonal)
- ✓ 2 cups baby potatoes, halved
- ✓ 2 cups broccoli florets
- ✓ 1 cup onions cut to 1-inch chunks
- ✓ 2 cups small mushrooms -half or quarter the large ones for uniform size

Directions:

- ❖ Preheat the oven to 400 degrees F
- ❖ In a large bowl, add the baby potatoes, broccoli florets, onions, small mushrooms, and baby carrots
- ❖ Add in the olive oil, salt, pepper, garlic powder and Italian seasoning and toss to evenly coat
- ❖ Spread the vegetables onto a sheet pan in one even layer
- ❖ Arrange the sausage slices on the pan over the vegetables
- ❖ Bake for 30 minutes – make sure to sake halfway through to prevent sticking
- ❖ Allow to cool
- ❖ Distribute the Italian sausages and vegetables among the containers and store in the fridge for 2-3 days
- ❖ To Serve: Reheat in the microwave for 1-2 minutes, or until heated through and enjoy!
- ❖ Recipe Notes: If you would like crispier potatoes, place them on the pan and bake for 15 minutes before adding the other ingredients to the pan.

Nutrition: Calories:321;Total Fat: 16g;Total Carbs: 23g;Fiber: 4g;Protein: 22g

3) BREAKFAST GREEK QUINOA BOWL

Cooking Time: 20 Minutes   **Servings: 6**

Ingredients:

- ✓ 1 tsp olive oil
- ✓ 1 (5 oz) bag baby spinach
- ✓ 1 pint cherry tomatoes, halved
- ✓ 1 cup feta cheese
- ✓ 2 cups cooked quinoa

- ✓ 12 eggs
- ✓ ¼ cup plain Greek yogurt
- ✓ 1 tsp onion powder
- ✓ 1 tsp granulated garlic
- ✓ ½ tsp salt
- ✓ ½ tsp pepper

Directions:

- ❖ In a large bowl whisk together eggs, Greek yogurt, onion powder, granulated garlic, salt, and pepper, set aside
- ❖ In a large skillet, heat olive oil and add spinach, cook the spinach until it is slightly wilted, about 3-4 minutes
- ❖ Add in cherry tomatoes, cook until tomatoes are softened, 4 minutes
- ❖ Stir in egg mixture and cook until the eggs are set, about 7-9 minutes, stir in the eggs as they cook to scramble
- ❖ Once the eggs have set stir in the feta and quinoa, cook until heated through
- ❖ Distribute evenly among the containers, store for 2-3 days
- ❖ To serve: Reheat in the microwave for 30 seconds to 1 minute or heated through

Nutrition: Calories:357;Total Carbohydrates: ;Total Fat: 20g;Protein: 23g

4) EGG, HAM WITH CHEESE FREEZER SANDWICHES

Cooking Time: 20 Minutes   **Servings: 6**

Ingredients:

- ✓ Cooking spray or oil to grease the baking dish
- ✓ 7 large eggs
- ✓ ½ cup low-fat (2%) milk
- ✓ ½ tsp garlic powder
- ✓ ½ tsp onion powder
- ✓ 1 tbsp Dijon mustard
- ✓ ½ tsp honey
- ✓ 6 whole-wheat English muffins
- ✓ 6 slices thinly sliced prosciutto
- ✓ 6 slices Swiss cheese

Directions:

- ❖ Preheat the oven to 375°F. Lightly oil or spray an 8-by--inch glass or ceramic baking dish with cooking spray.
- ❖ In a large bowl, whisk together the eggs, milk, garlic powder, and onion powder. Pour the mixture into the baking dish and bake for minutes, until the eggs are set and no longer jiggling. Cool.
- ❖ While the eggs are baking, mix the mustard and honey in a small bowl. Lay out the English muffin halves to start assembly.
- ❖ When the eggs are cool, use a biscuit cutter or drinking glass about the same size as the English muffin diameter to cut 6 egg circles. Divide the leftover egg scraps evenly to be added to each sandwich.
- ❖ Spread ½ tsp of honey mustard on each of the bottom English muffin halves. Top each with 1 slice of prosciutto, 1 egg circle and scraps, 1 slice of cheese, and the top half of the muffin.
- ❖ Wrap each sandwich tightly in foil.
- ❖ STORAGE: Store tightly wrapped sandwiches in the freezer for up to 1 month. To reheat, remove the foil, place the sandwich on a microwave-safe plate, and wrap with a damp paper towel. Microwave on high for 1½ minutes, flip over, and heat again for another 1½ minutes. Because cooking time can vary greatly between microwaves, you may need to experiment with a few sandwiches before you find the perfect amount of time to heat the whole item through.

Nutrition: Total calories: 361; Total fat: 17g; Saturated fat: 7g; Sodium: 953mg; Carbohydrates: 26g; Fiber: 3g; Protein: 24g

5) HEALTHY SALAD ZUCCHINI KALE TOMATO

Cooking Time: 20 Minutes   **Servings: 4**

Ingredients:

- ✓ 1 lb kale, chopped
- ✓ 2 tbsp fresh parsley, chopped
- ✓ 1 tbsp vinegar
- ✓ 1/2 cup can tomato, crushed
- ✓ 1 tsp paprika
- ✓ 1 cup zucchini, cut into cubes
- ✓ 1 cup grape tomatoes, halved
- ✓ 2 tbsp olive oil
- ✓ 1 onion, chopped
- ✓ 1 leek, sliced
- ✓ Pepper
- ✓ Salt

Directions:

- ❖ Add oil into the inner pot of instant pot and set the pot on sauté mode.
- ❖ Add leek and onion and sauté for 5 minutes.
- ❖ Add kale and remaining ingredients and stir well.
- ❖ Seal pot with lid and cook on high for 15 minutes.
- ❖ Once done, allow to release pressure naturally for 10 minutes then release remaining using quick release. Remove lid.
- ❖ Stir and serve.

Nutrition: Calories: 162; Fat: 3 g; Carbohydrates: 22.2 g; Sugar: 4.8 g; Protein: 5.2 g; Cholesterol: 0 mg

6) CHEESE WITH CAULIFLOWER FRITTATA AND PEPPERS

Cooking Time: 30 Minutes   **Servings: 6**

Ingredients:

- ✓ 10 eggs
- ✓ 1 seeded and chopped bell pepper
- ✓ ½ cup grated Parmigiano-Reggiano
- ✓ ½ cup milk, skim
- ✓ ½ tsp cayenne pepper
- ✓ 1 pound cauliflower, floret
- ✓ ½ tsp saffron
- ✓ 2 tbsp chopped chives
- ✓ Salt and black pepper as desired

Directions:

- ❖ Prepare your oven by setting the temperature to 370 degrees Fahrenheit. You should also grease a skillet suitable for the oven.
- ❖ In a medium-sized bowl, add the milk and eggs. Whisk them until they are frothy.
- ❖ Sprinkle the grated Parmigiano-Reggiano cheese into the frothy mixture and fold the ingredients together.
- ❖ Pour in the salt, saffron, cayenne pepper, and black pepper and gently stir.
- ❖ Add in the chopped bell pepper and gently stir until the ingredients are fully incorporated.
- ❖ Pour the egg mixture into the skillet and cook on medium heat over your stovetop for 4 minutes.
- ❖ Steam the cauliflower florets in a pan. To do this, add ½ inch of water and ½ tsp sea salt. Pour in the cauliflower and cover for 3 to 8 minutes. Drain any extra water.
- ❖ Add the cauliflower into the mixture and gently stir.
- ❖ Set the skillet into the preheated oven and turn your timer to 13 minutes. Once the mixture is golden brown in the middle, remove the frittata from the oven.
- ❖ Set your skillet aside for a couple of minutes so it can cool.
- ❖ Slice and garnish with chives before you serve.

Nutrition: calories: 207, fats: grams, carbohydrates: 8 grams, protein: 17 grams.

7) AVOCADO KALE OMELETTE

Cooking Time: 5 Minutes   **Servings: 1**

Ingredients:

- ✓ 2 eggs
- ✓ 1 tsp milk
- ✓ 2 tsp olive oil
- ✓ 1 cup kale (chopped)
- ✓ 1 tbsp lime juice
- ✓ 1 tbsp cilantro (chopped)
- ✓ 1 tsp sunflower seeds
- ✓ Pinch of red pepper (crushed)
- ✓ ¼ avocado (sliced)
- ✓ sea salt or plain salt
- ✓ freshly ground black pepper

Directions:

- ❖ Toss all the Ingredients: (except eggs and milk) to make the kale salad.
- ❖ Beat the eggs and milk in a bowl.
- ❖ Heat oil in a pan over medium heat. Then pour in the egg mixture and cook it until the bottom settles. Cook for 2 minutes and then flip it over and further cook for 20 seconds.
- ❖ Finally, put the Omelette in containers.
- ❖ Top the Omelette with the kale salad.
- ❖ Serve warm.

Nutrition: Calories: 399, Total Fat: 28.8g, Saturated Fat: 6.2, Cholesterol: 328 mg, Sodium: 162 mg, Total Carbohydrate: 25.2g, Dietary Fiber: 6.3 g, Total Sugars: 9 g, Protein: 15.8 g, Vitamin D: 31 mcg, Calcium: 166 mg, Iron: 4 mg, Potassium: 980 mg

8) BREAKFAST WITH MEDITERRANEAN-STYLE BURRITO

Cooking Time: 5 Minutes   **Servings:** 6

Ingredients:

- 9 eggs whole
- 6 tortillas whole 10 inch, regular or sun-dried tomato
- 3 tbsp sun-dried tomatoes, chopped
- 1/2 cup feta cheese I use light/low-fat feta
- 2 cups baby spinach washed and dried
- 3 tbsp black olives, sliced
- 3/4 cup refried beans, canned
- Garnish:
- Salsa

Directions:

- Spray a medium frying pan with non-stick spray, add the eggs and scramble and toss for about 5 minutes, or until eggs are no longer liquid
- Add in the spinach, black olives, sun-dried tomatoes and continue to stir and toss until no longer wet
- Add in the feta cheese and cover, cook until cheese is melted
- Add 2 tbsp of refried beans to each tortilla
- Top with egg mixture, dividing evenly between all burritos, and wrap
- Frying in a pan until lightly browned
- Allow to cool completely before slicing
- Wrap the slices in plastic wrap and then aluminum foil and place in the freezer for up to 2 months or fridge for 2 days
- To Serve: Remove the aluminum foil and plastic wrap, and microwave for 2 minutes, then allow to rest for 30 seconds, enjoy! Enjoy hot with salsa and fruit

Nutrition: Calories:252;Total Carbohydrates: 21g;Total Fat: 11g;Protein: 14g |

9) SHAKSHUKA AND FETA

Cooking Time: 40 Minutes   **Servings:** 4-6

Ingredients:

- 6 large eggs
- 3 tbsp extra-virgin olive oil
- 1 large onion, halved and thinly sliced
- 1 large red bell pepper, seeded and thinly sliced
- 3 garlic cloves, thinly sliced
- 1 tsp ground cumin
- 1 tsp sweet paprika
- ⅛ tsp cayenne, or to taste
- 1 (28-ounce) can whole plum tomatoes with juices, coarsely chopped
- ¾ tsp salt, more as needed
- ¼ tsp black pepper, more as needed
- 5 oz feta cheese, crumbled, about 1 1/4 cups
- To Serve:
- Chopped cilantro
- Hot sauce

Directions:

- Preheat oven to 375 degrees F
- In a large skillet over medium-low heat, add the oil
- Once heated, add the onion and bell pepper, cook gently until very soft, about 20 minutes
- Add in the garlic and cook until tender, 1 to 2 minutes, then stir in cumin, paprika and cayenne, and cook 1 minute
- Pour in tomatoes, season with 3/4 tsp salt and 1/4 tsp pepper, simmer until tomatoes have thickened, about 10 minutes
- Then stir in crumbled feta
- Gently crack eggs into skillet over tomatoes, season with salt and pepper
- Transfer skillet to oven
- Bake until eggs have just set, 7 to 10 minutes
- Allow to cool and distribute among the containers, store in the fridge for 2-3 days
- To Serve: Reheat in the oven at 360 degrees F for 5 minutes or until heated through

Nutrition: Calories:337;Carbs: 17g;Total Fat: 25g;Protein

10) SPINACH, FETA WITH EGG BREAKFAST QUESADILLAS

Cooking Time: 15 Minutes   **Servings: 5**

Ingredients:

- ✓ 8 eggs (optional)
- ✓ 2 tsp olive oil
- ✓ 1 red bell pepper
- ✓ 1/2 red onion
- ✓ 1/4 cup milk

- ✓ 4 handfuls of spinach leaves
- ✓ 1 1/2 cup mozzarella cheese
- ✓ 5 sun-dried tomato tortillas
- ✓ 1/2 cup feta
- ✓ 1/4 tsp salt
- ✓ 1/4 tsp pepper
- ✓ Spray oil

Directions:

- ❖ In a large non-stick pan over medium heat, add the olive oil
- ❖ Once heated, add the bell pepper and onion, cook for 4-5 minutes until soft
- ❖ In the meantime, whisk together the eggs, milk, salt and pepper in a bowl
- ❖ Add in the egg/milk mixture into the pan with peppers and onions, stirring frequently, until eggs are almost cooked through
- ❖ Add in the spinach and feta, fold into the eggs, stirring until spinach is wilted and eggs are cooked through
- ❖ Remove the eggs from heat and plate
- ❖ Spray a separate large non-stick pan with spray oil, and place over medium heat
- ❖ Add the tortilla, on one half of the tortilla, spread about ½ cup of the egg mixture
- ❖ Top the eggs with around ⅓ cup of shredded mozzarella cheese
- ❖ Fold the second half of the tortilla over, then cook for 2 minutes, or until golden brown
- ❖ Flip and cook for another minute until golden brown
- ❖ Allow the quesadilla to cool completely, divide among the container, store for 2 days or wrap in plastic wrap and foil, and freeze for up to 2 months
- ❖ To Serve: Reheat in oven at 375 for 3-5 minutes or until heated through

Nutrition: (1/2 quesadilla): Calories:213;Total Fat: 11g;Total Carbs: 15g;Protein: 15g

11) BREAKFAST COBBLER

Cooking Time: 12 Minutes   **Servings: 4**

Ingredients:

- ✓ 2 lbs apples, cut into chunks
- ✓ 1 1/2 cups water
- ✓ 1/4 tsp nutmeg
- ✓ 1 1/2 tsp cinnamon

- ✓ 1/2 cup dry buckwheat
- ✓ 1/2 cup dates, chopped
- ✓ Pinch of ground ginger

Directions:

- ❖ Spray instant pot from inside with cooking spray.
- ❖ Add all ingredients into the instant pot and stir well.
- ❖ Seal pot with a lid and select manual and set timer for 12 minutes.
- ❖ Once done, release pressure using quick release. Remove lid.
- ❖ Stir and serve.

Nutrition: Calories: 195;Fat: 0.9 g;Carbohydrates: 48.3 g;Sugar: 25.8 g;Protein: 3.3 g;Cholesterol: 0 mg

13) EGG-TOPPED QUINOA BOWL AND KALE

Cooking Time: 5 Minutes   **Servings: 2**

Ingredients:

- ✓ 1-ounce pancetta, chopped
- ✓ 1 bunch kale, sliced
- ✓ ½ cup cherry tomatoes, halved
- ✓ 1 tsp red wine vinegar

- ✓ 1 cup cooked quinoa
- ✓ 1 tsp olive oil
- ✓ 2 eggs
- ✓ 1/3 cup avocado, sliced
- ✓ sea salt or plain salt
- ✓ fresh black pepper

Directions:

- ❖ Start by heating pancetta in a skillet until golden brown. Add in kale and further cook for 2 minutes.
- ❖ Then, stir in tomatoes, vinegar, and salt and remove from heat.
- ❖ Now, divide this mixture into 2 bowls, add avocado to both, and then set aside.
- ❖ Finally, cook both the eggs and top each bowl with an egg.
- ❖ Serve hot with toppings of your choice.

Nutrition: Calories: 547, Total Fat: 22., Saturated Fat: 5.3, Cholesterol: 179 mg, Sodium: 412 mg, Total Carbohydrate: 62.5 g, Dietary Fiber: 8.6 g, Total Sugars: 1.7 g, Protein: 24.7 g, Vitamin D: 15 mcg, Calcium: 117 mg, Iron: 6 mg, Potassium: 1009 mg

14) STRAWBERRY GREEK COLD YOGURT

Cooking Time: 2-4 Hours   **Servings: 5**

Ingredients:

- ✓ 3 cups plain Greek low-fat yogurt
- ✓ 1 cup sugar
- ✓ ¼ cup lemon juice, freshly squeezed
- ✓ 2 tsp vanilla
- ✓ 1/8 tsp salt
- ✓ 1 cup strawberries, sliced

Directions:

- ❖ In a medium-sized bowl, add yogurt, lemon juice, sugar, vanilla, and salt.
- ❖ Whisk the whole mixture well.
- ❖ Freeze the yogurt mix in a 2-quart ice cream maker according to the given instructions.
- ❖ During the final minute, add the sliced strawberries.
- ❖ Transfer the yogurt to an airtight container.
- ❖ Place in the freezer for 2-4 hours.
- ❖ Remove from the freezer and allow it to stand for 5-15 minutes.
- ❖ Serve and enjoy!

Nutrition: Calories: 251, Total Fat: 0.5 g, Saturated Fat: 0.1 g, Cholesterol: 3 mg, Sodium: 130 mg, Total Carbohydrate: 48.7 g, Dietary Fiber: 0.6 g, Total Sugars: 47.3 g, Protein: 14.7 g, Vitamin D: 1 mcg, Calcium: 426 mg, Iron: 0 mg, Potassium: 62 mg

15) PEACH ALMOND OATMEAL

Cooking Time: 10 Minutes   **Servings: 2**

Ingredients:

- ✓ 1 cup unsweetened almond milk
- ✓ 2 cups of water
- ✓ 1 cup oats
- ✓ 2 peaches, diced
- ✓ Pinch of salt

Directions:

- ❖ Spray instant pot from inside with cooking spray.
- ❖ Add all ingredients into the instant pot and stir well.
- ❖ Seal pot with a lid and select manual and set timer for 10 minutes.
- ❖ Once done, allow to release pressure naturally for 10 minutes then release remaining using quick release. Remove lid.
- ❖ Stir and serve.

Nutrition: Calories: 234;Fat: 4.8 g;Carbohydrates: 42.7 g;Sugar: 9 g;Protein: 7.3 g;Cholesterol: 0 mg

16) BANANA PEANUT BUTTER PUDDING

Cooking Time: 25 Minutes   **Servings: 1**

Ingredients:

- ✓ 2 bananas, halved
- ✓ ¼ cup smooth peanut butter
- ✓ Coconut for garnish, shredded

Directions:

- ❖ Start by blending bananas and peanut butter in a blender and mix until smooth or desired texture obtained.
- ❖ Pour into a bowl and garnish with coconut if desired.
- ❖ Enjoy.

Nutrition: Calories: 589, Total Fat: 33.3g, Saturated Fat: 6.9, Cholesterol: 0 mg, Sodium: 13 mg, Total Carbohydrate: 66.5 g, Dietary Fiber: 10 g, Total Sugars: 38 g, Protein: 18.8 g, Vitamin D: 0 mcg, Calcium: 40 mg, Iron: 2 mg, Potassium: 1264 mg

17) COCONUT BANANA MIX

Cooking Time: 4 Minutes   **Servings: 4**

Ingredients:

- ✓ 1 cup coconut milk
- ✓ 1 banana
- ✓ 1 cup dried coconut
- ✓ 2 tbsp ground flax seed
- ✓ 3 tbsp chopped raisins
- ✓ ⅛ tsp nutmeg
- ✓ ⅛ tsp cinnamon
- ✓ Salt to taste

Directions:

- ❖ Set a large skillet on the stove and set it to low heat.
- ❖ Chop up the banana.
- ❖ Pour the coconut milk, nutmeg, and cinnamon into the skillet.
- ❖ Pour in the ground flaxseed while stirring continuously.
- ❖ Add the dried coconut and banana. Mix the ingredients until combined well.
- ❖ Allow the mixture to simmer for 2 to 3 minutes while stirring occasionally.
- ❖ Set four airtight containers on the counter.
- ❖ Remove the pan from heat and sprinkle enough salt for your taste buds.
- ❖ Divide the mixture into the containers and place them into the fridge overnight. They can remain in the fridge for up to 3 days.
- ❖ Before you set this tasty mixture in the microwave to heat up, you need to let it thaw on the counter for a bit.

Nutrition: calories: 279, fats: 22 grams, carbohydrates: 25 grams, protein: 6.4 grams

18) OLIVE OIL RASPBERRY-LEMON MUFFINS

Cooking Time: 20 Minutes   **Servings: 12**

Ingredients:

- ✓ Cooking spray to grease baking liners
- ✓ 1 cup all-purpose flour
- ✓ 1 cup whole-wheat flour
- ✓ ½ cup tightly packed light brown sugar
- ✓ ½ tsp baking soda
- ✓ ½ tsp aluminum-free baking powder
- ✓ ⅛ tsp kosher salt
- ✓ 1¼ cups buttermilk
- ✓ 1 large egg
- ✓ ¼ cup extra-virgin olive oil
- ✓ 1 tbsp freshly squeezed lemon juice
- ✓ Zest of 2 lemons
- ✓ 1¼ cups frozen raspberries (do not thaw)

Directions:

- ❖ Preheat the oven to 400°F and line a muffin tin with baking liners. Spray the liners lightly with cooking spray.
- ❖ In a large mixing bowl, whisk together the all-purpose flour, whole-wheat flour, brown sugar, baking soda, baking powder, and salt.
- ❖ In a medium bowl, whisk together the buttermilk, egg, oil, lemon juice, and lemon zest.
- ❖ Pour the wet ingredients into the dry ingredients and stir just until blended. Do not overmix.
- ❖ Fold in the frozen raspberries.
- ❖ Scoop about ¼ cup of batter into each muffin liner and bake for 20 minutes, or until the tops look browned and a paring knife comes out clean when inserted. Remove the muffins from the tin to cool.
- ❖ STORAGE: Store covered containers at room temperature for up to 4 days. To freeze muffins for up to 3 months, wrap them in foil and place in an airtight resealable bag.

Nutrition: Total calories: 166; Total fat: 5g; Saturated fat: 1g; Sodium: 134mg; Carbohydrates: 30g; Fiber: 3g; Protein: 4g

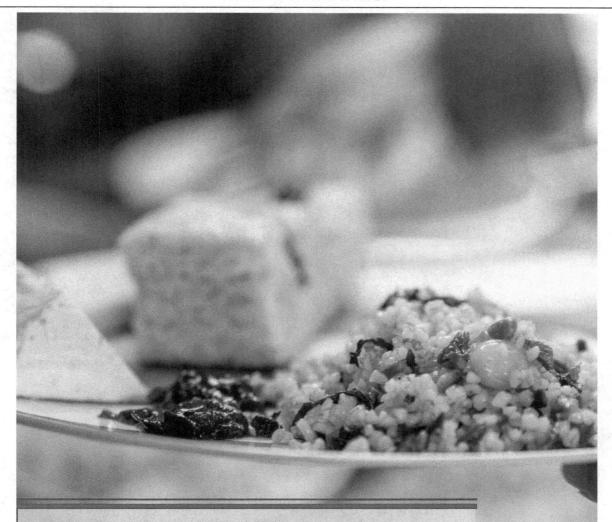

LUNCH & DINNER

19) MARINATED TUNA STEAK SPECIAL

Cooking Time: 15-20 Minutes   **Servings: 4**

Ingredients:

- ✓ Olive oil (2 tbsp.)
- ✓ Orange juice (.25 cup)
- ✓ Soy sauce (.25 cup)
- ✓ Lemon juice (1 tbsp.)
- ✓ Fresh parsley (2 tbsp.)
- ✓ Garlic clove (1)
- ✓ Ground black pepper (.5 tsp.)
- ✓ Fresh oregano (.5 tsp.)
- ✓ Tuna steaks (4 - 4 oz. Steaks)

Directions:

- ❖ Mince the garlic and chop the oregano and parsley.
- ❖ In a glass container, mix the pepper, oregano, garlic, parsley, lemon juice, soy sauce, olive oil, and orange juice.
- ❖ Warm the grill using the high heat setting. Grease the grate with oil.
- ❖ Add to tuna steaks and cook for five to six minutes. Turn and baste with the marinated sauce.
- ❖ Cook another five minutes or until it's the way you like it. Discard the remaining marinade.

Nutrition: Calories: 200;Protein: 27.4 grams;Fat: 7.9 grams

20) SHRIMP AND GARLIC PASTA

Cooking Time: 15 Minutes   **Servings: 4**

Ingredients:

- ✓ 6 ounces whole wheat spaghetti
- ✓ 12 ounces raw shrimp, peeled and deveined, cut into 1-inch pieces
- ✓ 1 bunch asparagus, trimmed
- ✓ 1 large bell pepper, thinly sliced
- ✓ 1 cup fresh peas
- ✓ 3 garlic cloves, chopped
- ✓ 1 and ¼ tsp kosher salt
- ✓ ½ and ½ cups non-fat plain yogurt
- ✓ 3 tbsp lemon juice
- ✓ 1 tbsp extra-virgin olive oil
- ✓ ½ tsp fresh ground black pepper
- ✓ ¼ cup pine nuts, toasted

Directions:

- ❖ Take a large sized pot and bring water to a boil
- ❖ Add your spaghetti and cook them for about minutes less than the directed package instruction
- ❖ Add shrimp, bell pepper, asparagus and cook for about 2- 4 minutes until the shrimp are tender
- ❖ Drain the pasta and the contents well
- ❖ Take a large bowl and mash garlic until a paste form
- ❖ Whisk in yogurt, parsley, oil, pepper and lemon juice into the garlic paste
- ❖ Add pasta mix and toss well
- ❖ Serve by sprinkling some pine nuts!
- ❖ Enjoy!
- ❖ Meal Prep/Storage Options: Store in airtight containers in your fridge for 1-3 days.

Nutrition: Calories: 406;Fat: 22g;Carbohydrates: 28g;Protein: 26g

21) BUTTER PAPRIKA SHRIMPS

Cooking Time: 30 Minutes   **Servings: 2**

Ingredients:

- ✓ ¼ tbsp smoked paprika
- ✓ 1/8 cup sour cream
- ✓ ½ pound tiger shrimps
- ✓ 1/8 cup butter
- ✓ Salt and black pepper, to taste

Directions:

- ❖ Preheat the oven to 390 degrees F and grease a baking dish.
- ❖ Mix together all the ingredients in a large bowl and transfer into the baking dish.
- ❖ Place in the oven and bake for about 15 minutes.
- ❖ Place paprika shrimp in a dish and set aside to cool for meal prepping. Divide it in 2 containers and cover the lid. Refrigerate for 1-2 days and reheat in microwave before serving.

Nutrition: Calories: 330 ;Carbohydrates: 1.;Protein: 32.6g;Fat: 21.5g;Sugar: 0.2g;Sodium: 458mg

22) MEDITERRANEAN-STYLE SALMON AVOCADO SALAD

Cooking Time: 10 Minutes　　　　　　　**Servings: 4**

Ingredients:

- ✓ 1 lb skinless salmon fillets
- ✓ Marinade/Dressing:
- ✓ 3 tbsp olive oil
- ✓ 2 tbsp lemon juice fresh, squeezed
- ✓ 1 tbsp red wine vinegar, optional
- ✓ 1 tbsp fresh chopped parsley
- ✓ 2 tsp garlic minced
- ✓ 1 tsp dried oregano
- ✓ 1 tsp salt
- ✓ Cracked pepper, to taste

- ✓ Salad:
- ✓ 4 cups Romaine (or Cos) lettuce leaves, washed and dried
- ✓ 1 large cucumber, diced
- ✓ 2 Roma tomatoes, diced
- ✓ 1 red onion, sliced
- ✓ 1 avocado, sliced
- ✓ 1/2 cup feta cheese crumbled
- ✓ 1/3 cup pitted Kalamata olives or black olives, sliced
- ✓ Lemon wedges to serve

Directions:

- ❖ In a jug, whisk together the olive oil, lemon juice, red wine vinegar, chopped parsley, garlic minced, oregano, salt and pepper
- ❖ Pour out half of the marinade into a large, shallow dish, refrigerate the remaining marinade to use as the dressing
- ❖ Coat the salmon in the rest of the marinade
- ❖ Place a skillet pan or grill over medium-high, add 1 tbsp oil and sear salmon on both sides until crispy and cooked through
- ❖ Allow the salmon to cool
- ❖ Distribute the salmon among the containers, store in the fridge for 2-3 days
- ❖ To Serve: Prepare the salad by placing the romaine lettuce, cucumber, roma tomatoes, red onion, avocado, feta cheese, and olives in a large salad bowl. Reheat the salmon in the microwave for 30seconds to 1 minute or until heated through.
- ❖ Slice the salmon and arrange over salad. Drizzle the salad with the remaining untouched dressing, serve with lemon wedges.

Nutrition: Calories:411;Carbs: 12g;Total Fat: 27g;Protein: 28g

23) KALE BEET SALAD

Cooking Time: 50 Minutes　　　　　　　**Servings: 6**

Ingredients:

- ✓ 1 bunch of kale, washed and dried, ribs removed, chopped
- ✓ 6 pieces washed beets, peeled and dried and cut into 1/2 inches
- ✓ 1/2 tsp dried rosemary
- ✓ 1/2 tsp garlic powder
- ✓ salt
- ✓ pepper
- ✓ olive oil
- ✓ 1/4 medium red onion, thinly sliced

- ✓ 1-2 tbsp slivered almonds, toasted
- ✓ 1/4 cup olive oil
- ✓ Juice of 1 1/2 lemon
- ✓ 1/4 cup honey
- ✓ 1/4 tsp garlic powder
- ✓ 1 tsp dried rosemary
- ✓ salt
- ✓ pepper

Directions:

- ❖ Preheat oven to 400 degrees F.
- ❖ Take a bowl and toss the kale with some salt, pepper, and olive oil.
- ❖ Lightly oil a baking sheet and add the kale.
- ❖ Roast in the oven for 5 minutes, and then remove and place to the side.
- ❖ Place beets in a bowl and sprinkle with a bit of rosemary, garlic powder, pepper, and salt; ensure beets are coated well.
- ❖ Spread the beets on the oiled baking sheet, place on the middle rack of your oven, and roast for 45 minutes, turning twice.
- ❖ Make the lemon vinaigrette by whisking all of the listed Ingredients: in a bowl.
- ❖ Once the beets are ready, remove from the oven and allow it to cool.
- ❖ Take a medium-sized salad bowl and add kale, onions, and beets.
- ❖ Dress with lemon honey vinaigrette and toss well.
- ❖ Garnish with toasted almonds.
- ❖ Enjoy!

Nutrition: Calories: 245, Total Fat: 17.6 g, Saturated Fat: 2.6 g, Cholesterol: 0 mg, Sodium: 77 mg, Total Carbohydrate: 22.9 g, Dietary Fiber: 3 g, Total Sugars:

17.7 g, Protein: 2.4 g, Vitamin D: 0 mcg, Calcium: 50 mg, Iron: 1 mg, Potassium: 416 mg

24) MOROCCAN FISH

Cooking Time: 1 Hour 25 Minutes   **Servings: 12**

Ingredients:

- ✓ Garbanzo beans (15 oz. Can)
- ✓ Red bell peppers (2)
- ✓ Large carrot (1)
- ✓ Vegetable oil (1 tbsp.)
- ✓ Onion (1)
- ✓ Garlic (1 clove)
- ✓ Tomatoes (3 chopped/14.5 oz can)
- ✓ Olives (4 chopped)
- ✓ Chopped fresh parsley (.25 cup)
- ✓ Ground cumin (.25 cup)
- ✓ Paprika (3 tbsp.)
- ✓ Chicken bouillon granules (2 tbsp.)
- ✓ Cayenne pepper (1 tsp.)
- ✓ Salt (to your liking)
- ✓ Tilapia fillets (5 lb.)

Directions:

- ❖ Drain and rinse the beans. Thinly slice the carrot and onion. Mince the garlic and chop the olives. Discard the seeds from the peppers and slice them into strips.
- ❖ Warm the oil in a frying pan using the medium temperature setting. Toss in the onion and garlic. Simmer them for approximately five minutes.
- ❖ Fold in the bell peppers, beans, tomatoes, carrots, and olives.
- ❖ Continue sautéing them for about five additional minutes.
- ❖ Sprinkle the veggies with the cumin, parsley, salt, chicken bouillon, paprika, and cayenne.
- ❖ Stir thoroughly and place the fish on top of the veggies.
- ❖ Pour in water to cover the veggies.
- ❖ Lower the heat setting and cover the pan to slowly cook until the fish is flaky (about 40 min..

Nutrition: Calories: 268;Protein: 42 grams;Fat: 5 grams

25) SARDINES WITH NIÇOISE-INSPIRED SALAD

Cooking Time: 15 Minutes   **Servings: 4**

Ingredients:

- ✓ 4 eggs
- ✓ 12 ounces baby red potatoes (about 12 potatoes)
- ✓ 6 ounces green beans, halved
- ✓ 4 cups baby spinach leaves or mixed greens
- ✓ 1 bunch radishes, quartered (about 1⅓ cups)
- ✓ 1 cup cherry tomatoes
- ✓ 20 kalamata or niçoise olives (about ⅓ cup)
- ✓ 3 (3.75-ounce) cans skinless, boneless sardines packed in olive oil, drained
- ✓ 8 tbsp Dijon Red Wine Vinaigrette

Directions:

- ❖ Place the eggs in a saucepan and cover with water. Bring the water to a boil. As soon as the water starts to boil, place a lid on the pan and turn the heat off. Set a timer for minutes.
- ❖ When the timer goes off, drain the hot water and run cold water over the eggs to cool. Peel the eggs when cool and cut in half.
- ❖ Prick each potato a few times with a fork. Place them on a microwave-safe plate and microwave on high for 4 to 5 minutes, until the potatoes are tender. Let cool and cut in half.
- ❖ Place green beans on a microwave-safe plate and microwave on high for 1½ to 2 minutes, until the beans are crisp-tender. Cool.
- ❖ Place 1 egg, ½ cup of green beans, 6 potato halves, 1 cup of spinach, ⅓ cup of radishes, ¼ cup of tomatoes, olives, and 3 sardines in each of 4 containers. Pour 2 tbsp of vinaigrette into each of 4 sauce containers.
- ❖ STORAGE: Store covered containers in the refrigerator for up to 4 days.

Nutrition: Total calories: 450; Total fat: 32g; Saturated fat: 5g; Sodium: 6mg; Carbohydrates: 22g; Fiber: 5g; Protein: 21g

26) POMODORO LETTUCE SALAD

Cooking Time: 15 Minutes   **Servings: 6**

Ingredients:

- ✓ 1 heart of Romaine lettuce, chopped
- ✓ 3 Roma tomatoes, diced
- ✓ 1 English cucumber, diced
- ✓ 1 small red onion, finely chopped
- ✓ ½ cup curly parsley, finely chopped
- ✓ 2 tbsp virgin olive oil
- ✓ lemon juice, ½ large lemon
- ✓ 1 tsp garlic powder
- ✓ salt
- ✓ pepper

Directions:

- ❖ Add all Ingredients: to a large bowl.
- ❖ Toss well and transfer them to containers.
- ❖ Enjoy!

Nutrition: Calories: 68, Total Fat: 9 g, Saturated Fat: 0.8 g, Cholesterol: 0 mg, Sodium: 7 mg, Total Carbohydrate: 6 g, Dietary Fiber: 1.5 g, Total Sugars: 3.3 g, Protein: 1.3 g, Vitamin D: 0 mcg, Calcium: 18 mg, Iron: 1 mg, Potassium: 309 mg

27) MEDITERRANEAN-STYLE CHICKEN PASTA BAKE

Cooking Time: 30 Minutes   **Servings:** 4

Ingredients:

- ✓ Marinade:
- ✓ 1½ lbs. boneless, skinless chicken thighs, cut into bite-sized pieces*
- ✓ 2 garlic cloves, thinly sliced
- ✓ 2-3 tbsp. marinade from artichoke hearts
- ✓ 4 sprigs of fresh oregano, leaves stripped
- ✓ Olive oil
- ✓ Red wine vinegar
- ✓ Pasta:
- ✓ 1 lb whole wheat fusilli pasta
- ✓ 1 red onion, thinly sliced
- ✓ 1 pint grape or cherry tomatoes, whole
- ✓ ½ cup marinated artichoke hearts, roughly chopped
- ✓ ½ cup white beans, rinsed + drained (I use northern white beans)
- ✓ ½ cup Kalamata olives, roughly chopped
- ✓ ⅓ cup parsley and basil leaves, roughly chopped
- ✓ 2-3 handfuls of part-skim shredded mozzarella cheese
- ✓ Salt, to taste
- ✓ Pepper, to taste
- ✓ Garnish:
- ✓ Parsley
- ✓ Basil leaves

Directions:

- ❖ Create the chicken marinade by drain the artichoke hearts reserving the juice
- ❖ In a large bowl, add the artichoke juice, garlic, chicken, and oregano leaves, drizzle with olive oil, a splash of red wine vinegar, and mix well to coat
- ❖ Marinate for at least 1 hour, maximum hours
- ❖ Cook the pasta in boiling salted water, drain and set aside
- ❖ Preheat your oven to 42degrees F
- ❖ In a casserole dish, add the sliced onions and tomatoes, toss with olive oil, salt and pepper. Then cook, stirring occasionally, until the onions are soft and the tomatoes start to burst, about 15-20 minutes
- ❖ In the meantime, in a large skillet over medium heat, add 1 tsp of olive oil
- ❖ Remove the chicken from the marinade, pat dry, and season with salt and pepper
- ❖ Working in batches, brown the chicken on both sides, leaving slightly undercooked
- ❖ Remove the casserole dish from the oven, add in the cooked pasta, browned chicken, artichoke hearts, beans, olives, and chopped herbs, stir to combine
- ❖ Top with grated cheese
- ❖ Bake for an additional 5-7 minutes, until the cheese is brown and bubbling
- ❖ Remove from the oven and allow the dish to cool completely
- ❖ Distribute among the containers, store for 2-3 days
- ❖ To Serve: Reheat in the microwave for 1-2 minutes or until heated through.
- ❖ Garnish with fresh herbs and serve

Nutrition: Calories:487;Carbs: 95g;Total Fat: 5g;Protein: 22g

28) VEGETABLE FLATBREAD ROAST

Cooking Time: 25 Minutes   **Servings:** 12

Ingredients:

- ✓ 16 oz pizza dough, homemade or frozen
- ✓ 6 oz soft goat cheese, divided
- ✓ ¾ cup grated Parmesan cheese divided
- ✓ 3 tbsp chopped fresh dill, divided
- ✓ 1 small red onion, sliced thinly
- ✓ 1 small zucchini, sliced thinly
- ✓ 2 small tomatoes, thinly sliced
- ✓ 1 small red pepper, thinly sliced into rings
- ✓ Olive oil
- ✓ Salt, to taste
- ✓ Pepper, to taste

Directions:

- ❖ Preheat the oven to 400 degrees F
- ❖ Roll the dough into a large rectangle, and then place it on a piece of parchment paper sprayed with non-stick spray
- ❖ Take a knife and spread half the goat cheese onto one half of the dough, then sprinkle with half the dill and half the Parmesan cheese
- ❖ Carefully fold the other half of the dough on top of the cheese, spread and sprinkle the remaining parmesan and goat cheese
- ❖ Layer the thinly sliced vegetables over the top
- ❖ Brush the olive oil over the top of the veggies and sprinkle with salt, pepper, and the remaining dill
- ❖ Bake for 22-25 minutes, until the edges are medium brown, cut in half, lengthwise
- ❖ Then slice the flatbread in long 2-inch slices and allow to cool
- ❖ Distribute among the containers, store for 2 days
- ❖ To Serve: Reheat in the oven at 375 degrees for 5 minutes or until hot. Enjoy with a fresh salad.

Nutrition: Calories:170;Carbs: 21g;Total Fat: 6g;Protein: 8g

29) COBB SALAD WITH STEAK

Cooking Time: 15 Minutes   **Servings: 4**

Ingredients:

- ✓ 6 large eggs
- ✓ 2 tbsp unsalted butter
- ✓ 1 lb steak
- ✓ 2 tbsp olive oil
- ✓ 6 cups baby spinach

- ✓ 1 cup cherry tomatoes, halved
- ✓ 1 cup pecan halves
- ✓ 1/2 cup crumbled feta cheese
- ✓ Kosher salt, to taste
- ✓ Freshly ground black pepper, to taste

Directions:

- ❖ In a large skillet over medium high heat, melt butter
- ❖ Using paper towels, pat the steak dry, then drizzle with olive oil and season with salt and pepper, to taste
- ❖ Once heated, add the steak to the skillet and cook, flipping once, until cooked through to desired doneness, - cook for 4 minutes per side for a medium-rare steak
- ❖ Transfer the steak to a plate and allow it to cool before dicing
- ❖ Place the eggs in a large saucepan and cover with cold water by 1 inch
- ❖ Bring to a boil and cook for 1 minute, cover the eggs with a tight-fitting lid and remove from heat, set aside for 8-10 minutes, then drain well and allow to cool before peeling and dicing
- ❖ Assemble the salad in the container by placing the spinach at the bottom of the container, top with arranged rows of steak, eggs, feta, tomatoes, and pecans
- ❖ To Serve: Top with the balsamic vinaigrette, or desired dressing
- ❖ Recipe Note: You can also use New York, rib-eye or filet mignon for this recipe

Nutrition: Calories:640;Total Fat: 51g;Total Carbs: 9.8g;Fiber: 5g;Protein: 38.8g

30) LAMB CHOPS GRILL

Cooking Time: 10 Minutes   **Servings: 4**

Ingredients:

- ✓ 4 8-ounce lamb shoulder chops
- ✓ 2 tbsp Dijon mustard
- ✓ 2 tbsp balsamic vinegar

- ✓ 1 tbsp chopped garlic
- ✓ ¼ tsp ground black pepper
- ✓ ½ cup olive oil
- ✓ 2 tbsp fresh basil, shredded

Directions:

- ❖ Pat the lamb chops dry and arrange them in a shallow glass-baking dish.
- ❖ Take a bowl and whisk in Dijon mustard, garlic, balsamic vinegar, and pepper.
- ❖ Mix well to make the marinade.
- ❖ Whisk oil slowly into the marinade until it is smooth.
- ❖ Stir in basil.
- ❖ Pour the marinade over the lamb chops, making sure to coat both sides.
- ❖ Cover, refrigerate and allow the chops to marinate for anywhere from 1-4 hours.
- ❖ Remove the chops from the refrigerator and leave out for 30 minutes or until room temperature.
- ❖ Preheat grill to medium heat and oil grate.
- ❖ Grill the lamb chops until the center reads 145 degrees F and they are nicely browned, about 5-minutes per side.
- ❖ Enjoy!

Nutrition: Calories: 1587, Total Fat: 97.5 g, Saturated Fat: 27.6 g, Cholesterol: 600 mg, Sodium: 729 mg, Total Carbohydrate: 1.3 g, Dietary Fiber: 0.4 g, Total

Sugars: 0.1 g, Protein: 176.5 g, Vitamin D: 0 mcg, Calcium: 172 mg, Iron: 15 mg, Potassium: 30 mg

31) CHILI BROILED CALAMARI

Cooking Time: 8 Minutes   **Servings: 4**

Ingredients:

- ✓ 2 tbsp extra virgin olive oil
- ✓ 1 tsp chili powder
- ✓ ½ tsp ground cumin
- ✓ Zest of 1 lime
- ✓ Juice of 1 lime
- ✓ Dash of sea salt
- ✓ 1 and ½ pounds squid, cleaned and split open, with tentacles cut into ½ inch rounds
- ✓ 2 tbsp cilantro, chopped
- ✓ 2 tbsp red bell pepper, minced

Directions:

- ❖ Take a medium bowl and stir in olive oil, chili powder, cumin, lime zest, sea salt, lime juice and pepper
- ❖ Add squid and let it marinade and stir to coat, coat and let it refrigerate for 1 hour
- ❖ Pre-heat your oven to broil
- ❖ Arrange squid on a baking sheet, broil for 8 minutes turn once until tender
- ❖ Garnish the broiled calamari with cilantro and red bell pepper
- ❖ Serve and enjoy!
- ❖ Meal Prep/Storage Options: Store in airtight containers in your fridge for 1-2 days.

Nutrition: Calories:159;Fat: 13g;Carbohydrates: 12g;Protein: 3g

32) SALMON AND CORN PEPPER SALSA

Cooking Time: 12 Minutes   **Servings: 2**

Ingredients:

- ✓ 1 garlic clove, grated
- ✓ ½ tsp mild chili powder
- ✓ ½ tsp ground coriander
- ✓ ¼ tsp ground cumin
- ✓ 2 limes – 1, zest and juice; 1 cut into wedges
- ✓ 2 tsp rapeseed oil
- ✓ 2 wild salmon fillets
- ✓ 1 ear of corn on the cob, husk removed
- ✓ 1 red onion, finely chopped
- ✓ 1 avocado, cored, peeled, and finely chopped
- ✓ 1 red pepper, deseeded and finely chopped
- ✓ 1 red chili, halved and deseeded
- ✓ ½ a pack of finely chopped coriander

Directions:

- ❖ Boil the corn in water for about 6-8 minutes until tender.
- ❖ Drain and cut off the kernels.
- ❖ In a bowl, combine garlic, spices, 1 tbsp of limejuice, and oil; mix well to prepare spice rub.
- ❖ Coat the salmon with the rub.
- ❖ Add the zest to the corn and give it a gentle stir.
- ❖ Heat a frying pan over medium heat.
- ❖ Add salmon and cook for about 2 minutes per side.
- ❖ Serve the cooked salmon with salsa and lime wedges.
- ❖ Enjoy!

Nutrition: Calories: 949, Total Fat: 57.4 g, Saturated Fat: 9.7 g, Cholesterol: 2mg, Sodium: 180 mg, Total Carbohydrate: 33.5 g, Dietary Fiber: 11.8 g, Total Sugars: 8.3 g, Protein: 76.8 g, Vitamin D: 0 mcg, Calcium: 100 mg, Iron: 3 mg, Potassium: 856 mg

33) ITALIAN-INSPIRED ROTISSERIE CHICKEN WITH BROCCOLI SLAW

Cooking Time: 15 Minutes   **Servings: 4**

Ingredients:

- ✓ 4 cups packaged broccoli slaw
- ✓ 1 cooked rotisserie chicken, meat removed (about 10 to 12 ounces)
- ✓ 1 bunch red radishes, stemmed, halved, and thickly sliced (about 1¼ cups)
- ✓ 1 cup sliced red onion
- ✓ ½ cup pitted kalamata or niçoise olives, roughly chopped
- ✓ ½ cup sliced pepperoncini
- ✓ 8 tbsp Dijon Red Wine Vinaigrette, divided

Directions:

- ❖ Place the broccoli slaw, chicken, radishes, onion, olives, and pepperoncini in a large mixing bowl. Toss to combine.
- ❖ Place cups of salad in each of 4 containers. Pour 2 tbsp of vinaigrette into each of 4 sauce containers.
- ❖ STORAGE: Store covered containers in the refrigerator for up to 5 days.

Nutrition: Total calories: 329; Total fat: 2; Saturated fat: 4g; Sodium: 849mg; Carbohydrates: 10g; Fiber: 3g; Protein: 20g

34) FLATBREAD AND ROASTED VEGETABLES

Cooking Time: 45 Minutes   **Servings: 12**

Ingredients:

- 5 ounces goat cheese
- 1 thinly sliced onion
- 2 thinly sliced tomatoes
- Olive oil
- ¼ tsp pepper
- ⅛ tsp salt
- 16 ounces homemade or frozen pizza dough
- ¾ tbsp chopped dill, fresh is better
- 1 thinly sliced zucchini
- 1 red pepper, cup into rings

Directions:

- Set your oven to 400 degrees Fahrenheit.
- Set the dough on a large piece of parchment paper. Use a rolling pin to roll the dough into a large rectangle.
- Spread half of the goat cheese on ½ of the pizza dough.
- Sprinkle half of the dill on the other half of the dough.
- Fold the dough so the half with the dill is on top of the cheese.
- Spread the remaining goat cheese on the pizza dough and then sprinkle the rest of the dill over the cheese.
- Layer the vegetables on top in any arrangement you like.
- Drizzle olive oil on top of the vegetables.
- Sprinkle salt and pepper over the olive oil.
- Set the piece of parchment paper on a pizza pan or baking pan and place it in the oven.
- Set the timer for 22 minutes. If the edges are not a medium brown, leave the flatbread in the oven for another couple of minutes.
- Remove the pizza from the oven when it is done and cut the flatbread in half lengthwise.
- Slice the flatbread into 2-inch long pieces and enjoy!

Nutrition: calories: 170, fats: 5 grams, carbohydrates: 20 grams, protein: 8 grams.

35) SEAFOOD RICE

Cooking Time: 40 Minutes   **Servings: 4-5**

Ingredients:

- 4 small lobster tails (6-12 oz each)
- Water
- 3 tbsp Extra Virgin Olive Oil
- 1 large yellow onion, chopped
- 2 cups Spanish rice or short grain rice, soaked in water for 15 minutes and then drained
- 4 garlic cloves, chopped
- 2 large pinches of Spanish saffron threads soaked in 1/2 cup water
- 1 tsp Sweet Spanish paprika
- 1 tsp cayenne pepper
- 1/2 tsp aleppo pepper flakes
- Salt, to taste
- 2 large Roma tomatoes, finely chopped
- 6 oz French green beans, trimmed
- 1 lb prawns or large shrimp or your choice, peeled and deveined
- 1/4 cup chopped fresh parsley

Directions:

- In a large pot, add 3 cups of water and bring it to a rolling boil
- Add in the lobster tails and allow boil briefly, about 1-minutes or until pink, remove from heat
- Using tongs transfer the lobster tails to a plate and Do not discard the lobster cooking water
- Allow the lobster is cool, then remove the shell and cut into large chunks.
- In a large deep pan or skillet over medium-high heat, add 3 tbsp olive oil
- Add the chopped onions, sauté the onions for 2 minutes and then add the rice, and cook for 3 more minutes, stirring regularly
- Then add in the lobster cooking water and the chopped garlic and, stir in the saffron and its soaking liquid, cayenne pepper, aleppo pepper, paprika, and salt
- Gently stir in the chopped tomatoes and green beans, bring to a boil and allow the liquid slightly reduce, then cover (with lid or tightly wrapped foil) and cook over low heat for 20 minutes
- Once done, uncover and spread the shrimp over the rice, push it into the rice slightly, add in a little water, if needed
- Cover and cook for another 15 minutes until the shrimp turn pink
- Then add in the cooked lobster chunks
- Once the lobster is warmed through, remove from heat allow the dish to cool completely
- Distribute among the containers, store for 2 days
- To Serve: Reheat in the microwave for 1-2 minutes or until heated through. Garnish with parsley and enjoy!
- Recipe Notes: Remember to soak your rice if needed to help with the cooking process

Nutrition: Calories:536;Carbs: 56g;Total Fat: 26g;Protein: 50g

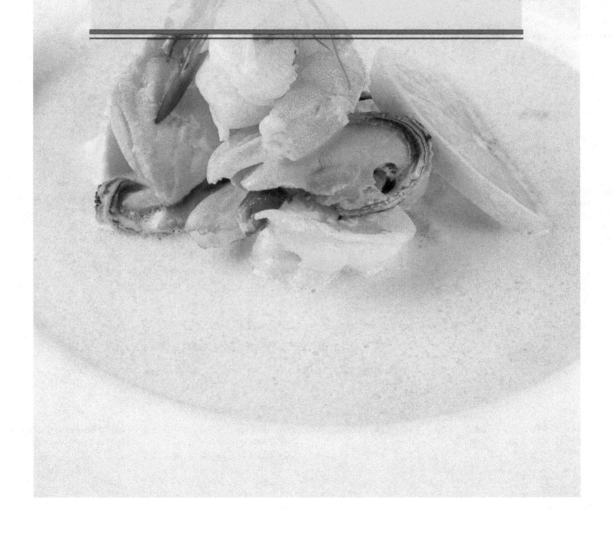

SOUPS & SALADS

36) MEXICAN-STYLE TORTILLA SOUP

Cooking Time: 40 Minutes   **Servings:** 4

Ingredients:

- ✓ 1-pound chicken breasts, boneless and skinless
- ✓ 1 can (15 ounces whole peeled tomatoes
- ✓ 1 can (10 ounces red enchilada sauce
- ✓ 1 and 1/2 tsp minced garlic
- ✓ 1 yellow onion, diced
- ✓ 1 can (4 ounces fire-roasted diced green chile
- ✓ 1 can (15 ounces black beans, drained and rinsed
- ✓ 1 can (15 ounces fire-roasted corn, undrained
- ✓ 1 container (32 ounces chicken stock or broth
- ✓ 1 tsp ground cumin
- ✓ 2 tsp chili powder
- ✓ 3/4 tsp paprika
- ✓ 1 bay leaf
- ✓ Salt and freshly cracked pepper, to taste
- ✓ 1 tbsp chopped cilantro Tortilla strips, Freshly squeezed lime juice, freshly grated cheddar cheese,

Directions:

- ❖ Set your Instant Pot on Sauté mode.
- ❖ Toss olive oil, onion and garlic into the insert of the Instant Pot.
- ❖ Sauté for 4 minutes then add chicken and remaining ingredients.
- ❖ Mix well gently then seal and lock the lid.
- ❖ Select Manual mode for 7 minutes at high pressure.
- ❖ Once done, release the pressure completely then remove the lid.
- ❖ Adjust seasoning as needed.
- ❖ Garnish with desired toppings.
- ❖ Enjoy.

Nutrition: Calories: 390;Carbohydrate: 5.6g;Protein: 29.5g;Fat: 26.5g;Sugar: 2.1g;Sodium: 620mg

37) MEDITERRANEAN CHICKEN NOODLE SOUP

Cooking Time: 35 Minutes   **Servings:** 6

Ingredients:

- ✓ 1 tbsp olive oil
- ✓ 1 1/2 cups peeled and diced carrots
- ✓ 1 1/2 cup diced celery
- ✓ 1 cup chopped yellow onion
- ✓ 3 tbsp minced garlic
- ✓ 8 cups low-sodium chicken broth
- ✓ 2 tsp minced fresh thyme
- ✓ 2 tsp minced fresh rosemary
- ✓ 1 bay leaf
- ✓ salt and freshly ground black pepper
- ✓ 2 1/2 lbs. bone-in, skin-on chicken thighs, skinned
- ✓ 3 cups wide egg noodles, such as American beauty
- ✓ 1 tbsp fresh lemon juice
- ✓ 1/4 cup chopped fresh parsley

Directions:

- ❖ Preheat olive oil in the insert of the Instant Pot on Sauté mode.
- ❖ Add onion, celery, and carrots and sauté them for minutes.
- ❖ Stir in garlic and sauté for 1 minute.
- ❖ Add bay leaf, thyme, broth, rosemary, salt, and pepper.
- ❖ Seal and secure the Instant Pot lid and select Manual mode for 10 minutes at high pressure.
- ❖ Once done, release the pressure completely then remove the lid.
- ❖ Add noodles to the insert and switch the Instant Pot to sauté mode.
- ❖ Cook the soup for 6 minutes until noodles are all done.
- ❖ Remove the chicken and shred it using a fork.
- ❖ Return the chicken to the soup then add lemon juice and parsley.
- ❖ Enjoy.

Nutrition: Calories: 333;Carbohydrate: 3.3g;Protein: 44.7g;Fat: 13.7g;Sugar: 1.1g;Sodium: 509mg

38) SPECIAL TURKEY ARUGULA SALAD

Cooking Time: 5 Minutes   **Servings:** 2

Ingredients:

- ✓ 4 oz turkey breast meat, diced into small pieces
- ✓ 3.5 oz arugula leaves
- ✓ 10 raspberries
- ✓ Juice from ½ a lime
- ✓ 2 tbsp extra virgin olive oil

Directions:

- ❖ Mix together the turkey with the rest of the ingredients in a large bowl until well combined.
- ❖ Dish out in a glass bowl and serve immediately.

Nutrition: Calories: 246;Carbs: 15.4g;Fats: 15.9g;Proteins: 12.2g;Sodium: 590mg;Sugar: 7.6g

39) SPECIAL CHEESY BROCCOLI SOUP

Cooking Time: 30 Minutes   **Servings: 4**

Ingredients:

- ½ cup heavy whipping cream
- 1 cup broccoli
- 1 cup cheddar cheese
- Salt, to taste
- 1½ cups chicken broth

Directions:

- ❖ Heat chicken broth in a large pot and add broccoli.
- ❖ Bring to a boil and stir in the rest of the ingredients.
- ❖ Allow the soup to simmer on low heat for about 20 minutes.
- ❖ Ladle out into a bowl and serve hot.

Nutrition: Calories: 188;Carbs: 2.6g;Fats: 15g;Proteins: 9.8g;Sodium: 514mg;Sugar: 0.8g

40) DELICIOUS RICH POTATO SOUP

Cooking Time: 30 Minutes   **Servings: 4**

Ingredients:

- 1 tbsp butter
- 1 medium onion, diced
- 3 cloves garlic, minced
- 3 cups chicken broth
- 1 can/box cream of chicken soup
- 7-8 medium-sized russet potatoes, peeled and chopped
- 1 1/2 tsp salt
- Black pepper to taste
- 1 cup milk
- 1 tbsp flour
- 2 cups shredded cheddar cheese
- Garnish:
- 5-6 slices bacon, chopped
- Sliced green onions
- Shredded cheddar cheese

Directions:

- ❖ Heat butter in the insert of the Instant Pot on sauté mode.
- ❖ Add onions and sauté for 4 minutes until soft.
- ❖ Stir in garlic and sauté it for 1 minute.
- ❖ Add potatoes, cream of chicken, broth, salt, and pepper to the insert.
- ❖ Mix well then seal and lock the lid.
- ❖ Cook this mixture for 10 minutes at Manual Mode with high pressure.
- ❖ Meanwhile, mix flour with milk in a bowl and set it aside.
- ❖ Once the instant pot beeps, release the pressure completely.
- ❖ Remove the Instant Pot lid and switch the instant pot to Sauté mode.
- ❖ Pour in flour slurry and stir cook the mixture for 5 minutes until it thickens.
- ❖ Add 2 cups of cheddar cheese and let it melt.
- ❖ Garnish it as desired.
- ❖ Serve.

Nutrition: Calories: 784;Carbohydrate: 54.8g;Protein: 34g;Fat: 46.5g;Sugar: 7.5g;Sodium: 849mg

41) MEDITERRANEAN-STYLE LENTIL SOUP

Cooking Time: 20 Minutes   **Servings: 4**

Ingredients:

- 1 tbsp olive oil
- 1/2 cup red lentils
- 1 medium yellow or red onion
- 2 garlic cloves, chopped
- 1/2 tsp ground cumin
- 1/2 tsp ground coriander
- 1/2 tsp ground sumac
- 1/2 tsp red chili flakes
- 1/2 tsp dried parsley
- 3/4 tsp dried mint flakes
- pinch of sugar
- 2.5 cups water
- salt, to taste
- black pepper, to taste
- juice of 1/2 lime
- parsley or cilantro, to garnish

Directions:

- ❖ Preheat oil in the insert of your Instant Pot on Sauté mode.
- ❖ Add onion and sauté until it turns golden brown.
- ❖ Toss in the garlic, parsley sugar, mint flakes, red chili flakes, sumac, coriander, and cumin.
- ❖ Stir cook this mixture for 2 minutes.
- ❖ Add water, lentils, salt, and pepper. Stir gently.
- ❖ Seal and lock the Instant Pot lid and select Manual mode for 8 minutes at high pressure.
- ❖ Once done, release the pressure completely then remove the lid.
- ❖ Stir well then add lime juice.
- ❖ Serve warm.

Nutrition: Calories: 525;Carbohydrate: 59.8g;Protein: 30.1g;Fat: 19.3g;Sugar: 17.3g;Sodium: 897mg

42) DELICIOUS CREAMY KETO CUCUMBER SALAD

Cooking Time: 5 Minutes   **Servings: 2**

Ingredients:

- ✓ 2 tbsp mayonnaise
- ✓ Salt and black pepper, to taste

- ✓ 1 cucumber, sliced and quartered
- ✓ 2 tbsp lemon juice

Directions:

- ❖ Mix together the mayonnaise, cucumber slices, and lemon juice in a large bowl.
- ❖ Season with salt and black pepper and combine well.
- ❖ Dish out in a glass bowl and serve while it is cold.

Nutrition: Calories: 8Carbs: 9.3g;Fats: 5.2g;Proteins: 1.2g;Sodium: 111mg;Sugar: 3.8g

43) SAUSAGE KALE SOUP AND MUSHROOMS

Cooking Time: 1 Hour 10 Minutes   **Servings: 6**

Ingredients:

- ✓ 2 cups fresh kale, cut into bite sized pieces
- ✓ 6.5 ounces mushrooms, sliced
- ✓ 6 cups chicken bone broth

- ✓ 1 pound sausage, cooked and sliced
- ✓ Salt and black pepper, to taste

Directions:

- ❖ Heat chicken broth with two cans of water in a large pot and bring to a boil.
- ❖ Stir in the rest of the ingredients and allow the soup to simmer on low heat for about 1 hour.
- ❖ Dish out and serve hot.

Nutrition: Calories: 259;Carbs: ;Fats: 20g;Proteins: 14g;Sodium: 995mg;Sugar: 0.6g

44) CLASSIC MINESTRONE SOUP

Cooking Time: 25 Minutes   **Servings: 6**

Ingredients:

- ✓ 2 tbsp olive oil
- ✓ 3 cloves garlic, minced
- ✓ 1 onion, diced
- ✓ 2 carrots, peeled and diced
- ✓ 2 stalks celery, diced
- ✓ 1 1/2 tsp dried basil
- ✓ 1 tsp dried oregano
- ✓ 1/2 tsp fennel seed
- ✓ 6 cups low sodium chicken broth
- ✓ 1 (28-ounce can diced tomatoes

- ✓ 1 (16-ounce can kidney beans, drained and rinsed
- ✓ 1 zucchini, chopped
- ✓ 1 (3-inch Parmesan rind
- ✓ 1 bay leaf
- ✓ 1 bunch kale leaves, chopped
- ✓ 2 tsp red wine vinegar
- ✓ Kosher salt and black pepper, to taste
- ✓ 1/3 cup freshly grated Parmesan
- ✓ 2 tbsp chopped fresh parsley leaves

Directions:

- ❖ Preheat olive oil in the insert of the Instant Pot on Sauté mode.
- ❖ Add carrots, celery, and onion, sauté for 3 minutes.
- ❖ Stir in fennel seeds, oregano, and basil. Stir cook for 1 minute.
- ❖ Add stock, beans, tomatoes, parmesan, bay leaf, and zucchini.
- ❖ Secure and seal the Instant Pot lid then select Manual mode to cook for minutes at high pressure.
- ❖ Once done, release the pressure completely then remove the lid.
- ❖ Add kale and let it sit for 2 minutes in the hot soup.
- ❖ Stir in red wine, vinegar, pepper, and salt.
- ❖ Garnish with parsley and parmesan.
- ❖ Enjoy.

Nutrition: Calories: 805;Carbohydrate: 2.5g;Protein: 124.1g;Fat: 34g;Sugar: 1.4g;Sodium: 634mg

45) SPECIAL KOMBU SEAWEED SALAD

Cooking Time: 40 Minutes   **Servings: 6**

Ingredients:

- ✓ 4 garlic cloves, crushed
- ✓ 1 pound fresh kombu seaweed, boiled and cut into strips

- ✓ 2 tbsp apple cider vinegar
- ✓ Salt, to taste
- ✓ 2 tbsp coconut aminos

Directions:

- ❖ Mix together the kombu, garlic, apple cider vinegar, and coconut aminos in a large bowl.
- ❖ Season with salt and combine well.
- ❖ Dish out in a glass bowl and serve immediately.

Nutrition: Calories: 257;Carbs: 16.9g;Fats: 19.;Proteins: 6.5g;Sodium: 294mg;Sugar: 2.7g

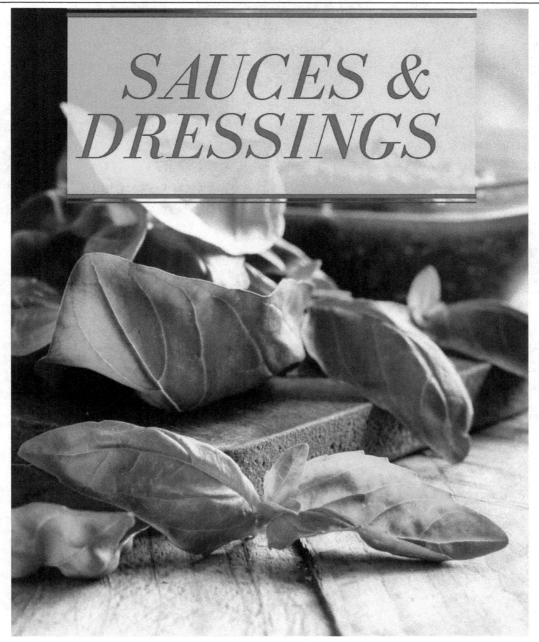

SAUCES &
DRESSINGS

46) SPECIAL POMEGRANATE VINAIGRETTE

Cooking Time: 5 Minutes   **Servings:** ½ Cup

Ingredients:

- ⅓ cup pomegranate juice
- 1 tsp Dijon mustard
- 1 tbsp apple cider vinegar
- ½ tsp dried mint
- 2 tbsp plus 2 tsp olive oil

Directions:

- ❖ Place the pomegranate juice, mustard, vinegar, and mint in a small bowl and whisk to combine.
- ❖ Whisk in the oil, pouring it into the bowl in a thin steam.
- ❖ Pour the vinaigrette into a container and refrigerate.
- ❖ STORAGE: Store the covered container in the refrigerator for up to 2 weeks. Bring the vinaigrette to room temperature and shake before serving.

Nutrition: (2 tbsp): Total calories: 94; Total fat: 10g; Saturated fat: 2g; Sodium: 30mg; Carbohydrates: 3g; Fiber: 0g; Protein: 0g

47) GREEN OLIVE WITH SPINACH TAPENADE

Cooking Time: 20 Minutes   **Servings:** 1½ Cups

Ingredients:

- 1 cup pimento-stuffed green olives, drained
- 3 packed cups baby spinach
- 1 tsp chopped garlic
- ½ tsp dried oregano
- ⅓ cup packed fresh basil
- 2 tbsp olive oil
- 2 tsp red wine vinegar

Directions:

- ❖ Place all the ingredients in the bowl of a food processor and pulse until the mixture looks finely chopped but not puréed.
- ❖ Scoop the tapenade into a container and refrigerate.
- ❖ STORAGE: Store the covered container in the refrigerator for up to 5 days.

Nutrition: (¼ cup): Total calories: 80; Total fat: 8g; Saturated fat: 1g; Sodium: 6mg; Carbohydrates: 1g; Fiber: 1g; Protein: 1g

48) BULGUR PILAF AND ALMONDS

Cooking Time: 20 Minutes   **Servings:** 4

Ingredients:

- ⅔ cup uncooked bulgur
- 1⅓ cups water
- ¼ cup sliced almonds
- 1 cup small diced red bell pepper
- ⅓ cup chopped fresh cilantro
- 1 tbsp olive oil
- ¼ tsp salt

Directions:

- ❖ Place the bulgur and water in a saucepan and bring the water to a boil. Once the water is at a boil, cover the pot with a lid and turn off the heat. Let the covered pot stand for 20 minutes.
- ❖ Transfer the cooked bulgur to a large mixing bowl and add the almonds, peppers, cilantro, oil, and salt. Stir to combine.
- ❖ Place about 1 cup of bulgur in each of 4 containers.
- ❖ STORAGE: Store covered containers in the refrigerator for up to 5 days. Bulgur can be either reheated or eaten at room temperature.

Nutrition: Total calories: 17 Total fat: 7g; Saturated fat: 1g; Sodium: 152mg; Carbohydrates: 25g; Fiber: 6g; Protein: 4g

49) SPANISH GARLIC YOGURT SAUCE

Cooking Time: 5 Minutes   **Servings:** 1 Cup

Ingredients:

- 1 cup low-fat (2%) plain Greek yogurt
- ½ tsp garlic powder
- 1 tbsp freshly squeezed lemon juice
- 1 tbsp olive oil
- ¼ tsp kosher salt

Directions:

- ❖ Mix all the ingredients in a medium bowl until well combined.
- ❖ Spoon the yogurt sauce into a container and refrigerate.
- ❖ STORAGE: Store the covered container in the refrigerator for up to 7 days

Nutrition: (¼ cup): Total calories: 75; Total fat: 5g; Saturated fat: 1g; Sodium: 173mg; Carbohydrates: 3g; Fiber: 0g; Protein: 6g.

50) ORANGE WITH CINNAMON–SCENTED WHOLE-WHEAT COUSCOUS

Cooking Time: 10 Minutes　　　　　**Servings: 4**

Ingredients:

- ✓ 2 tsp olive oil
- ✓ ¼ cup minced shallot
- ✓ ½ cup freshly squeezed orange juice (from 2 oranges)
- ✓ ½ cup water
- ✓ ⅛ tsp ground cinnamon
- ✓ ¼ tsp kosher salt
- ✓ 1 cup whole-wheat couscous

Directions:

- ❖ Heat the oil in a saucepan over medium heat. Once the oil is shimmering, add the shallot and cook for 2 minutes, stirring frequently. Add the orange juice, water, cinnamon, and salt, and bring to a boil.
- ❖ Once the liquid is boiling, add the couscous, cover the pan, and turn off the heat. Leave the couscous covered for 5 minutes. When the couscous is done, fluff with a fork.
- ❖ Place ¾ cup of couscous in each of 4 containers.
- ❖ STORAGE: Store covered containers in the refrigerator for up to 5 days. Freeze for up to 2 months.

Nutrition: Total calories: 21 Total fat: 4g; Saturated fat: <1g; Sodium: 147mg; Carbohydrates: 41g; Fiber: 5g; Protein: 8g

51) CHUNKY ROASTED CHERRY TOMATO WITH BASIL SAUCE

Cooking Time: 40 Minutes　　　　　**Servings: 1⅓ Cups**

Ingredients:

- ✓ 2 pints cherry tomatoes (20 ounces total)
- ✓ 2 tsp olive oil, plus 3 tbsp
- ✓ ¼ tsp kosher salt
- ✓ ½ tsp chopped garlic
- ✓ ¼ cup fresh basil leaves

Directions:

- ❖ Preheat the oven to 350°F. Line a sheet pan with a silicone baking mat or parchment paper.
- ❖ Place the tomatoes on the lined sheet pan and toss with tsp of oil. Roast for 40 minutes, shaking the pan halfway through.
- ❖ While the tomatoes are still warm, place them in a medium mixing bowl and add the salt, the garlic, and the remaining tbsp of oil. Mash the tomatoes with the back of a fork. Stir in the fresh basil.
- ❖ Scoop the sauce into a container and refrigerate.
- ❖ STORAGE: Store the covered container in the refrigerator for up to days.

Nutrition: (⅓ cup): Total calories: 141; Total fat: 13g; Saturated fat: 2g; Sodium: 158mg; Carbohydrates: 7g; Fiber: 2g; Protein: 1g

52) CELERY HEART, BASIL, AND ALMOND PESTO

Cooking Time: 10 Minutes　　　　　**Servings: 1 Cup**

Ingredients:

- ✓ ½ cup raw, unsalted almonds
- ✓ 3 cups fresh basil leaves, (about 1½ ounces)
- ✓ ½ cup chopped celery hearts with leaves
- ✓ ¼ tsp kosher salt
- ✓ 1 tbsp freshly squeezed lemon juice
- ✓ ¼ cup olive oil
- ✓ 3 tbsp water

Directions:

- ❖ Place the almonds in the bowl of a food processor and process until they look like coarse sand.
- ❖ Add the basil, celery hearts, salt, lemon juice, oil and water and process until smooth. The sauce will be somewhat thick. If you would like a thinner sauce, add more water, oil, or lemon juice, depending on your taste preference.
- ❖ Scoop the pesto into a container and refrigerate.
- ❖ STORAGE: Store the covered container in the refrigerator for up to 2 weeks. Pesto may be frozen for up to 6 months.

Nutrition: (¼ cup): Total calories: 231; Total fat: 22g; Saturated fat: 3g; Sodium: 178mg; Carbohydrates: 6g; Fiber: 3g; Protein: 4g

53) SAUTÉED KALE AND GARLIC WITH LEMON

Cooking Time: 7 Minutes　　　　　**Servings: 4**

Ingredients:

- ✓ 1 tbsp olive oil
- ✓ 3 bunches kale, stemmed and roughly chopped
- ✓ 2 tsp chopped garlic
- ✓ ¼ tsp kosher salt
- ✓ 1 tbsp freshly squeezed lemon juice

Directions:

- ❖ Heat the oil in a -inch skillet over medium-high heat. Once the oil is shimmering, add as much kale as will fit in the pan. You will probably only fit half the leaves into the pan at first. Mix the kale with tongs so that the leaves are coated with oil and start to wilt. As the kale wilts, keep adding more of the raw kale, continuing to use tongs to mix. Once all the kale is in the pan, add the garlic and salt and continue to cook until the kale is tender. Total cooking time from start to finish should be about 7 minutes.
- ❖ Mix the lemon juice into the kale. Add additional salt and/or lemon juice if necessary. Place 1 cup of kale in each of 4 containers and refrigerate.
- ❖ STORAGE: Store covered containers in the refrigerator for up to 5 days

Nutrition: Total calories: 8 Total fat: 1g; Saturated fat: <1g; Sodium: 214mg; Carbohydrates: 17g; Fiber: 6g; Protein: 6g

54) CREAMY POLENTA AND CHIVES WITH PARMESAN
Cooking Time: 15 Minutes   **Servings: 5**

Ingredients:

- ✓ 1 tsp olive oil
- ✓ ¼ cup minced shallot
- ✓ ½ cup white wine
- ✓ 3¼ cups water
- ✓ ¾ cup cornmeal
- ✓ 3 tbsp grated Parmesan cheese
- ✓ ½ tsp kosher salt
- ✓ ¼ cup chopped chives

Directions:

- ❖ Heat the oil in a saucepan over medium heat. Once the oil is shimmering, add the shallot and sauté for 2 minutes. Add the wine and water and bring to a boil.
- ❖ Pour the cornmeal in a thin, even stream into the liquid, stirring continuously until the mixture starts to thicken.
- ❖ Reduce the heat to low and continue to cook for 10 to 12 minutes, whisking every 1 to 2 minutes.
- ❖ Turn the heat off and stir in the cheese, salt, and chives. Cool.
- ❖ Place about ¾ cup of polenta in each of containers.
- ❖ STORAGE: Store covered containers in the refrigerator for up to 5 days.

Nutrition: Total calories: 110; Total fat: 3g; Saturated fat: 1g; Sodium: 29g; Carbohydrates: 16g; Fiber: 1g; Protein: 3g

55) SPECIAL MOCHA-NUT STUFFED DATES
Cooking Time: 10 Minutes   **Servings: 5**

Ingredients:

- ✓ 2 tbsp creamy, unsweetened, unsalted almond butter
- ✓ 1 tsp unsweetened cocoa powder
- ✓ 3 tbsp walnut pieces
- ✓ 2 tbsp water
- ✓ ¼ tsp honey
- ✓ ¾ tsp instant espresso powder
- ✓ 10 Medjool dates, pitted

Directions:

- ❖ In a small bowl, combine the almond butter, cocoa powder, and walnut pieces.
- ❖ Place the water in a small microwaveable mug and heat on high for 30 seconds. Add the honey and espresso powder to the water and stir to dissolve.
- ❖ Add the espresso water to the cocoa bowl and combine thoroughly until a creamy, thick paste forms.
- ❖ Stuff each pitted date with 1 tsp of mocha filling.
- ❖ Place 2 dates in each of small containers.
- ❖ STORAGE: Store covered containers in the refrigerator for up to 5 days.

Nutrition: Total calories: 205; Total fat: ; Saturated fat: 1g; Sodium: 1mg; Carbohydrates: 39g; Fiber: 4g; Protein: 3g

56) EGGPLANT DIP ROAST (BABA GHANOUSH)
Cooking Time: 45 Minutes   **Servings: 2 Cups**

Ingredients:

- ✓ 2 eggplants (close to 1 pound each)
- ✓ 1 tsp chopped garlic
- ✓ 3 tbsp unsalted tahini
- ✓ ¼ cup freshly squeezed lemon juice
- ✓ 1 tbsp olive oil
- ✓ ½ tsp kosher salt

Directions:

- ❖ Preheat the oven to 450°F and line a sheet pan with a silicone baking mat or parchment paper.
- ❖ Prick the eggplants in many places with a fork, place on the sheet pan, and roast in the oven until extremely soft, about 45 minutes. The eggplants should look like they are deflating.
- ❖ When the eggplants are cool, cut them open and scoop the flesh into a large bowl. You may need to use your hands to pull the flesh away from the skin. Discard the skin. Mash the flesh very well with a fork.
- ❖ Add the garlic, tahini, lemon juice, oil, and salt. Taste and adjust the seasoning with additional lemon juice, salt, or tahini if needed.
- ❖ Scoop the dip into a container and refrigerate.
- ❖ STORAGE: Store the covered container in the refrigerator for up to 5 days.

Nutrition: (¼ cup): Total calories: 8 Total fat: 5g; Saturated fat: 1g; Sodium: 156mg; Carbohydrates: 10g; Fiber: 4g; Protein: 2g

57) DELICIOUS HONEY-LEMON VINAIGRETTE

Cooking Time: 5 Minutes   **Servings:** ½ Cup

Ingredients:

- ✓ ¼ cup freshly squeezed lemon juice
- ✓ 1 tsp honey
- ✓ 2 tsp Dijon mustard
- ✓ ⅛ tsp kosher salt
- ✓ ¼ cup olive oil

Directions:

- ❖ Place the lemon juice, honey, mustard, and salt in a small bowl and whisk to combine.
- ❖ Whisk in the oil, pouring it into the bowl in a thin steam.
- ❖ Pour the vinaigrette into a container and refrigerate.
- ❖ STORAGE: Store the covered container in the refrigerator for up to 2 weeks. Allow the vinaigrette to come to room temperature and shake before serving.

Nutrition: (2 tbsp): Total calories: 131; Total fat: 14g; Saturated fat: 2g; Sodium: 133mg; Carbohydrates: 3g; Fiber: <1g; Protein: <1g

58) SPANISH-STYLE ROMESCO SAUCE

Cooking Time: 10 Minutes   **Servings:** 1⅔ Cups

Ingredients:

- ✓ ½ cup raw, unsalted almonds
- ✓ 4 medium garlic cloves (do not peel)
- ✓ 1 (12-ounce) jar of roasted red peppers, drained
- ✓ ½ cup canned diced fire-roasted tomatoes, drained
- ✓ 1 tsp smoked paprika
- ✓ ½ tsp kosher salt
- ✓ Pinch cayenne pepper
- ✓ 2 tsp red wine vinegar
- ✓ 2 tbsp olive oil

Directions:

- ❖ Preheat the oven to 350°F.
- ❖ Place the almonds and garlic cloves on a sheet pan and toast in the oven for 10 minutes. Remove from the oven and peel the garlic when cool enough to handle.
- ❖ Place the almonds in the bowl of a food processor. Process the almonds until they resemble coarse sand, to 45 seconds. Add the garlic, peppers, tomatoes, paprika, salt, and cayenne. Blend until smooth.
- ❖ Once the mixture is smooth, add the vinegar and oil and blend until well combined. Taste and add more vinegar or salt if needed.
- ❖ Scoop the romesco sauce into a container and refrigerate.
- ❖ STORAGE: Store the covered container in the refrigerator for up to 7 days.

Nutrition: (⅓ cup): Total calories: 158; Total fat: 13g; Saturated fat: 1g; Sodium: 292mg; Carbohydrates: 10g; Fiber: 3g; Protein: 4g

59) CARDAMOM MASCARPONE AND STRAWBERRIES

Cooking Time: 10 Minutes   **Servings:** 4

Ingredients:

- ✓ 1 (8-ounce) container mascarpone cheese
- ✓ 2 tsp honey
- ✓ ¼ tsp ground cardamom
- ✓ 2 tbsp milk
- ✓ 1 pound strawberries (should be 24 strawberries in the pack)

Directions:

- ❖ Combine the mascarpone, honey, cardamom, and milk in a medium mixing bowl.
- ❖ Mix the ingredients with a spoon until super creamy, about 30 seconds.
- ❖ Place 6 strawberries and 2 tbsp of the mascarpone mixture in each of 4 containers.
- ❖ STORAGE: Store covered containers in the refrigerator for up to 5 days.

Nutrition: Total calories: 289; Total fat: 2; Saturated fat: 10g; Sodium: 26mg; Carbohydrates: 11g; Fiber: 3g; Protein: 1g

60) SWEET SPICY GREEN PUMPKIN SEEDS

Cooking Time: 15 Minutes   **Servings:** 2 Cups

Ingredients:

- ✓ 2 cups raw green pumpkin seeds (pepitas)
- ✓ 1 egg white, beaten until frothy
- ✓ 3 tbsp honey
- ✓ 1 tbsp chili powder
- ✓ ¼ tsp cayenne pepper
- ✓ 1 tsp ground cinnamon
- ✓ ¼ tsp kosher salt

Directions:

- ❖ Preheat the oven to 350°F. Line a sheet pan with a silicone baking mat or parchment paper.
- ❖ In a medium bowl, mix all the ingredients until the seeds are well coated. Place on the lined sheet pan in a single, even layer.
- ❖ Bake for 15 minutes. Cool the seeds on the sheet pan, then peel clusters from the baking mat and break apart into small pieces.
- ❖ Place ¼ cup of seeds in each of 8 small containers or resealable sandwich bags.
- ❖ STORAGE: Store covered containers or resealable bags at room temperature for up to days.

Nutrition: (¼ cup): Total calories: 209; Total fat: 15g; Saturated fat: 3g; Sodium: 85mg; Carbohydrates: 11g; Fiber: 2g; Protein: 10g

61) DELICIOUS RASPBERRY RED WINE SAUCE

Cooking Time: 20 Minutes   **Servings: 1 Cup**

Ingredients:

- ✓ 2 tsp olive oil
- ✓ 2 tbsp finely chopped shallot
- ✓ 1½ cups frozen raspberries
- ✓ 1 cup dry, fruity red wine
- ✓ 1 tsp thyme leaves, roughly chopped
- ✓ 1 tsp honey
- ✓ ¼ tsp kosher salt
- ✓ ½ tsp unsweetened cocoa powder

Directions:

- ❖ In a -inch skillet, heat the oil over medium heat. Add the shallot and cook until soft, about 2 minutes.
- ❖ Add the raspberries, wine, thyme, and honey and cook on medium heat until reduced, about 15 minutes. Stir in the salt and cocoa powder.
- ❖ Transfer the sauce to a blender and blend until smooth. Depending on how much you can scrape out of your blender, this recipe makes ¾ to 1 cup of sauce.
- ❖ Scoop the sauce into a container and refrigerate.
- ❖ STORAGE: Store the covered container in the refrigerator for up to 7 days.

Nutrition: (¼ cup): Total calories: 107; Total fat: 3g; Saturated fat: <1g; Sodium: 148mg; Carbohydrates: 1g; Fiber: 4g; Protein: 1g

62) ANTIPASTO SHRIMP SKEWERS

Cooking Time: 10 Minutes   **Servings: 4**

Ingredients:

- ✓ 16 pitted kalamata or green olives
- ✓ 16 fresh mozzarella balls (ciliegine)
- ✓ 16 cherry tomatoes
- ✓ 16 medium (41 to 50 per pound) precooked peeled, deveined shrimp
- ✓ 8 (8-inch) wooden or metal skewers

Directions:

- ❖ Alternate 2 olives, 2 mozzarella balls, 2 cherry tomatoes, and 2 shrimp on 8 skewers.
- ❖ Place skewers in each of 4 containers.
- ❖ STORAGE: Store covered containers in the refrigerator for up to 4 days.

Nutrition: Total calories: 108; Total fat: 6g; Saturated fat: 1g; Sodium: 328mg; Carbohydrates: ; Fiber: 1g; Protein: 9g

63) SMOKED PAPRIKA WITH OLIVE OIL–MARINATED CARROTS

Cooking Time: 5 Minutes   **Servings: 4**

Ingredients:

- ✓ 1 (1-pound) bag baby carrots (not the petite size)
- ✓ 2 tbsp olive oil
- ✓ 2 tbsp red wine vinegar
- ✓ ¼ tsp garlic powder
- ✓ ¼ tsp ground cumin
- ✓ ¼ tsp smoked paprika
- ✓ ⅛ tsp red pepper flakes
- ✓ ¼ cup chopped parsley
- ✓ ¼ tsp kosher salt

Directions:

- ❖ Pour enough water into a saucepan to come ¼ inch up the sides. Turn the heat to high, bring the water to a boil, add the carrots, and cover with a lid. Steam the carrots for 5 minutes, until crisp tender.
- ❖ After the carrots have cooled, mix with the oil, vinegar, garlic powder, cumin, paprika, red pepper, parsley, and salt.
- ❖ Place ¾ cup of carrots in each of 4 containers.
- ❖ STORAGE: Store covered containers in the refrigerator for up to 5 days.

Nutrition: Total calories: 109; Total fat: 7g; Saturated fat: 1g; Sodium: 234mg; Carbohydrates: 11g; Fiber: 3g; Protein: 2g

64) GREEK TZATZIKI SAUCE

Cooking Time: 15 Minutes   **Servings: 2½ Cups**

Ingredients:

- ✓ 1 English cucumber
- ✓ 2 cups low-fat (2%) plain Greek yogurt
- ✓ 1 tbsp olive oil
- ✓ 2 tsp freshly squeezed lemon juice
- ✓ ½ tsp chopped garlic
- ✓ ½ tsp kosher salt
- ✓ ⅛ tsp freshly ground black pepper
- ✓ 2 tbsp chopped fresh dill
- ✓ 2 tbsp chopped fresh mint

Directions:

- ❖ Place a sieve over a medium bowl. Grate the cucumber, with the skin, over the sieve. Press the grated cucumber into the sieve with the flat surface of a spatula to press as much liquid out as possible.
- ❖ In a separate medium bowl, place the yogurt, oil, lemon juice, garlic, salt, pepper, dill, and mint and stir to combine.
- ❖ Press on the cucumber one last time, then add it to the yogurt mixture. Stir to combine. Taste and add more salt and lemon juice if necessary.
- ❖ Scoop the sauce into a container and refrigerate.
- ❖ STORAGE: Store the covered container in the refrigerator for up to days.

Nutrition: (¼ cup): Total calories: 51; Total fat: 2g; Saturated fat: 1g; Sodium: 137mg; Carbohydrates: 3g; Fiber: <1g; Protein: 5g

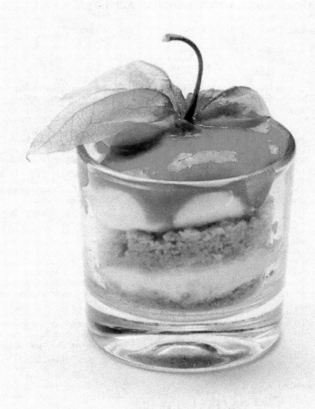

DESSERTS & SNACKS

65) CHERRY BROWNIES AND WALNUTS

Cooking Time: 25 To 30 Minutes   **Servings: 9**

Ingredients:

- 9 fresh cherries that are stemmed and pitted or 9 frozen cherries
- ½ cup sugar or sweetener substitute
- ¼ cup extra virgin olive oil
- 1 tsp vanilla extract
- ¼ tsp sea salt
- ½ cup whole-wheat pastry flour
- ¼ tsp baking powder
- ⅓ cup walnuts, chopped
- 2 eggs
- ½ cup plain Greek yogurt
- ⅓ cup cocoa powder, unsweetened

Directions:

- ❖ Make sure one of the metal racks in your oven is set in the middle.
- ❖ Turn the temperature on your oven to 375 degrees Fahrenheit.
- ❖ Using cooking spray, grease a 9-inch square pan.
- ❖ Take a large bowl and add the oil and sugar or sweetener substitute. Whisk the ingredients well.
- ❖ Add the eggs and use a mixer to beat the ingredients together.
- ❖ Pour in the yogurt and continue to beat the mixture until it is smooth.
- ❖ Take a medium bowl and combine the cocoa powder, flour, sea salt, and baking powder by whisking them together.
- ❖ Combine the powdered ingredients into the wet ingredients and use your electronic mixer to incorporate the ingredients together thoroughly.
- ❖ Add in the walnuts and stir.
- ❖ Pour the mixture into the pan.
- ❖ Sprinkle the cherries on top and push them into the batter. You can use any design, but it is best to make three rows and three columns with the cherries. This ensures that each piece of the brownie will have one cherry.
- ❖ Put the batter into the oven and turn your timer to 20 minutes.
- ❖ Check that the brownies are done using the toothpick test before removing them from the oven. Push the toothpick into the middle of the brownies and once it comes out clean, remove the brownies.
- ❖ Let the brownies cool for 5 to 10 minutes before cutting and serving.

Nutrition: calories: 225, fats: 10 grams, carbohydrates: 30 grams, protein: 5 grams

66) SPECIAL FRUIT DIP

Cooking Time: 10 To 15 Minutes   **Servings: 10**

Ingredients:

- ¼ cup coconut milk, full-fat is best
- ¼ cup vanilla yogurt
- ⅓ cup marshmallow creme
- 1 cup cream cheese, set at room temperature
- 2 tbsp maraschino cherry juice

Directions:

- ❖ In a large bowl, add the coconut milk, vanilla yogurt, marshmallow creme, cream cheese, and cherry juice.
- ❖ Using an electric mixer, set to low speed and blend the ingredients together until the fruit dip is smooth.
- ❖ Serve the dip with some of your favorite fruits and enjoy!

Nutrition: calories: 110, fats: 11 grams, carbohydrates: 3 grams, protein: 3 grams

67) DELICIOUS LEMONY TREAT

Cooking Time: 30 Minutes   **Servings: 4**

Ingredients:

- ✓ 1 lemon, medium in size
- ✓ 1 ½ tsp cornstarch
- ✓ 1 cup Greek yogurt, plain is best
- ✓ Fresh fruit
- ✓ ¼ cup cold water
- ✓ ⅔ cup heavy whipped cream
- ✓ 3 tbsp honey
- ✓ Optional: mint leaves

Directions:

- ❖ Take a large glass bowl and your metal, electric mixer and set them in the refrigerator so they can chill.
- ❖ In a separate bowl, add the yogurt and set that in the fridge.
- ❖ Zest the lemon into a medium bowl that is microwavable.
- ❖ Cut the lemon in half and then squeeze 1 tbsp of lemon juice into the bowl.
- ❖ Combine the cornstarch and water. Mix the ingredients thoroughly.
- ❖ Pour in the honey and whisk the ingredients together.
- ❖ Put the mixture into the microwave for 1 minute on high.
- ❖ Once the microwave stops, remove the mixture and stir.
- ❖ Set it back into the microwave for 15 to 30 seconds or until the mixture starts to bubble and thicken.
- ❖ Take the bowl of yogurt from the fridge and pour in the warm mixture while whisking.
- ❖ Put the yogurt mixture back into the fridge.
- ❖ Take the large bowl and beaters out of the fridge.
- ❖ Put your electronic mixer together and pour the whipped cream into the chilled bowl.
- ❖ Beat the cream until soft peaks start to form. This can take up to 3 minutes, depending on how fresh your cream is.
- ❖ Remove the yogurt from the fridge.
- ❖ Fold the yogurt into the cream using a rubber spatula. Remember to lift and turn the mixture so it doesn't deflate.
- ❖ Place back into the fridge until you are serving the dessert or for 15 minutes. The dessert should not be in the fridge for longer than 1 hour.
- ❖ When you serve the lemony goodness, you will spoon it into four dessert dishes and drizzle with extra honey or even melt some chocolate to drizzle on top.
- ❖ Add a little fresh mint and enjoy!

Nutrition: calories: 241, fats: 16 grams, carbohydrates: 21 grams, protein: 7 grams

68) MELON AND GINGER

Cooking Time: 10 To 15 Minutes   **Servings: 4**

Ingredients:

- ✓ ½ cantaloupe, cut into 1-inch chunks
- ✓ 2 cups of watermelon, cut into 1-inch chunks
- ✓ 2 cups honeydew melon, cut into 1-inch chunks
- ✓ 2 tbsp of raw honey
- ✓ Ginger, 2 inches in size, peeled, grated, and preserve the juice

Directions:

- ❖ In a large bowl, combine your cantaloupe, honeydew melon, and watermelon. Gently mix the ingredients.
- ❖ Combine the ginger juice and stir.
- ❖ Drizzle on the honey, serve, and enjoy! You can also chill the mixture for up to an hour before serving.

Nutrition: calories: 91, fats: 0 grams, carbohydrates: 23 grams, protein: 1 gram.

69) DELICIOUS ALMOND SHORTBREAD COOKIES

Cooking Time: 25 Minutes   **Servings:** 16

Ingredients:

- ½ cup coconut oil
- 1 tsp vanilla extract
- 2 egg yolks
- 1 tbsp brandy
- 1 cup powdered sugar
- 1 cup finely ground almonds
- 3 ½ cups cake flour
- ½ cup almond butter
- 1 tbsp water or rose flower water

Directions:

- In a large bowl, combine the coconut oil, powdered sugar, and butter. If the butter is not soft, you want to wait until it softens up. Use an electric mixer to beat the ingredients together at high speed.
- In a small bowl, add the egg yolks, brandy, water, and vanilla extract. Whisk well.
- Fold the egg yolk mixture into the large bowl.
- Add the flour and almonds. Fold and mix with a wooden spoon.
- Place the mixture into the fridge for at least 1 hour and 30 minutes.
- Preheat your oven to 325 degrees Fahrenheit.
- Take the mixture, which now looks like dough, and divide it into 1-inch balls.
- With a piece of parchment paper on a baking sheet, arrange the cookies and flatten them with a fork or your fingers.
- Place the cookies in the oven for 13 minutes, but watch them so they don't burn.
- Transfer the cookies onto a rack to cool for a couple of minutes before enjoying!

Nutrition: calories: 250, fats: 14 grams, carbohydrates: 30 grams, protein: 3 grams

70) CLASSIC CHOCOLATE FRUIT KEBABS

Cooking Time: 30 Minutes   **Servings:** 6

Ingredients:

- 24 blueberries
- 12 strawberries with the green leafy top part removed
- 12 green or red grapes, seedless
- 12 pitted cherries
- 8 ounces chocolate

Directions:

- Line a baking sheet with a piece of parchment paper and place 6, -inch long wooden skewers on top of the paper.
- Start by threading a piece of fruit onto the skewers. You can create and follow any pattern that you like with the ingredients. An example pattern is 1 strawberry, 1 cherry, blueberries, 2 grapes. Repeat the pattern until all of the fruit is on the skewers.
- In a saucepan on medium heat, melt the chocolate. Stir continuously until the chocolate has melted completely.
- Carefully scoop the chocolate into a plastic sandwich bag and twist the bag closed starting right above the chocolate.
- Snip the corner of the bag with scissors.
- Drizzle the chocolate onto the kebabs by squeezing it out of the bag.
- Put the baking pan into the freezer for 20 minutes.
- Serve and enjoy!

Nutrition: calories: 254, fats: 15 grams, carbohydrates: 28 grams, protein: 4 grams. 71)

72) PEACHES AND BLUE CHEESE CREAM

Cooking Time: 20 Hours 10 Minutes   **Servings:** 4

Ingredients:

- 4 peaches
- 1 cinnamon stick
- 4 ounces sliced blue cheese
- ⅓ cup orange juice, freshly squeezed is best
- 3 whole cloves
- 1 tsp of orange zest, taken from the orange peel
- ¼ tsp cardamom pods
- ⅔ cup red wine
- 2 tbsp honey, raw or your preferred variety
- 1 vanilla bean
- 1 tsp allspice berries
- 4 tbsp dried cherries

Directions:

- Set a saucepan on top of your stove range and add the cinnamon stick, cloves, orange juice, cardamom, vanilla, allspice, red wine, and orange zest. Whisk the ingredients well. Add your peaches to the mixture and poach them for hours or until they become soft.
- Take a spoon to remove the peaches and boil the rest of the liquid to make the syrup. You want the liquid to reduce itself by at least half.
- While the liquid is boiling, combine the dried cherries, blue cheese, and honey into a bowl. Once your peaches are cooled, slice them into halves.
- Top each peach with the blue cheese mixture and then drizzle the liquid onto the top. Serve and enjoy!

Nutrition: calories: 211, fats: 24 grams, carbohydrates: 15 grams, protein: 6 grams

73) MEDITERRANEAN-STYLE BLACKBERRY ICE CREAM

Cooking Time: 15 Minutes   **Servings: 6**

Ingredients:

- ✓ 3 egg yolks
- ✓ 1 container of Greek yogurt
- ✓ 1 pound mashed blackberries
- ✓ ½ tsp vanilla essence
- ✓ 1 tsp arrowroot powder
- ✓ ¼ tsp ground cloves
- ✓ 5 ounces sugar or sweetener substitute
- ✓ 1 pound heavy cream

Directions:

- ❖ In a small bowl, add the arrowroot powder and egg yolks. Whisk or beat them with an electronic mixture until they are well combined.
- ❖ Set a saucepan on top of your stove and turn your heat to medium.
- ❖ Add the heavy cream and bring it to a boil.
- ❖ Turn off the heat and add the egg mixture into the cream through folding.
- ❖ Turn the heat back on to medium and pour in the sugar. Cook the mixture for 10 minutes or until it starts to thicken.
- ❖ Remove the mixture from heat and place it in the fridge so it can completely cool. This should take about one hour.
- ❖ Once the mixture is cooled, add in the Greek yogurt, ground cloves, blackberries, and vanilla by folding in the ingredients.
- ❖ Transfer the ice cream into a container and place it in the freezer for at least two hours.
- ❖ Serve and enjoy!

Nutrition: calories: 402, fats: 20 grams, carbohydrates: 52 grams, protein: 8 grams

74) CLASSIC STUFFED FIGS

Cooking Time: 20 Minutes   **Servings: 6**

Ingredients:

- ✓ 10 halved fresh figs
- ✓ 20 chopped almonds
- ✓ 4 ounces goat cheese, divided
- ✓ 2 tbsp of raw honey

Directions:

- ❖ Turn your oven to broiler mode and set it to a high temperature.
- ❖ Place your figs, cut side up, on a baking sheet. If you like to place a piece of parchment paper on top you can do this, but it is not necessary.
- ❖ Sprinkle each fig with half of the goat cheese.
- ❖ Add a tbsp of chopped almonds to each fig.
- ❖ Broil the figs for 3 to 4 minutes.
- ❖ Take them out of the oven and let them cool for 5 to 7 minutes.
- ❖ Sprinkle with the remaining goat cheese and honey.

Nutrition: calories: 209, fats: 9 grams, carbohydrates: 26 grams, protein: grams.

75) CHIA PUDDING AND STRAWBERRIES

Cooking Time: 4 Hours 5 Minutes   **Servings: 4**

Ingredients:

- ✓ 2 cups unsweetened almond milk
- ✓ 1 tbsp vanilla extract
- ✓ 2 tbsp raw honey
- ✓ ¼ cup chia seeds
- ✓ 2 cups fresh and sliced strawberries

Directions:

- ❖ In a medium bowl, combine the honey, chia seeds, vanilla, and unsweetened almond milk. Mix well.
- ❖ Set the mixture in the refrigerator for at least 4 hours.
- ❖ When you serve the pudding, top it with strawberries. You can even create a design in a glass serving bowl or dessert dish by adding a little pudding on the bottom, a few strawberries, top the strawberries with some more pudding, and then top the dish with a few strawberries.

Nutrition: calories: 108, fats: grams, carbohydrates: 17 grams, protein: 3 grams

MEAT
RECIPES

76) CLASSIC AIOLI BAKED CHICKEN WINGS

Cooking Time: 35 Minutes   **Servings:** 4

Ingredients:

- ✓ 4 chicken wings
- ✓ 1 cup Halloumi cheese, cubed
- ✓ 1 tbsp garlic, finely minced
- ✓ 1 tbsp fresh lime juice
- ✓ 1 tbsp fresh coriander, chopped
- ✓ 6 black olives, pitted and halved
- ✓ 1 ½ tbsp butter
- ✓ 1 hard-boiled egg yolk
- ✓ 1 tbsp balsamic vinegar
- ✓ 1/2 cup extra-virgin olive oil
- ✓ 1/4 tsp flaky sea salt
- ✓ Sea salt and pepper, to season

Directions:

- ❖ In a saucepan, melt the butter until sizzling. Sear the chicken wings for 5 minutes per side. Season with salt and pepper to taste.
- ❖ Place the chicken wings on a parchment-lined baking pan
- ❖ Mix the egg yolk, garlic, lime juice, balsamic vinegar, olive oil, and salt in your blender until creamy, uniform and smooth.
- ❖ Spread the Aioli over the fried chicken. Now, scatter the coriander and black olives on top of the chicken wings.
- ❖ Bake in the preheated oven at 380 degrees F for 20 to 2minutes. Top with the cheese and bake an additional 5 minutes until hot and bubbly.
- ❖ Storing
- ❖ Place the chicken wings in airtight containers or Ziploc bags; keep in your refrigerator for up 3 to 4 days.
- ❖ For freezing, place the chicken wings in airtight containers or heavy-duty freezer bags. Freeze up to 3 months. Once thawed in the refrigerator, heat in the preheated oven at 375 degrees F for 20 to 25 minutes or until heated through. Enjoy!

Nutrition: 562 Calories; 43.8g Fat; 2.1g Carbs; 40.8g Protein; 0.4g Fiber

77) SPECIAL SMOKED PORK SAUSAGE KETO BOMBS

Cooking Time: 15 Minutes   **Servings:** 6

Ingredients:

- ✓ 3/4 pound smoked pork sausage, ground
- ✓ 1 tsp ginger-garlic paste
- ✓ 2 tbsp scallions, minced
- ✓ 1 tbsp butter, room temperature
- ✓ 1 tomato, pureed
- ✓ 4 ounces mozzarella cheese, crumbled
- ✓ 2 tbsp flaxseed meal
- ✓ 8 ounces cream cheese, room temperature
- ✓ Sea salt and ground black pepper, to taste

Directions:

- ❖ Melt the butter in a frying pan over medium-high heat. Cook the sausage for about 4 minutes, crumbling with a spatula.
- ❖ Add in the ginger-garlic paste, scallions, and tomato; continue to cook over medium-low heat for a further 6 minutes. Stir in the remaining ingredients.
- ❖ Place the mixture in your refrigerator for 1 to 2 hours until firm. Roll the mixture into bite-sized balls.
- ❖ Storing
- ❖ Transfer the balls to the airtight containers and place in your refrigerator for up to 3 days.
- ❖ For freezing, place in a freezer safe containers and freeze up to 1 month. Enjoy!

Nutrition: 383 Calories; 32. Fat; 5.1g Carbs; 16.7g Protein; 1.7g Fiber

78) TURKEY MEATBALLS AND TANGY BASIL CHUTNEY

Cooking Time: 30 Minutes   **Servings:** 6

Ingredients:

- ✓ 2 tbsp sesame oil
- ✓ For the Meatballs:
- ✓ 1/2 cup Romano cheese, grated
- ✓ 1 tsp garlic, minced
- ✓ 1/2 tsp shallot powder
- ✓ 1/4 tsp dried thyme
- ✓ 1/2 tsp mustard seeds
- ✓ 2 small-sized eggs, lightly beaten
- ✓ 1 ½ pounds ground turkey
- ✓ 1/2 tsp sea salt
- ✓ 1/4 tsp ground black pepper, or more to taste
- ✓ 3 tbsp almond meal
- ✓ For the Basil Chutney:
- ✓ 2 tbsp fresh lime juice
- ✓ 1/4 cup fresh basil leaves
- ✓ 1/4 cup fresh parsley
- ✓ 1/2 cup cilantro leaves
- ✓ 1 tsp fresh ginger root, grated
- ✓ 2 tbsp olive oil
- ✓ 2 tbsp water
- ✓ 1 tbsp habanero chili pepper, deveined and minced

Directions:

- ❖ In a mixing bowl, combine all ingredients for the meatballs. Roll the mixture into meatballs and reserve.
- ❖ Heat the sesame oil in a frying pan over a moderate flame. Sear the meatballs for about 8 minutes until browned on all sides.
- ❖ Make the chutney by mixing all the ingredients in your blender or food processor.
- ❖ Storing
- ❖ Place the meatballs in airtight containers or Ziploc bags; keep in your refrigerator for up to 3 to 4 days.
- ❖ Freeze the meatballs in airtight containers or heavy-duty freezer bags. Freeze up to 3 to 4 months. To defrost, slowly reheat in a frying pan.
- ❖ Store the basil chutney in the refrigerator for up to a week. Bon appétit!

Nutrition: 390 Calories; 27.2g Fat; 1. Carbs; 37.4g Protein; 0.3g Fiber

79) ROASTED CHICKEN AND CASHEW PESTO

Cooking Time: 35 Minutes

Servings: 4

Ingredients:

- ✓ 1 cup leeks, chopped
- ✓ 1 pound chicken legs, skinless
- ✓ Salt and ground black pepper, to taste
- ✓ 1/2 tsp red pepper flakes
- ✓ For the Cashew-Basil Pesto:

- ✓ 1/2 cup cashews
- ✓ 2 garlic cloves, minced
- ✓ 1/2 cup fresh basil leaves
- ✓ 1/2 cup Parmigiano-Reggiano cheese, preferably freshly grated
- ✓ 1/2 cup olive oil

Directions:

- ❖ Place the chicken legs in a parchment-lined baking pan. Season with salt and pepper, Then, scatter the leeks around the chicken legs.
- ❖ Roast in the preheated oven at 390 degrees F for 30 to 35 minutes, rotating the pan occasionally.
- ❖ Pulse the cashews, basil, garlic, and cheese in your blender until pieces are small. Continue blending while adding olive oil to the mixture. Mix until the desired consistency is reached.
- ❖ Storing
- ❖ Place the chicken in airtight containers or Ziploc bags; keep in your refrigerator for up 3 to 4 days.
- ❖ To freeze the chicken legs, place them in airtight containers or heavy-duty freezer bags. Freeze up to 3 months. Once thawed in the refrigerator, heat in the preheated oven at 375 degrees F for 20 to 25 minutes.
- ❖ Store your pesto in the refrigerator for up to a week. Bon appétit!

Nutrition: 5 Calories; 44.8g Fat; 5g Carbs; 38.7g Protein; 1g Fiber

80) SPECIAL DUCK BREASTS IN BOOZY SAUCE

Cooking Time: 20 Minutes

Servings: 4

Ingredients:

- ✓ 1 ½ pounds duck breasts, butterflied
- ✓ 1 tbsp tallow, room temperature
- ✓ 1 ½ cups chicken consommé
- ✓ 3 tbsp soy sauce

- ✓ 2 ounces vodka
- ✓ 1/2 cup sour cream
- ✓ 4 scallion stalks, chopped
- ✓ Salt and pepper, to taste

Directions:

- ❖ Melt the tallow in a frying pan over medium-high flame. Sear the duck breasts for about 5 minutes, flipping them over occasionally to ensure even cooking.
- ❖ Add in the scallions, salt, pepper, chicken consommé, and soy sauce. Partially cover and continue to cook for a further 8 minutes.
- ❖ Add in the vodka and sour cream; remove from the heat and stir to combine well.
- ❖ Storing
- ❖ Place the duck breasts in airtight containers or Ziploc bags; keep in your refrigerator for up to 3 to 4 days.
- ❖ For freezing, place duck breasts in airtight containers or heavy-duty freezer bags. Freeze up to 2 to 3 months. Once thawed in the refrigerator, reheat in a saucepan. Bon appétit!

Nutrition: 351 Calories; 24. Fat; 6.6g Carbs; 22.1g Protein; 0.6g Fiber

81) WHITE CAULIFLOWER WITH CHICKEN CHOWDER

Cooking Time: 30 Minutes

Servings: 6

Ingredients:

- ✓ 1 cup leftover roast chicken breasts
- ✓ 1 head cauliflower, broken into small-sized florets
- ✓ Sea salt and ground white pepper, to taste
- ✓ 2 ½ cups water
- ✓ 3 cups chicken consommé

- ✓ 1 ¼ cups sour cream
- ✓ 1/2 stick butter
- ✓ 1/2 cup white onion, finely chopped
- ✓ 1 tsp fresh garlic, finely minced
- ✓ 1 celery, chopped

Directions:

- ❖ In a heavy bottomed pot, melt the butter over a moderate heat. Cook the onion, garlic and celery for about 5 minutes or until they've softened.
- ❖ Add in the salt, white pepper, water, chicken consommé, chicken, and cauliflower florets; bring to a boil. Reduce the temperature to simmer and continue to cook for 30 minutes.
- ❖ Puree the soup with an immersion blender. Fold in sour cream and stir to combine well.
- ❖ Storing
- ❖ Spoon your chowder into airtight containers or Ziploc bags; keep in your refrigerator for up to 3 to 4 days.
- ❖ For freezing, place your chowder in airtight containers. It will maintain the best quality for about 4 to months. Defrost in the refrigerator. Bon appétit!

Nutrition: 231 Calories; 18.2g Fat; 5.9g Carbs; 11.9g Protein; 1.4g Fiber

82) Taro Leaf with Chicken Soup

Cooking Time: 45 Minutes   **Servings:** 4

Ingredients:

- ✓ 1 pound whole chicken, boneless and chopped into small chunks
- ✓ 1/2 cup onions, chopped
- ✓ 1/2 cup rutabaga, cubed
- ✓ 2 carrots, peeled
- ✓ 2 celery stalks
- ✓ Salt and black pepper, to taste

- ✓ 1 cup chicken bone broth
- ✓ 1/2 tsp ginger-garlic paste
- ✓ 1/2 cup taro leaves, roughly chopped
- ✓ 1 tbsp fresh coriander, chopped
- ✓ 3 cups water
- ✓ 1 tsp paprika

Directions:

- ❖ Place all ingredients in a heavy-bottomed pot. Bring to a boil over the highest heat.
- ❖ Turn the heat to simmer. Continue to cook, partially covered, an additional 40 minutes.
- ❖ Storing
- ❖ Spoon the soup into four airtight containers or Ziploc bags; keep in your refrigerator for up to 3 to days.
- ❖ For freezing, place the soup in airtight containers. It will maintain the best quality for about to 6 months. Defrost in the refrigerator. Bon appétit!

Nutrition: 25Calories; 12.9g Fat; 3.2g Carbs; 35.1g Protein; 2.2g Fiber

83) CREAMY GREEK-STYLE SOUP

Cooking Time: 30 Minutes   **Servings:** 4

Ingredients:

- ✓ 1/2 stick butter
- ✓ 1/2 cup zucchini, diced
- ✓ 2 garlic cloves, minced
- ✓ 4 ½ cups roasted vegetable broth

- ✓ Sea salt and ground black pepper, to season
- ✓ 1 ½ cups leftover turkey, shredded
- ✓ 1/3 cup double cream
- ✓ 1/2 cup Greek-style yogurt

Directions:

- ❖ In a heavy-bottomed pot, melt the butter over medium-high heat. Once hot, cook the zucchini and garlic for 2 minutes until they are fragrant.
- ❖ Add in the broth, salt, black pepper, and leftover turkey. Cover and cook for minutes, stirring periodically.
- ❖ Then, fold in the cream and yogurt. Continue to cook for 5 minutes more or until thoroughly warmed.
- ❖ Storing
- ❖ Spoon the soup into four airtight containers or Ziploc bags; keep in your refrigerator for up to 3 to 4 days.
- ❖ For freezing, place the soup in airtight containers. It will maintain the best quality for about 4 to months. Defrost in the refrigerator. Enjoy!

Nutrition: 256 Calories; 18.8g Fat; 5.4g Carbs; 15.8g Protein; 0.2g Fiber

84) LOW-CARB PORK WRAPS

Cooking Time: 15 Minutes   **Servings:** 4

Ingredients:

- ✓ 1 pound ground pork
- ✓ 2 garlic cloves, finely minced
- ✓ 1 chili pepper, deveined and finely minced
- ✓ 1 tsp mustard powder
- ✓ 1 tbsp sunflower seeds

- ✓ 2 tbsp champagne vinegar
- ✓ 1 tbsp coconut aminos
- ✓ Celery salt and ground black pepper, to taste
- ✓ 2 scallion stalks, sliced
- ✓ 1 head lettuce

Directions:

- ❖ Sear the ground pork in the preheated pan for about 8 minutes. Stir in the garlic, chili pepper, mustard seeds, and sunflower seeds; continue to sauté for minute longer or until aromatic.
- ❖ Add in the vinegar, coconut aminos, salt, black pepper, and scallions. Stir to combine well.
- ❖ Storing
- ❖ Place the ground pork mixture in airtight containers or Ziploc bags; keep in your refrigerator for up to 3 to days.
- ❖ For freezing, place the ground pork mixture it in airtight containers or heavy-duty freezer bags. Freeze up to 2 to 3 months. Defrost in the refrigerator and reheat in the skillet.
- ❖ Add spoonfuls of the pork mixture to the lettuce leaves, wrap them and serve.

Nutrition: 281 Calories; 19.4g Fat; 5.1g Carbs; 22.1g Protein; 1.3g Fiber

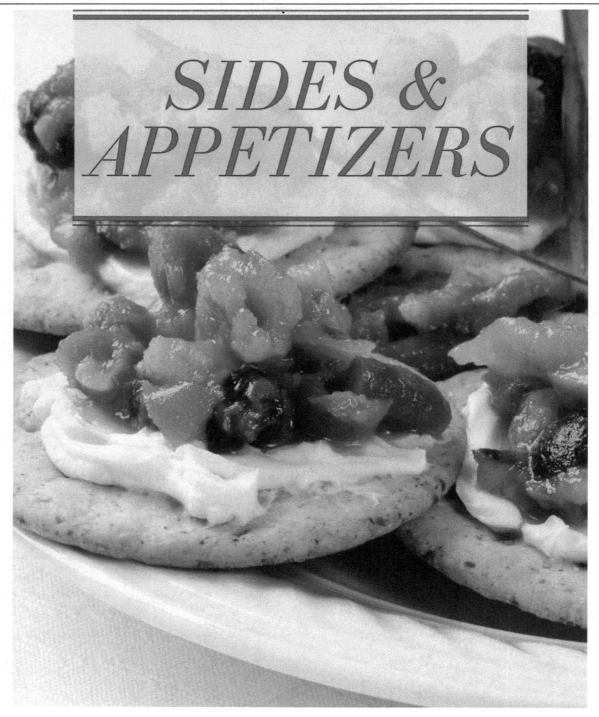

SIDES &
APPETIZERS

85) ITALIAN CHICKEN BACON PASTA

Cooking Time: 35 Minutes   **Servings: 4**

Ingredients:

- ✓ 8 ounces linguine pasta
- ✓ 3 slices of bacon
- ✓ 1 pound boneless chicken breast, cooked and diced
- ✓ Salt
- ✓ 1 6-ounce can artichoke hearts
- ✓ 2 ounce can diced tomatoes, undrained
- ✓ ¼ tsp dried rosemary
- ✓ 1/3 cup crumbled feta cheese, plus extra for topping
- ✓ 2/3 cup pitted black olives

Directions:

- ❖ Fill a large pot with salted water and bring to a boil.
- ❖ Add linguine and cook for 8-10 minutes until al dente.
- ❖ Cook bacon until brown, and then crumble.
- ❖ Season chicken with salt.
- ❖ Place chicken and bacon into a large skillet.
- ❖ Add tomatoes and rosemary and simmer the mixture for about 20 minutes.
- ❖ Stir in feta cheese, artichoke hearts, and olives, and cook until thoroughly heated.
- ❖ Toss the freshly cooked pasta with chicken mixture and cool.
- ❖ Spread over the containers.
- ❖ Before eating, garnish with extra feta if your heart desires!

Nutrition: 755, Total Fat: 22.5 g, Saturated Fat: 6.5 g, Cholesterol: 128 mg, Sodium: 852 mg, Total Carbohydrate: 75.4 g, Dietary Fiber: 7.3 g, Total Sugars: 3.4 g, Protein: 55.6 g, Vitamin D: 0 mcg, Calcium: 162 mg, Iron: 7 mg, Potassium: 524 mg

86) LOVELY CREAMY GARLIC SHRIMP PASTA

Cooking Time: 15 Minutes   **Servings: 4**

Ingredients:

- ✓ 6 ounces whole-wheat spaghetti, your favorite
- ✓ 12 ounces raw shrimp, peeled, deveined, and cut into 1-inch pieces
- ✓ 1 bunch asparagus, trimmed and thinly sliced
- ✓ 1 large bell pepper, thinly sliced
- ✓ 3 cloves garlic, chopped
- ✓ 1¼ tsp kosher salt
- ✓ 1½ cups non-fat plain yogurt
- ✓ ¼ cup flat-leaf parsley, chopped
- ✓ 3 tbsp lemon juice
- ✓ 1 tbsp extra virgin olive oil
- ✓ ½ tsp fresh ground black pepper
- ✓ ¼ cup toasted pine nuts

Directions:

- ❖ Bring water to a boil in a large pot.
- ❖ Add spaghetti and cook for about minutes less than called for by the package instructions.
- ❖ Add shrimp, bell pepper, asparagus and cook for about 2-4 minutes until the shrimp are tender.
- ❖ Drain the pasta.
- ❖ In a large bowl, mash the garlic until paste forms.
- ❖ Whisk yogurt, parsley, oil, pepper, and lemon juice into the garlic paste.
- ❖ Add pasta mixture and toss well.
- ❖ Cool and spread over the containers.
- ❖ Sprinkle with pine nuts.
- ❖ Enjoy!

Nutrition: 504, Total Fat: 15.4 g, Saturated Fat: 4.9 g, Cholesterol: 199 mg, Sodium: 2052 mg, Total Carbohydrate: 42.2 g, Dietary Fiber: 3.5 g, Total Sugars: 26.6 g, Protein: 43.2 g, Vitamin D: 0 mcg, Calcium: 723 mg, Iron: 3 mg, Potassium: 3 mg

87) SPECIAL MUSHROOM FETTUCCINE

Cooking Time: 15 Minutes   **Servings: 5**

Ingredients:

- ✓ 12 ounces whole-wheat fettuccine (or any other)
- ✓ 1 tbsp extra virgin olive oil
- ✓ 4 cups mixed mushrooms, such as oyster, cremini, etc., sliced
- ✓ 4 cups broccoli, divided
- ✓ 1 tbsp minced garlic
- ✓ ½ cup dry sherry
- ✓ 2 cups low-fat milk
- ✓ 2 tbsp all-purpose flour
- ✓ ½ tsp salt
- ✓ ½ tsp freshly ground pepper
- ✓ 1 cup finely shredded Asiago cheese, plus some for topping

Directions:

- ❖ Cook pasta in a large pot of boiling water for about 8- minutes.
- ❖ Drain pasta and set it to the side. Add oil to large skillet and heat over medium heat.
- ❖ Add mushrooms and broccoli, and cook for about 8-10 minutes until the mushrooms have released the liquid.
- ❖ Add garlic and cook for about 1 minute until fragrant. Add sherry, making sure to scrape up any brown bits.
- ❖ Bring the mix to a boil and cook for about 1 minute until evaporated.
- ❖ In a separate bowl, whisk flour and milk. Add the mix to your skillet, and season with salt and pepper.
- ❖ Cook well for about 2 minutes until the sauce begins to bubble and is thickened. Stir in Asiago cheese until it has fully melted.
- ❖ Add the sauce to your pasta and give it a gentle toss. Spread over the containers. Serve with extra cheese.

Nutrition: 503, Total Fat: 19.6 g, Saturated Fat: 6.3 g, Cholesterol: 25 mg, Sodium: 1136 mg, Total Carbohydrate: 57.5 g, Dietary Fiber: 12.4 g, Total Sugars: 6.4 g, Protein: 24.5 g, Vitamin D: 51 mcg, Calcium: 419 mg, Iron: 5 mg, Potassium: 390 mg

88) ORIGINAL LEMON GARLIC SARDINE FETTUCCINE

Cooking Time: 15 Minutes   **Servings: 4**

Ingredients:

- ✓ 8 ounces whole-wheat fettuccine
- ✓ 4 tbsp extra-virgin olive oil, divided
- ✓ 4 cloves garlic, minced
- ✓ 1 cup fresh breadcrumbs
- ✓ ¼ cup lemon juice
- ✓ 1 tsp freshly ground pepper
- ✓ ½ tsp of salt
- ✓ 2 4-ounce cans boneless and skinless sardines, dipped in tomato sauce
- ✓ ½ cup fresh parsley, chopped
- ✓ ¼ cup finely shredded parmesan cheese

Directions:

- ❖ Fill a large pot with water and bring to a boil.
- ❖ Cook pasta according to package instructions until tender (about 10 minutes).
- ❖ In a small skillet, heat 2 tbsp of oil over medium heat.
- ❖ Add garlic and cook for about 20 seconds, until sizzling and fragrant.
- ❖ Transfer the garlic to a large bowl.
- ❖ Add the remaining 2 tbsp of oil to skillet and heat over medium heat.
- ❖ Add breadcrumbs and cook for 5-6 minutes until golden and crispy.
- ❖ Whisk lemon juice, salt, and pepper into the garlic bowl.
- ❖ Add pasta to the garlic bowl, along with garlic, sardines, parmesan, and parsley; give it a gentle stir.
- ❖ Cool and spread over the containers.
- ❖ Before eating, sprinkle with breadcrumbs.
- ❖ Enjoy!

Nutrition: 633, Total Fat: 27.7 g, Saturated Fat: 6.4 g, Cholesterol: 40 mg, Sodium: 771 mg, Total Carbohydrate: 55.9 g, Dietary Fiber: 7.7 g, Total Sugars: 2.1 g, Protein: 38.6 g, Vitamin D: 0 mcg, Calcium: 274 mg, Iron: 7 mg, Potassium: mg

89) DELICIOUS SPINACH ALMOND STIR-FRY

Cooking Time: 10 Minutes   **Servings: 2**

Ingredients:

- ✓ 2 ounces spinach
- ✓ 1 tbsp coconut oil
- ✓ 3 tbsp almond, slices
- ✓ sea salt or plain salt
- ✓ freshly ground black pepper

Directions:

- ❖ Start by heating a skillet with coconut oil; add spinach and let it cook.
- ❖ Then, add salt and pepper as the spinach is cooking.
- ❖ Finally, add in the almond slices.
- ❖ Serve warm.

Nutrition: 117, Total Fat: 11.4 g, Saturated Fat: 6.2 g, Cholesterol: 0 mg, Sodium: 23 mg, Total Carbohydrate: 2.9 g, Dietary Fiber: 1.7 g, Total Sugars: 0.g, Protein: 2.7 g, Vitamin D: 0 mcg, Calcium: 52 mg, Iron: 1 mg, Potassium: 224 mg

90) ITALIAN BBQ CARROTS

Cooking Time: 30 Minutes   **Servings: 8**

Ingredients:

- ✓ 2 pounds baby carrots (organic)
- ✓ 1 tbsp olive oil
- ✓ 1 tbsp garlic powder
- ✓ 1 tbsp onion powder
- ✓ sea salt or plain salt
- ✓ freshly ground black pepper

Directions:

- ❖ Mix all the Ingredients: in a plastic bag so that the carrots are well coated with the mixture.
- ❖ Then, on the BBQ grill place a piece of aluminum foil and spread the carrots in a single layer.
- ❖ Finally, grill for 30 minutes or until tender.
- ❖ Serve warm.

Nutrition: 388, Total Fat: 1.9 g, Saturated Fat: 0.3 g, Cholesterol: 0 mg, Sodium: 89 mg, Total Carbohydrate: 10.8 g, Dietary Fiber: 3.4 g, Total Sugars: 6 g, Protein: 1 g, Vitamin D: 0 mcg, Calcium: 40 mg, Iron: 1 mg, Potassium: 288 mg

91) MEDITERRANEAN-STYLE BAKED ZUCCHINI STICKS

Cooking Time: 20 Minutes   **Servings: 8**

Ingredients:

- ✓ ¼ cup feta cheese, crumbled
- ✓ 4 zucchini
- ✓ ¼ cup parsley, chopped
- ✓ ½ cup tomatoes, minced
- ✓ ½ cup kalamata olives, pitted and minced
- ✓ 1 cup red bell pepper, minced
- ✓ 1 tbsp oregano
- ✓ ¼ cup garlic, minced
- ✓ 1 tbsp basil
- ✓ sea salt or plain salt
- ✓ freshly ground black pepper

Directions:

- ❖ Start by cutting zucchini in half (lengthwise) and scoop out the middle.
- ❖ Then, combine garlic, black pepper, bell pepper, oregano, basil, tomatoes, and olives in a bowl.
- ❖ Now, fill in the middle of each zucchini with this mixture. Place these on a prepared baking dish and bake the dish at 0 degrees F for about 15 minutes.
- ❖ Finally, top with feta cheese and broil on high for 3 minutes or until done. Garnish with parsley.
- ❖ Serve warm.

Nutrition: 53, Total Fat: 2.2 g, Saturated Fat: 0.9 g, Cholesterol: 4 mg, Sodium: 138 mg, Total Carbohydrate: 7.5 g, Dietary Fiber: 2.1 g, Total Sugars: 3 g, Protein: 2.g, Vitamin D: 0 mcg, Calcium: 67 mg, Iron: 1 mg, Potassium: 353 mg

92) ARTICHOKE OLIVE PASTA

Cooking Time: 25 Minutes   **Servings: 4**

Ingredients:

- ✓ salt
- ✓ pepper
- ✓ 2 tbsp olive oil, divided
- ✓ 2 garlic cloves, thinly sliced
- ✓ 1 can artichoke hearts, drained, rinsed, and quartered lengthwise
- ✓ 1-pint grape tomatoes, halved lengthwise, divided
- ✓ ½ cup fresh basil leaves, torn apart
- ✓ 12 ounces whole-wheat spaghetti
- ✓ ½ medium onion, thinly sliced
- ✓ ½ cup dry white wine
- ✓ 1/3 cup pitted Kalamata olives, quartered lengthwise
- ✓ ¼ cup grated Parmesan cheese, plus extra for serving

Directions:

- ❖ Fill a large pot with salted water.
- ❖ Pour the water to a boil and cook your pasta according to package instructions until al dente.
- ❖ Drain the pasta and reserve 1 cup of the cooking water.
- ❖ Return the pasta to the pot and set aside.
- ❖ Heat 1 tbsp of olive oil in a large skillet over medium-high heat.
- ❖ Add onion and garlic, season with pepper and salt, and cook well for about 3-4 minutes until nicely browned.
- ❖ Add wine and cook for 2 minutes until evaporated.
- ❖ Stir in artichokes and keep cooking 2-3 minutes until brown.
- ❖ Add olives and half of your tomatoes.
- ❖ Cook well for 1-2 minutes until the tomatoes start to break down.
- ❖ Add pasta to the skillet.
- ❖ Stir in the rest of the tomatoes, cheese, basil, and remaining oil.
- ❖ Thin the mixture with the reserved pasta water if needed.
- ❖ Place in containers and sprinkle with extra cheese.
- ❖ Enjoy!

Nutrition: 340, Total Fat: 11.9 g, Saturated Fat: 3.3 g, Cholesterol: 10 mg, Sodium: 278 mg, Total Carbohydrate: 35.8 g, Dietary Fiber: 7.8 g, Total Sugars: 4.8 g, Protein: 11.6 g, Vitamin D: 0 mcg, Calcium: 193 mg, Iron: 3 mg, Potassium: 524 mg

93) MEDITERRANEAN OLIVE TUNA PASTA

Cooking Time: 20 Minutes   **Servings: 4**

Ingredients:

- ✓ 8 ounces of tuna steak, cut into 3 pieces
- ✓ ¼ cup green olives, chopped
- ✓ 3 cloves garlic, minced
- ✓ 2 cups grape tomatoes, halved
- ✓ ½ cup white wine
- ✓ 2 tbsp lemon juice
- ✓ 6 ounces pasta - whole wheat gobetti, rotini, or penne
- ✓ 1 10-ounce package frozen artichoke hearts, thawed and squeezed dry
- ✓ 4 tbsp extra-virgin olive oil, divided
- ✓ 2 tsp fresh grated lemon zest
- ✓ 2 tsp fresh rosemary, chopped, divided
- ✓ ½ tsp salt, divided
- ✓ ¼ tsp fresh ground pepper
- ✓ ¼ cup fresh basil, chopped

Directions:

- ❖ Preheat grill to medium-high heat.
- ❖ Take a large pot of water and put it on to boil.
- ❖ Place the tuna pieces in a bowl and add 1 tbsp of oil, 1 tsp of rosemary, lemon zest, a ¼ tsp of salt, and pepper.
- ❖ Grill the tuna for about 3 minutes per side.
- ❖ Transfer tuna to a plate and allow it to cool.
- ❖ Place the pasta in boiling water and cook according to package instructions.
- ❖ Drain the pasta.
- ❖ Flake the tuna into bite-sized pieces.
- ❖ In a large skillet, heat remaining oil over medium heat.
- ❖ Add artichoke hearts, garlic, olives, and remaining rosemary.
- ❖ Cook for about 3-4 minutes until slightly browned.
- ❖ Add tomatoes, wine, and bring the mixture to a boil.
- ❖ Cook for about 3 minutes until the tomatoes are broken down.
- ❖ Stir in pasta, lemon juice, tuna, and remaining salt.
- ❖ Cook for 1-2 minutes until nicely heated.
- ❖ Spread over the containers.
- ❖ Before eating, garnish with some basil and enjoy!

Nutrition: 455, Total Fat: 21.2 g, Saturated Fat: 3.5 g, Cholesterol: 59 mg, Sodium: 685 mg, Total Carbohydrate: 38.4 g, Dietary Fiber: 6.1 g, Total Sugars: 3.5 g, Protein: 25.5 g, Vitamin D: 0 mcg, Calcium: 100 mg, Iron: 5 mg, Potassium: 800 mg

94) SPECIAL BRAISED ARTICHOKES

Cooking Time: 30 Minutes   **Servings: 6**

Ingredients:

- ✓ 6 tbsp olive oil
- ✓ 2 pounds baby artichokes, trimmed
- ✓ ½ cup lemon juice
- ✓ 4 garlic cloves, thinly sliced
- ✓ ½ tsp salt
- ✓ 1½ pounds tomatoes, seeded and diced
- ✓ ½ cup almonds, toasted and sliced

Directions:

- ❖ Heat oil in a skillet over medium heat.
- ❖ Add artichokes, garlic, and lemon juice, and allow the garlic to sizzle.
- ❖ Season with salt.
- ❖ Reduce heat to medium-low, cover, and simmer for about 15 minutes.
- ❖ Uncover, add tomatoes, and simmer for another 10 minutes until the tomato liquid has mostly evaporated.
- ❖ Season with more salt and pepper.
- ❖ Sprinkle with toasted almonds.
- ❖ Enjoy!

Nutrition: Calories: 265, Total Fat: 1g, Saturated Fat: 2.6 g, Cholesterol: 0 mg, Sodium: 265 mg, Total Carbohydrate: 23 g, Dietary Fiber: 8.1 g, Total Sugars: 12.4 g, Protein: 7 g, Vitamin D: 0 mcg, Calcium: 81 mg, Iron: 2 mg, Potassium: 1077 mg

95) DELICIOUS FRIED GREEN BEANS

Cooking Time: 15 Minutes   **Servings: 2**

Ingredients:

- ✓ ½ pound green beans, trimmed
- ✓ 1 egg
- ✓ 2 tbsp olive oil
- ✓ 1¼ tbsp almond flour
- ✓ 2 tbsp parmesan cheese
- ✓ ½ tsp garlic powder
- ✓ sea salt or plain salt
- ✓ freshly ground black pepper

Directions:

- ❖ Start by beating the egg and olive oil in a bowl.
- ❖ Then, mix the remaining Ingredients: in a separate bowl and set aside.
- ❖ Now, dip the green beans in the egg mixture and then coat with the dry mix.
- ❖ Finally, grease a baking pan, then transfer the beans to the pan and bake at 5 degrees F for about 12-15 minutes or until crisp.
- ❖ Serve warm.

Nutrition: Calories: 334, Total Fat: 23 g, Saturated Fat: 8.3 g, Cholesterol: 109 mg, Sodium: 397 mg, Total Carbohydrate: 10.9 g, Dietary Fiber: 4.3 g, Total Sugars: 1.9 g, Protein: 18.1 g, Vitamin D: 8 mcg, Calcium: 398 mg, Iron: 2 mg, Potassium: 274 mg

96) VEGGIE MEDITERRANEAN-STYLE PASTA

Cooking Time: 2 Hours   **Servings: 4**

Ingredients:

- ✓ 1 tbsp olive oil
- ✓ 1 small onion, finely chopped
- ✓ 2 small garlic cloves, finely chopped
- ✓ 2 14-ounce cans diced tomatoes
- ✓ 1 tbsp sun-dried tomato paste
- ✓ 1 bay leaf
- ✓ 1 tsp dried thyme
- ✓ 1 tsp dried basil
- ✓ 1 tsp oregano
- ✓ 1 tsp dried parsley
- ✓ bread of your choice

- ✓ ½ tsp salt
- ✓ ½ tsp brown sugar
- ✓ freshly ground black pepper
- ✓ 1 piece aubergine
- ✓ 2 pieces courgettes
- ✓ 2 pieces red peppers, de-seeded
- ✓ 2 garlic cloves, peeled
- ✓ 2-3 tbsp olive oil
- ✓ 12 small vine-ripened tomatoes
- ✓ 16 ounces of pasta of your preferred shape, such as Gigli, conchiglie, etc.
- ✓ 3½ ounces parmesan cheese

Directions:

- ❖ Heat oil in a pan over medium heat.
- ❖ Add onions and fry them until tender.
- ❖ Add garlic and stir-fry for 1 minute.
- ❖ Add the remaining Ingredients: listed under the sauce and bring to a boil.
- ❖ Reduce the heat, cover, and simmer for 60 minutes.
- ❖ Season with black pepper and salt as needed. Set aside.
- ❖ Preheat oven to 350 degrees F.
- ❖ Chop up courgettes, aubergine and red peppers into 1-inch pieces.
- ❖ Place them on a roasting pan along with whole garlic cloves.
- ❖ Drizzle with olive oil and season with salt and black pepper.
- ❖ Mix the veggies well and roast in the oven for 45 minutes until they are tender.
- ❖ Add tomatoes just before 20 minutes to end time.
- ❖ Cook your pasta according to package instructions.
- ❖ Drain well and stir into the sauce.
- ❖ Divide the pasta sauce between 4 containers and top with vegetables.
- ❖ Grate some parmesan cheese on top and serve with bread.
- ❖ Enjoy!

Nutrition: Calories: 211, Total Fat: 14.9 g, Saturated Fat: 2.1 g, Cholesterol: 0 mg, Sodium: 317 mg, Total Carbohydrate: 20.1 g, Dietary Fiber: 5.7 g, Total Sugars: 11.7 g, Protein: 4.2 g, Vitamin D: 0 mcg, Calcium: 66 mg, Iron: 2 mg, Potassium: 955 mg

97) CLASSIC BASIL PASTA

Cooking Time: 40 Minutes   **Servings: 4**

Ingredients:

- ✓ 2 red peppers, de-seeded and cut into chunks
- ✓ 2 red onions cut into wedges
- ✓ 2 mild red chilies, de-seeded and diced
- ✓ 3 garlic cloves, coarsely chopped
- ✓ 1 tsp golden caster sugar
- ✓ 2 tbsp olive oil, plus extra for serving

- ✓ 2 pounds small ripe tomatoes, quartered
- ✓ 12 ounces pasta
- ✓ a handful of basil leaves, torn
- ✓ 2 tbsp grated parmesan
- ✓ salt
- ✓ pepper

Directions:

- ❖ Preheat oven to 390 degrees F.
- ❖ On a large roasting pan, spread peppers, red onion, garlic, and chilies.
- ❖ Sprinkle sugar on top.
- ❖ Drizzle olive oil and season with salt and pepper.
- ❖ Roast the veggies for 1minutes.
- ❖ Add tomatoes and roast for another 15 minutes.
- ❖ In a large pot, cook your pasta in salted boiling water according to instructions.
- ❖ Once ready, drain pasta.
- ❖ Remove the veggies from the oven and carefully add pasta.
- ❖ Toss everything well and let it cool.
- ❖ Spread over the containers.
- ❖ Before eating, place torn basil leaves on top, and sprinkle with parmesan.
- ❖ Enjoy!

Nutrition: Calories: 384, Total Fat: 10.8 g, Saturated Fat: 2.3 g, Cholesterol: 67 mg, Sodium: 133 mg, Total Carbohydrate: 59.4 g, Dietary Fiber: 2.3 g, Total Sugars: 5.7 g, Protein: 1 g, Vitamin D: 0 mcg, Calcium: 105 mg, Iron: 4 mg, Potassium: 422 mg

98) ORIGINAL RED ONION KALE PASTA

Cooking Time: 25 Minutes   **Servings:** 4

Ingredients:

- 2½ cups vegetable broth
- ¾ cup dry lentils
- ½ tsp of salt
- 1 bay leaf
- ¼ cup olive oil
- 1 large red onion, chopped
- 1 tsp fresh thyme, chopped
- ½ tsp fresh oregano, chopped
- 1 tsp salt, divided
- ½ tsp black pepper
- 8 ounces vegan sausage, sliced into ¼-inch slices
- 1 bunch kale, stems removed and coarsely chopped
- 1 pack rotini

Directions:

- ❖ Add vegetable broth, ½ tsp of salt, bay leaf, and lentils to a saucepan over high heat and bring to a boil.
- ❖ Reduce the heat to medium-low and allow to cook for about minutes until tender.
- ❖ Discard the bay leaf.
- ❖ Take another skillet and heat olive oil over medium-high heat.
- ❖ Stir in thyme, onions, oregano, ½ a tsp of salt, and pepper; cook for 1 minute.
- ❖ Add sausage and reduce heat to medium-low.
- ❖ Cook for 10 minutes until the onions are tender.
- ❖ Bring water to a boil in a large pot, and then add rotini pasta and kale.
- ❖ Cook for about 8 minutes until al dente.
- ❖ Remove a bit of the cooking water and put it to the side.
- ❖ Drain the pasta and kale and return to the pot.
- ❖ Stir in both the lentils mixture and the onions mixture.
- ❖ Add the reserved cooking liquid to add just a bit of moistness.
- ❖ Spread over containers.

Nutrition: Calories: 508, Total Fat: 17 g, Saturated Fat: 3 g, Cholesterol: 0 mg, Sodium: 2431 mg, Total Carbohydrate: 59.3 g, Dietary Fiber: 6 g, Total Sugars: 4.8 g, Protein: 30.9 g, Vitamin D: 0 mcg, Calcium: 256 mg, Iron: 8 mg, Potassium: 1686 mg

99) ITALIAN SCALLOPS PEA FETTUCCINE

Cooking Time: 15 Minutes   **Servings:** 5

Ingredients:

- 8 ounces whole-wheat fettuccine (pasta, macaroni)
- 1 pound large sea scallops
- ¼ tsp salt, divided
- 1 tbsp extra virgin olive oil
- 1 8-ounce bottle of clam juice
- 1 cup low-fat milk
- ¼ tsp ground white pepper
- 3 cups frozen peas, thawed
- ¾ cup finely shredded Romano cheese, divided
- 1/3 cup fresh chives, chopped
- ½ tsp freshly grated lemon zest
- 1 tsp lemon juice

Directions:

- ❖ Boil water in a large pot and cook fettuccine according to package instructions.
- ❖ Drain well and put it to the side.
- ❖ Heat oil in a large, non-stick skillet over medium-high heat.
- ❖ Pat the scallops dry and sprinkle them with 1/8 tsp of salt.
- ❖ Add the scallops to the skillet and cook for about 2-3 minutes per side until golden brown. Remove scallops from pan.
- ❖ Add clam juice to the pan you removed the scallops from.
- ❖ In another bowl, whisk in milk, white pepper, flour, and remaining 1/8 tsp of salt.
- ❖ Once the mixture is smooth, whisk into the pan with the clam juice.
- ❖ Bring the entire mix to a simmer and keep stirring for about 1-2 minutes until the sauce is thick.
- ❖ Return the scallops to the pan and add peas. Bring it to a simmer.
- ❖ Stir in fettuccine, chives, ½ a cup of Romano cheese, lemon zest, and lemon juice.
- ❖ Mix well until thoroughly combined.
- ❖ Cool and spread over containers.
- ❖ Before eating, serve with remaining cheese sprinkled on top.
- ❖ Enjoy!

Nutrition: Calories: 388, Total Fat: 9.2 g, Saturated Fat: 3.7 g, Cholesterol: 33 mg, Sodium: 645 mg, Total Carbohydrate: 50.1 g, Dietary Fiber: 10.4 g, Total Sugars: 8.7 g, Protein: 24.9 g, Vitamin D: 25 mcg, Calcium: 293 mg, Iron: 4 mg, Potassium: 247 mg

100) ORIGINAL RED ONION KALE PASTA
Cooking Time: 25 Minutes   Servings: 4

Ingredients:

- ✓ 2½ cups vegetable broth
- ✓ ¾ cup dry lentils
- ✓ ½ tsp of salt
- ✓ 1 bay leaf
- ✓ ¼ cup olive oil
- ✓ 1 large red onion, chopped
- ✓ 1 tsp fresh thyme, chopped
- ✓ ½ tsp fresh oregano, chopped

- ✓ 1 tsp salt, divided
- ✓ ½ tsp black pepper
- ✓ 8 ounces vegan sausage, sliced into ¼-inch slices
- ✓ 1 bunch kale, stems removed and coarsely chopped
- ✓ 1 pack rotini

Directions:

- ❖ Add vegetable broth, ½ tsp of salt, bay leaf, and lentils to a saucepan over high heat and bring to a boil.
- ❖ Reduce the heat to medium-low and allow to cook for about minutes until tender.
- ❖ Discard the bay leaf.
- ❖ Take another skillet and heat olive oil over medium-high heat.
- ❖ Stir in thyme, onions, oregano, ½ a tsp of salt, and pepper; cook for 1 minute.
- ❖ Add sausage and reduce heat to medium-low.
- ❖ Cook for 10 minutes until the onions are tender.
- ❖ Bring water to a boil in a large pot, and then add rotini pasta and kale.
- ❖ Cook for about 8 minutes until al dente.
- ❖ Remove a bit of the cooking water and put it to the side.
- ❖ Drain the pasta and kale and return to the pot.
- ❖ Stir in both the lentils mixture and the onions mixture.
- ❖ Add the reserved cooking liquid to add just a bit of moistness.
- ❖ Spread over containers.

Nutrition: Calories: 508, Total Fat: 17 g, Saturated Fat: 3 g, Cholesterol: 0 mg, Sodium: 2431 mg, Total Carbohydrate: 59.3 g, Dietary Fiber: 6 g, Total Sugars: 4.8 g, Protein: 30.9 g, Vitamin D: 0 mcg, Calcium: 256 mg, Iron: 8 mg, Potassium: 1686 mg

101) ITALIAN SCALLOPS PEA FETTUCCINE
Cooking Time: 15 Minutes   Servings: 5

Ingredients:

- ✓ 8 ounces whole-wheat fettuccine (pasta, macaroni)
- ✓ 1 pound large sea scallops
- ✓ ¼ tsp salt, divided
- ✓ 1 tbsp extra virgin olive oil
- ✓ 1 8-ounce bottle of clam juice
- ✓ 1 cup low-fat milk

- ✓ ¼ tsp ground white pepper
- ✓ 3 cups frozen peas, thawed
- ✓ ¾ cup finely shredded Romano cheese, divided
- ✓ 1/3 cup fresh chives, chopped
- ✓ ½ tsp freshly grated lemon zest
- ✓ 1 tsp lemon juice

Directions:

- ❖ Boil water in a large pot and cook fettuccine according to package instructions.
- ❖ Drain well and put it to the side.
- ❖ Heat oil in a large, non-stick skillet over medium-high heat.
- ❖ Pat the scallops dry and sprinkle them with 1/8 tsp of salt.
- ❖ Add the scallops to the skillet and cook for about 2-3 minutes per side until golden brown. Remove scallops from pan.
- ❖ Add clam juice to the pan you removed the scallops from.
- ❖ In another bowl, whisk in milk, white pepper, flour, and remaining 1/8 tsp of salt.
- ❖ Once the mixture is smooth, whisk into the pan with the clam juice.
- ❖ Bring the entire mix to a simmer and keep stirring for about 1-2 minutes until the sauce is thick.
- ❖ Return the scallops to the pan and add peas. Bring it to a simmer.
- ❖ Stir in fettuccine, chives, ½ a cup of Romano cheese, lemon zest, and lemon juice.
- ❖ Mix well until thoroughly combined.
- ❖ Cool and spread over containers.
- ❖ Before eating, serve with remaining cheese sprinkled on top.
- ❖ Enjoy!

Nutrition: Calories: 388, Total Fat: 9.2 g, Saturated Fat: 3.7 g, Cholesterol: 33 mg, Sodium: 645 mg, Total Carbohydrate: 50.1 g, Dietary Fiber: 10.4 g, Total Sugars: 8.7 g, Protein: 24.9 g, Vitamin D: 25 mcg, Calcium: 293 mg, Iron: 4 mg, Potassium: 247 mg

PART II: INTRODUCTION

What is the Mediterranean diet, you may ask, and can a vegetarian diet be both Mediterranean and vegetarian?

A well-balanced food program can be defined as such when all food groups are included according to the body's physiological needs so that it can function at its best. Consequently, you can feel (and look) at your best, healthy, full of energy, and vital!

The main food groups consist of the right amount of carbohydrates, proteins, and fats. Within these groups, you will find various foods that provide nutrients, fiber, vitamins s, and minerals depending on their quality. Let me further explain this fundamental concept: within fats, there are good and not good fats; within carbohydrates, there are the simple and the complex, and within proteins, there are mainly two sources: animal or vegetable.

And this is the exciting part because to be a vegetarian; you do not exclude the protein group from your diet. You simply choose a different source.

The Mediterranean diet's enormous success is partly since it is one of the most complete and balanced diets available. The Mediterranean diet includes various foods in all food groups, so the answer to our first question is: yes! It is possible to follow a Mediterranean diet that is also vegetarian.

Let's explore a little more about what to eat, when and where...and why...

Scientists have created blue zones around the world. These are areas where citizens live longer and healthier lives than in other regions. Reasons for this vary but are often health-related. In Italy, Sardinia is home to one of the oldest living denizens. Farming are very importantly to their lifestyles, and they have an excellent reputation worldwide. Gardening for Mediterranean diets provides easy acess to the fruits and vegetables necessary tollo followow theis lifestyle. Fruits and vegetables are for a Mediterrnean diet tend prefer temperate conditions, but many are hardy. Items like olive oil, fresh fish, and fresh veggies are the highlight. Even if you can't great a fish, you can plant fodods that will make you feel better about your Mediterranean lifestyle. Suggested products for the Mediterranean garden are Olives Cucumbers Celery Artichokes Tomatoes Figs Beans Date Citrus Grapes Peppers Squash Mint Thyme.

THE MEDITERRANEAN & VEGETARIAN DIETS

The vegetarian diet excludes meat and fish consumption but, unlike the vegan diet, allows animal products such as eggs and dairy products.

Suppose you are vegetarian and you are interested in following the Mediterranean diet. In that case, you can still eat many of the traditional foods that are widely used in Mediterranean recipes, such as some high-quality cheeses like ricotta, parmesan, and pecorino or fresh mozzarella. However, if you need to lose weight, you still need to limit these foods' consumption as they are genuine and carry a high-fat content.

The foods consist of manly vegetable ingredients such as legumes, seeds, nuts, vegetables, and fruits in the vegan program. There are also foods derived from animals in a vegetarian diet, such as yogurt, all kinds of dairy products, and eggs. In the vegetarian program, the meat of the animal itself is prohibited. That is, you can still eat animal products and benefit from them without actually taking their life.

What is essential to know is that eating healthier is not just a matter of food choices, but the quality of the food you choose. You may favor organic, free-range eggs instead of cage-farmed eggs; the same goes for dairy. You can choose good quality hormone-free dairy products. When you buy yogurt - or when you purchase anything really - read the labels and always opt for the most straightforward, highest quality selection.

Let's talk about butter - how delicious is that? Butter has a much higher quality than faux-artificial products like margarine. Choose organic, grass-fed, eat small amounts, and it's beautiful!

Foods like eggs, certain dairy products, kefir are rich in vitamin B12, a type of vitamin that vegans should take with supplements because it is not found in most plant products.

A common thread in vegetarian, vegan, and Mediterranean diets is the consumption of many plant-based foods.

Choose good quality seasonal fruits and vegetables. Other extremely healthy products which are vegetarian and widely spread in the Mediterranean diet include garlic, onions, extra virgin olive oil, fresh Mediterranean herbs (like basil, oregano, sage, rosemary, marjoram, thyme, etc.), tomatoes, eggplants, olives, and many more.

Mediterranean herbs are really special because they provide health benefits and allow you to reduce the consumption of salt because they give taste and flavor to most of your recipes.

Nuts, almonds, and seeds (like flax seeds, hemp, sunflower, chia) are healthful foods that you can eat as a healthy snack or breakfast. Almonds are very popular in Sicily and Southern Italy, which is in the middle of the Mediterranean Sea. These ingredients are widely spread worldwide. Nuts and honey are used in many dessert recipes. You can simply add them to your natural yogurt and enjoy them.

All legumes (there are countless varieties) are to be included in the Mediterranean diet for vegetarians. They represent a healthful source of protein and other nutrients that can replace animal meat.

Buy a selection of fresh, raw (the dried version, not the pre-cooked or canned version) legumes, all different kinds of beans, chickpeas, and broad beans. Remember to soak them in water overnight – or at least for 6/8 hours - before cooking them.

If you want to make a legume soup, simply prepare a mixture of minced carrot, onion, and garlic, sauté with extra virgin olive oil, add legumes and water, and cook for about two hours, or until thoroughly cooked. All water is reduced, and the soup is creamy.

If you want to use legumes to prepare other recipes like salads or rice and vegetable dishes, soak them, cook them in boiling water and drain them. It is really simple, easy, healthy and delicious. *It just requires some patience and practice of new eating and cooking habits!*

Lentils are a delicious type of legumes, and they are even easier to prepare because they don't need to be soaked in water and cook much faster (30 or 40 minutes according to the quality and the size).

Extra virgin olive oil is a beneficial and healthy product rich in good quality fats. Rather than using various hyper-caloric sauces, rich in sugar and artificial flavor, by following the Mediterranean diet for vegetarians, you can easily replace them with extra virgin olive oil, pure and simple.

A most common condiment in the Mediterranean diet's innumerable recipes is the Mediterranean emulsion, a straightforward compound made of extra virgin olive oil, freshly squeezed lemon juice, salt, and pepper. This emulsion is used to season any type of salad or vegetable dish.

The only precaution is choosing the best quality possible and prefers tin or glass bottles rather than plastic.

The Mediterranean diet also includes cakes and sure desserts as long as they are made of good quality ingredients, preferably homemade, and consumed in small amounts.

To substitute white flour to bake a cake, you could use whole grain flour or almond flour or spelled flour or any sort of flour that was not treated and bleached artificially. Instead of sugar, you could use raw, organic honey and no other artificial flavorings and colorings.

The basic rule of the Mediterranean diet is quality, the authenticity of the foods. Authenticity because the simpler, the better, and most genuine. Choose foods that grow in nature naturally.

If you are trying to lose weight, you can still have some chocolate now and then; you could favor dark chocolate instead of milk chocolate to make it less fattening. If you are vegan, make sure that you buy the kind that is entirely milk-free.

These were some basic guidelines to help you know a little more about the Mediterranean diet for vegetarians.

Now let's look at some more information about the health benefits and the meal plan solution.

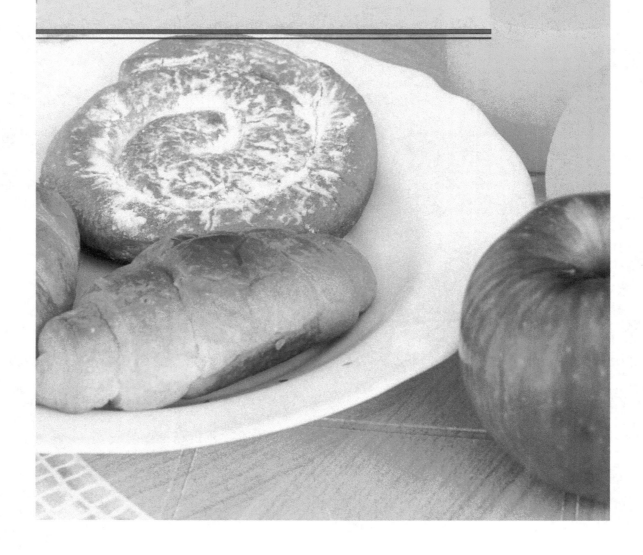

BREAKFAST

102) CAULIFLOWER FRITTERS AND HUMMUS

Cooking Time: 15 Minutes   **Servings: 4**

Ingredients:

- ✓ 2 (15 oz) cans chickpeas, divided
- ✓ 2 1/2 tbsp olive oil, divided, plus more for frying
- ✓ 1 cup onion, chopped, about 1/2 a small onion
- ✓ 2 tbsp garlic, minced
- ✓ 2 cups cauliflower, cut into small pieces, about 1/2 a large head
- ✓ 1/2 tsp salt
- ✓ black pepper
- ✓ Topping:
- ✓ Hummus, of choice
- ✓ Green onion, diced

Directions:

❖ Preheat oven to 400°F

❖ Rinse and drain 1 can of the chickpeas, place them on a paper towel to dry off well

❖ Then place the chickpeas into a large bowl, removing the loose skins that come off, and toss with 1 tbsp of olive oil, spread the chickpeas onto a large pan (being careful not to over-crowd them) and sprinkle with salt and pepper

❖ Bake for 20 minutes, then stir, and then bake an additional 5-10 minutes until very crispy

❖ Once the chickpeas are roasted, transfer them to a large food processor and process until broken down and crumble - Don't over process them and turn it into flour, as you need to have some texture. Place the mixture into a small bowl, set aside

❖ In a large pan over medium-high heat, add the remaining 1 1/2 tbsp of olive oil

❖ Once heated, add in the onion and garlic, cook until lightly golden brown, about 2 minutes. Then add in the chopped cauliflower, cook for an additional 2 minutes, until the cauliflower is golden

❖ Turn the heat down to low and cover the pan, cook until the cauliflower is fork tender and the onions are golden brown and caramelized, stirring often, about 3-5 minutes

❖ Transfer the cauliflower mixture to the food processor, drain and rinse the remaining can of chickpeas and add them into the food processor, along with the salt and a pinch of pepper. Blend until smooth, and the mixture starts to ball, stop to scrape down the sides as needed

❖ Transfer the cauliflower mixture into a large bowl and add in 1/2 cup of the roasted chickpea crumbs (you won't use all of the crumbs, but it is easier to break them down when you have a larger amount.), stir until well combined

❖ In a large bowl over medium heat, add in enough oil to lightly cover the bottom of a large pan

❖ Working in batches, cook the patties until golden brown, about 2-3 minutes, flip and cook again

❖ Distribute among the container, placing parchment paper in between the fritters. Store in the fridge for 2-3 days

❖ To Serve: Heat through in the oven at 350F for 5-8 minutes. Top with hummus, green onion and enjoy!

❖ Recipe Notes: Don't add too much oil while frying the fritter or they will end up soggy. Use only enough to cover the pan. Use a fork while frying and resist the urge to flip them every minute to see if they are golden

Nutrition: Calories:333;Total Carbohydrates: 45g;Total Fat: 13g;Protein: 14g

103) BREAKFAST GREEK QUINOA BOWL

Cooking Time: 20 Minutes   **Servings: 6**

Ingredients:

- ✓ 12 eggs
- ✓ ¼ cup plain Greek yogurt
- ✓ 1 tsp onion powder
- ✓ 1 tsp granulated garlic
- ✓ ½ tsp salt
- ✓ ½ tsp pepper
- ✓ 1 tsp olive oil
- ✓ 1 (5 oz) bag baby spinach
- ✓ 1 pint cherry tomatoes, halved
- ✓ 1 cup feta cheese
- ✓ 2 cups cooked quinoa

Directions:

- ❖ In a large bowl whisk together eggs, Greek yogurt, onion powder, granulated garlic, salt, and pepper, set aside
- ❖ In a large skillet, heat olive oil and add spinach, cook the spinach until it is slightly wilted, about 3-4 minutes
- ❖ Add in cherry tomatoes, cook until tomatoes are softened, 4 minutes
- ❖ Stir in egg mixture and cook until the eggs are set, about 7-9 minutes, stir in the eggs as they cook to scramble
- ❖ Once the eggs have set stir in the feta and quinoa, cook until heated through
- ❖ Distribute evenly among the containers, store for 2-3 days
- ❖ To serve: Reheat in the microwave for 30 seconds to 1 minute or heated through

Nutrition: Calories:357;Total Carbohydrates: ;Total Fat: 20g;Protein: 23g

104) Healthy Salad Zucchini Kale Tomato

Cooking Time: 20 Minutes   **Servings: 4**

Ingredients:

- ✓ 1 lb kale, chopped
- ✓ 2 tbsp fresh parsley, chopped
- ✓ 1 tbsp vinegar
- ✓ 1/2 cup can tomato, crushed
- ✓ 1 tsp paprika
- ✓ 1 cup zucchini, cut into cubes
- ✓ 1 cup grape tomatoes, halved
- ✓ 2 tbsp olive oil
- ✓ 1 onion, chopped
- ✓ 1 leek, sliced
- ✓ Pepper
- ✓ Salt

Directions:

- ❖ Add oil into the inner pot of instant pot and set the pot on sauté mode.
- ❖ Add leek and onion and sauté for 5 minutes.
- ❖ Add kale and remaining ingredients and stir well.
- ❖ Seal pot with lid and cook on high for 15 minutes.
- ❖ Once done, allow to release pressure naturally for 10 minutes then release remaining using quick release. Remove lid.
- ❖ Stir and serve.

Nutrition: Calories: 162;Fat: 3 g;Carbohydrates: 22.2 g;Sugar: 4.8 g;Protein: 5.2 g;Cholesterol: 0 mg

105) Cheese with Cauliflower Frittata and Peppers

Cooking Time: 30 Minutes   **Servings: 6**

Ingredients:

- ✓ 10 eggs
- ✓ 1 seeded and chopped bell pepper
- ✓ ½ cup grated Parmigiano-Reggiano
- ✓ ½ cup milk, skim
- ✓ ½ tsp cayenne pepper
- ✓ 1 pound cauliflower, floret
- ✓ ½ tsp saffron
- ✓ 2 tbsp chopped chives
- ✓ Salt and black pepper as desired

Directions:

- ❖ Prepare your oven by setting the temperature to 370 degrees Fahrenheit. You should also grease a skillet suitable for the oven.
- ❖ In a medium-sized bowl, add the milk and eggs. Whisk them until they are frothy.
- ❖ Sprinkle the grated Parmigiano-Reggiano cheese into the frothy mixture and fold the ingredients together.
- ❖ Pour in the salt, saffron, cayenne pepper, and black pepper and gently stir.
- ❖ Add in the chopped bell pepper and gently stir until the ingredients are fully incorporated.
- ❖ Pour the egg mixture into the skillet and cook on medium heat over your stovetop for 4 minutes.
- ❖ Steam the cauliflower florets in a pan. To do this, add ½ inch of water and ½ tsp sea salt. Pour in the cauliflower and cover for 3 to 8 minutes. Drain any extra water.
- ❖ Add the cauliflower into the mixture and gently stir.
- ❖ Set the skillet into the preheated oven and turn your timer to 13 minutes. Once the mixture is golden brown in the middle, remove the frittata from the oven.

- ❖ Set your skillet aside for a couple of minutes so it can cool.
- ❖ Slice and garnish with chives before you serve.

Nutrition: calories: 207, fats: grams, carbohydrates: 8 grams, protein: 17 grams.

106) AVOCADO KALE OMELETTE

Cooking Time: 5 Minutes   **Servings: 1**

Ingredients:

- ✓ 2 eggs
- ✓ 1 tsp milk
- ✓ 2 tsp olive oil
- ✓ 1 cup kale (chopped)
- ✓ 1 tbsp lime juice
- ✓ 1 tbsp cilantro (chopped)
- ✓ 1 tsp sunflower seeds
- ✓ Pinch of red pepper (crushed)
- ✓ ¼ avocado (sliced)
- ✓ sea salt or plain salt
- ✓ freshly ground black pepper

Directions:

- ❖ Toss all the Ingredients: (except eggs and milk) to make the kale salad.
- ❖ Beat the eggs and milk in a bowl.
- ❖ Heat oil in a pan over medium heat. Then pour in the egg mixture and cook it until the bottom settles. Cook for 2 minutes and then flip it over and further cook for 20 seconds.
- ❖ Finally, put the Omelette in containers.
- ❖ Top the Omelette with the kale salad.
- ❖ Serve warm.

Nutrition: Calories: 399, Total Fat: 28.8g, Saturated Fat: 6.2, Cholesterol: 328 mg, Sodium: 162 mg, Total Carbohydrate: 25.2g, Dietary Fiber: 6.3 g, Total Sugars: 9 g, Protein: 15.8 g, Vitamin D: 31 mcg, Calcium: 166 mg, Iron: 4 mg, Potassium: 980 mg

107) PORRIDGE WITH STRAWBERRIES AND COCONUT

Preparation Time: 12 minutes   **Servings: 2**

Ingredients:

- ✓ 1 tbsp flax seed powder
- ✓ 1 oz olive oil
- ✓ 1 tbsp coconut flour
- ✓ 1 pinch ground chia seeds
- ✓ 5 tbsp coconut cream
- ✓ Thawed frozen strawberries

Directions:

- ❖ In a small bowl, mix the flax seed powder with the 3 tbsp water, and allow soaking for 5 minutes.
- ❖ Place a non-stick saucepan over low heat and pour in the olive oil, vegan "flax egg," coconut flour, chia seeds, and coconut cream.
- ❖ Cook the mixture while stirring continuously until your desired consistency is achieved. Turn the heat off and spoon the porridge into serving bowls.
- ❖ Top with 4 to 6 strawberries and serve immediately.

108) BROCCOLI BROWNS

Preparation Time: 35 minutes   **Servings: 4**

Ingredients:

- ✓ 3 tbsp flax seed powder
- ✓ 1 head broccoli, cut into florets
- ✓ ½ white onion, grated
- ✓ 1 tsp salt
- ✓ 1 tbsp freshly ground black pepper
- ✓ 5 tbsp plant butter, for frying

Directions:

- ❖ In a small bowl, mix the flax seed powder with 9 tbsp water, and allow soaking for 5 minutes. Pour the broccoli into a food processor and pulse a few times until smoothly grated.
- ❖ Transfer the broccoli into a bowl, add the vegan "flax egg," white onion, salt, and black pepper. Use a spoon to mix the ingredients evenly and set aside 5 to 10 minutes to firm up a bit. Place a large non-stick skillet over medium heat and drop 1/3 of the plant butter to melt until no longer shimmering.
- ❖ Ladle scoops of the broccoli mixture into the skillet (about 3 to 4 hash browns per batch). Flatten the pancakes to measure 3 to 4 inches in diameter, and fry until golden brown on one side, 4 minutes. Turn the pancakes with a spatula and cook the other side to brown too, another 5 minutes.
- ❖ Transfer the hash browns to a serving plate and repeat the frying process for the remaining broccoli mixture. Serve the hash browns warm with green salad.

109) AVOCADO SANDWICH WITHOUT BREAD

Preparation Time: 10 minutes

Servings: 2

Ingredients:

- ✓ 1 avocado, sliced
- ✓ 1 large red tomato, sliced
- ✓ 2 oz gem lettuce leaves
- ✓ ½ oz plant butter
- ✓ 1 oz tofu, sliced
- ✓ Freshly chopped parsley to garnish

Directions:

- ❖ Put the avocado on a plate and place the tomato slices by the avocado. Arrange the lettuce (with the inner side facing you) on a flat plate to serve as the base of the sandwich.
- ❖ To assemble the sandwich, smear each leaf of the lettuce with plant butter, and arrange some tofu slices in the leaves. Then, share the avocado and tomato slices on each cheese. Garnish with parsley and serve.

110) BERRY BOWL

Preparation Time: 10 minutes

Preparation Time:

Preparation Time: 2

Ingredients:

- ✓ 1 ½ cups coconut milk
- ✓ 2 small-sized bananas
- ✓ 1 cup mixed berries, frozen

Ingredients:

- ✓ 2 tbsp almond butter
- ✓ 1 tbsp chia seeds
- ✓ 2 tbsp granola

Directions:

- ❖ Add the coconut milk, bananas, berries, almond butter and chia seeds.
- ❖ Puree until creamy, uniform and smooth.
- ❖ Divide the blended mixture between serving bowls and top with granola. Serve immediately

111) BANANA AND FIGS OATMEAL

Preparation Time: 15 minutes

Preparation Time:

Preparation Time: 2

Ingredients:

- ✓ 1 ½ cups almond milk
- ✓ 1/2 cup rolled oats
- ✓ A pinch of sea salt
- ✓ A pinch of grated nutmeg

Ingredients:

- ✓ 1/3 tsp cinnamon
- ✓ 3 dried figs, chopped
- ✓ 2 bananas, peeled and sliced
- ✓ 1 tbsp maple syrup

Directions:

- ❖ In a deep saucepan, bring the milk to a rapid boil. Add in the oats, cover the saucepan and turn the heat to medium.
- ❖ Add in the salt, nutmeg and cinnamon. Continue to cook for about 12 minutes, stirring periodically.
- ❖ Spoon the mixture into serving bowls; top with figs and bananas; add a few drizzles of the maple syrup to each serving and serve warm. Enjoy

112) GRANOLA WITH DRIED CURRANTS

Preparation Time: 25 minutes   **Preparation Time:**   **Preparation Time:** 12

Ingredients:

- 1/2 cup coconut oil
- 1/3 cup maple syrup
- 1 tsp vanilla paste
- 1/2 tsp ground cardamom
- 1 tsp ground cinnamon
- 1/3 tsp Himalayan salt

Ingredients:

- 4 cups old-fashioned oats
- 1/2 cup pecans, chopped
- 1/2 cup walnuts, chopped
- 1/4 cup pepitas
- 1 cup dried currants

Directions:

- ❖ Begin by preheating your oven to 290 degrees F; line a large baking sheet with a piece parchment paper.
- ❖ Then, thoroughly combine the coconut oil, maple syrup, vanilla paste, cardamom, cinnamon and Himalayan salt.
- ❖ Gradually add in the oats, nuts and seeds; toss to coat well.
- ❖ Spread the mixture out onto the prepared baking sheet.
- ❖ Bake in the middle of the oven, stirring halfway through the cooking time, for about 20 minutes or until golden brown.
- ❖ Stir in the dried currants and let your granola cool completely before storing. Store in an airtight container.
- ❖ Serve with your favorite plant-based milk or yogurt. Enjoy

113) FRUIT SALAD WITH LEMON AND GINGER SYRUP

Preparation Time: 10 minutes+ chilling time   **Preparation Time:**   **Servings: 4**

Ingredients:

- 1/2 cup fresh lemon juice
- 1/4 cup agave syrup
- 1 tsp fresh ginger, grated
- 1/2 tsp vanilla extract

Ingredients:

- 1 banana, sliced
- 2 cups mixed berries
- 1 cup seedless grapes
- 2 cups apples, cored and diced

Directions:

- ❖ Bring the lemon juice, agave syrup and ginger to a boil over medium-high heat. Then, turn the heat to medium-low and let it simmer for about 6 minutes until it has slightly thickened.
- ❖ Remove from the heat and stir in the vanilla extract. Allow it to cool.
- ❖ Layer the fruits in serving bowls. Pour the cooled sauce over the fruit and serve well chilled. Enjoy!

114) STRAWBERRY GREEK COLD YOGURT

Cooking Time: 2-4 Hours   **Servings: 5**

Ingredients:

- ✓ 3 cups plain Greek low-fat yogurt
- ✓ 1 cup sugar
- ✓ ¼ cup lemon juice, freshly squeezed
- ✓ 2 tsp vanilla
- ✓ 1/8 tsp salt
- ✓ 1 cup strawberries, sliced

Directions:

- ❖ In a medium-sized bowl, add yogurt, lemon juice, sugar, vanilla, and salt.
- ❖ Whisk the whole mixture well.
- ❖ Freeze the yogurt mix in a 2-quart ice cream maker according to the given instructions.
- ❖ During the final minute, add the sliced strawberries.
- ❖ Transfer the yogurt to an airtight container.
- ❖ Place in the freezer for 2-4 hours.
- ❖ Remove from the freezer and allow it to stand for 5-15 minutes.
- ❖ Serve and enjoy!

Nutrition: Calories: 251, Total Fat: 0.5 g, Saturated Fat: 0.1 g, Cholesterol: 3 mg, Sodium: 130 mg, Total Carbohydrate: 48.7 g, Dietary Fiber: 0.6 g, Total Sugars: 47.3 g, Protein: 14.7 g, Vitamin D: 1 mcg, Calcium: 426 mg, Iron: 0 mg, Potassium: 62 mg

115) PEACH ALMOND OATMEAL

Cooking Time: 10 Minutes   **Servings: 2**

Ingredients:

- ✓ 1 cup unsweetened almond milk
- ✓ 2 cups of water
- ✓ 1 cup oats
- ✓ 2 peaches, diced
- ✓ Pinch of salt

Directions:

- ❖ Spray instant pot from inside with cooking spray.
- ❖ Add all ingredients into the instant pot and stir well.
- ❖ Seal pot with a lid and select manual and set timer for 10 minutes.
- ❖ Once done, allow to release pressure naturally for 10 minutes then release remaining using quick release. Remove lid.
- ❖ Stir and serve.

Nutrition: Calories: 234;Fat: 4.8 g;Carbohydrates: 42.7 g;Sugar: 9 g;Protein: 7.3 g;Cholesterol: 0 mg

116) BANANA PEANUT BUTTER PUDDING

Cooking Time: 25 Minutes   **Servings: 1**

Ingredients:

- ✓ 2 bananas, halved
- ✓ ¼ cup smooth peanut butter
- ✓ Coconut for garnish, shredded

Directions:

- ❖ Start by blending bananas and peanut butter in a blender and mix until smooth or desired texture obtained.
- ❖ Pour into a bowl and garnish with coconut if desired.
- ❖ Enjoy.

Nutrition: Calories: 589, Total Fat: 33.3g, Saturated Fat: 6.9, Cholesterol: 0 mg, Sodium: 13 mg, Total Carbohydrate: 66.5 g, Dietary Fiber: 10 g, Total Sugars: 38 g, Protein: 18.8 g, Vitamin D: 0 mcg, Calcium: 40 mg, Iron: 2 mg, Potassium: 1264 mg

117) Coconut Banana Mix

Cooking Time: 4 Minutes   **Servings: 4**

Ingredients:

- ✓ 1 cup coconut milk
- ✓ 1 banana
- ✓ 1 cup dried coconut
- ✓ 2 tbsp ground flax seed
- ✓ 3 tbsp chopped raisins
- ✓ ⅛ tsp nutmeg
- ✓ ⅛ tsp cinnamon
- ✓ Salt to taste

Directions:

- ❖ Set a large skillet on the stove and set it to low heat.
- ❖ Chop up the banana.
- ❖ Pour the coconut milk, nutmeg, and cinnamon into the skillet.
- ❖ Pour in the ground flaxseed while stirring continuously.
- ❖ Add the dried coconut and banana. Mix the ingredients until combined well.
- ❖ Allow the mixture to simmer for 2 to 3 minutes while stirring occasionally.
- ❖ Set four airtight containers on the counter.
- ❖ Remove the pan from heat and sprinkle enough salt for your taste buds.
- ❖ Divide the mixture into the containers and place them into the fridge overnight. They can remain in the fridge for up to 3 days.
- ❖ Before you set this tasty mixture in the microwave to heat up, you need to let it thaw on the counter for a bit.

Nutrition: calories: 279, fats: 22 grams, carbohydrates: 25 grams, protein: 6.4 grams

118) OLIVE OIL RASPBERRY-LEMON MUFFINS

Cooking Time: 20 Minutes   **Servings: 12**

Ingredients:

- ✓ Cooking spray to grease baking liners
- ✓ 1 cup all-purpose flour
- ✓ 1 cup whole-wheat flour
- ✓ ½ cup tightly packed light brown sugar
- ✓ ½ tsp baking soda
- ✓ ½ tsp aluminum-free baking powder
- ✓ ⅛ tsp kosher salt
- ✓ 1¼ cups buttermilk
- ✓ 1 large egg
- ✓ ¼ cup extra-virgin olive oil
- ✓ 1 tbsp freshly squeezed lemon juice
- ✓ Zest of 2 lemons
- ✓ 1¼ cups frozen raspberries (do not thaw)

Directions:

- ❖ Preheat the oven to 400°F and line a muffin tin with baking liners. Spray the liners lightly with cooking spray.
- ❖ In a large mixing bowl, whisk together the all-purpose flour, whole-wheat flour, brown sugar, baking soda, baking powder, and salt.
- ❖ In a medium bowl, whisk together the buttermilk, egg, oil, lemon juice, and lemon zest.
- ❖ Pour the wet ingredients into the dry ingredients and stir just until blended. Do not overmix.
- ❖ Fold in the frozen raspberries.
- ❖ Scoop about ¼ cup of batter into each muffin liner and bake for 20 minutes, or until the tops look browned and a paring knife comes out clean when inserted. Remove the muffins from the tin to cool.
- ❖ STORAGE: Store covered containers at room temperature for up to 4 days. To freeze muffins for up to 3 months, wrap them in foil and place in an airtight resealable bag.

Nutrition: Total calories: 166; Total fat: 5g; Saturated fat: 1g; Sodium: 134mg; Carbohydrates: 30g; Fiber: 3g; Protein: 4g

119) Creamy Bread with Sesame

Preparation Time: 40 minutes   **Preparation Time:**   **Preparation Time:** 6

Ingredients:

- ✓ 4 tbsp flax seed powder
- ✓ 2/3 cup cashew cream cheese
- ✓ 4 tbsp sesame oil + for brushing
- ✓ 1 cup coconut flour

Ingredients:

- ✓ 2 tbsp psyllium husk powder
- ✓ 1 tsp salt
- ✓ 1 tsp baking powder
- ✓ 1 tbsp sesame seeds

Ingredients:

- ❖ In a bowl, mix the flax seed powder with 1 ½ cups water until smoothly combined and set aside to soak for 5 minutes. Preheat oven to 400 F. When the vegan "flax egg" is ready, beat in the cream cheese and sesame oil until well mixed.
- ❖ Whisk in the coconut flour, psyllium husk powder, salt, and baking powder until adequately blended.
- ❖ Grease a 9 x 5 inches baking tray with cooking spray, and spread the dough in the tray. Allow the mixture to stand for 5 minutes and then brush with some sesame oil.

❖ Sprinkle with the sesame seeds and bake the dough for 30 minutes or until golden brown on top and set within. Take out the bread and allow cooling for a few minutes. Slice and serve

120) DIFFERENT SEEDS BREAD

Preparation Time: 55 minutes

Preparation Time:

Preparation Time: 6

Ingredients:

- ✓ 3 tbsp ground flax seeds
- ✓ ¾ cup coconut flour
- ✓ 1 cup almond flour
- ✓ 3 tsp baking powder
- ✓ 5 tbsp sesame seeds
- ✓ ½ cup chia seeds
- ✓ 1 tsp ground caraway seeds
- ✓ 1 tsp hemp seeds

Ingredients:

- ✓ ¼ cup psyllium husk powder
- ✓ 1 tsp salt
- ✓ 2/3 cup cashew cream cheese
- ✓ ½ cup melted coconut oil
- ✓ ¾ cup coconut cream
- ✓ 1 tbsp poppy seeds

Ingredients:

- ❖ Preheat oven to 350 F and line a loaf pan with parchment paper.
- ❖ For the vegan "flax egg," whisk flax seed powder with ½ cup of water and let the mixture sit to soak for 5 minutes. In a bowl, evenly combine the coconut flour, almond flour, baking powder, sesame seeds, chia seeds, ground caraway seeds, hemp seeds, psyllium husk powder, and salt.
- ❖ In another bowl, use an electric hand mixer to whisk the cream cheese, coconut oil, coconut whipping cream, and vegan "flax egg." Pour the liquid ingredients into the dry ingredients, and continue whisking with the hand mixer until a dough forms. Transfer the dough to the loaf pan, sprinkle with poppy seeds, and bake in the oven for 45 minutes or until a knife inserted into the bread comes out clean. Remove the parchment paper with the bread, and allow cooling on a rack

121) NAAN BREAD

Preparation Time: 25 minutes

Preparation Time:

Preparation Time: 6

Ingredients:

- ✓ ¾ cup almond flour
- ✓ 2 tbsp psyllium husk powder
- ✓ ½ tsp salt
- ✓ ½ tsp baking powder
- ✓ 1/3 cup olive oil

Ingredients:

- ✓ Plant butter for frying
- ✓ 4 oz plant butter
- ✓ 2 garlic cloves, minced

Ingredients:

- ❖ In a bowl, mix the almond flour, psyllium husk powder, salt, and baking powder.
- ❖ Mix in some olive oil and 2 cups of boiling water to combine the ingredients, like a thick porridge. Stir thoroughly and allow the dough to rise for 5 minutes.
- ❖ Divide the dough into 6 to 8 pieces and mold into balls. Place the balls on parchment paper and flatten with your hands.
- ❖ Melt the plant butter in a frying pan and fry the naan on both sides to have a beautiful, golden color. Transfer the naan to a plate and keep warm in the oven. For the garlic butter, add the remaining plant butter to the frying pan and sauté the garlic until fragrant, about 3 minutes. Pour the garlic butter into a bowl and serve as a dip along with the naan

122)   Couscous Pearl Salad

Cooking Time: 10 Minutes   **Servings: 6**

Ingredients:

- ✓ lemon juice, 1 large lemon
- ✓ 1/3 cup extra-virgin olive oil
- ✓ 1 tsp dill weed
- ✓ 1 tsp garlic powder
- ✓ salt
- ✓ pepper
- ✓ 2 cups Pearl Couscous
- ✓ 2 tbsp extra virgin olive oil
- ✓ 2 cups grape tomatoes, halved
- ✓ water as needed

- ✓ 1/3 cup red onions, finely chopped
- ✓ ½ English cucumber, finely chopped
- ✓ 1 15-ounce can chickpeas
- ✓ 1 14-ounce can artichoke hearts, roughly chopped
- ✓ ½ cup pitted Kalamata olives
- ✓ 15-20 pieces fresh basil leaves, roughly torn and chopped
- ✓ 3 ounces fresh mozzarella

Directions:

- ❖ Start by preparing the vinaigrette by mixing all Ingredients: in a bowl. Set aside.
- ❖ Heat olive oil in a medium-sized heavy pot over medium heat.
- ❖ Add couscous and cook until golden brown.
- ❖ Add 3 cups of boiling water and cook the couscous according to package instructions.
- ❖ Once done, drain in a colander and put it to the side.
- ❖ In a large mixing bowl, add the rest of the Ingredients: except the cheese and basil.
- ❖ Add the cooked couscous, basil, and mix everything well.
- ❖ Give the vinaigrette a gentle stir and whisk it into the couscous salad. Mix well.
- ❖ Adjust/add seasoning as desired.
- ❖ Add mozzarella cheese.
- ❖ Garnish with some basil.
- ❖ Enjoy!

Nutrition: Calories: 578, Total Fat: 25.3g, Saturated Fat: 4.6, Cholesterol: 8 mg, Sodium: 268 mg, Total Carbohydrate: 70.1g, Dietary Fiber: 17.5 g, Total Sugars: 10.8 g, Protein: 23.4 g, Vitamin D: 0 mcg, Calcium: 150 mg, Iron: 6 mg, Potassium: 1093 mg

123)   **TOMATO MUSHROOM EGG CUPS**

Cooking Time: 5 Minutes   **Servings: 4**

Ingredients:

- ✓ 4 eggs
- ✓ 1/2 cup tomatoes, chopped
- ✓ 1/2 cup mushrooms, chopped
- ✓ 2 tbsp fresh parsley, chopped

- ✓ 1/4 cup half and half
- ✓ 1/2 cup cheddar cheese, shredded
- ✓ Pepper
- ✓ Salt

Directions:

- ❖ In a bowl, whisk the egg with half and half, pepper, and salt.
- ❖ Add tomato, mushrooms, parsley, and cheese and stir well.
- ❖ Pour egg mixture into the four small jars and seal jars with lid.
- ❖ Pour 1 1/2 cups of water into the instant pot then place steamer rack in the pot.
- ❖ Place jars on top of the steamer rack.
- ❖ Seal pot with lid and cook on high for 5 minutes.
- ❖ Once done, release pressure using quick release. Remove lid.
- ❖ Serve and enjoy.

Nutrition: Calories: 146;Fat: 10.g;Carbohydrates: 2.5 g;Sugar: 1.2 g;Protein: 10 g;Cholesterol: 184 mg

124)   **BREAKFAST MEDITERRANEAN-STYLE SALAD**

Cooking Time: 10 Minutes   **Servings: 2**

Ingredients:

- ✓ 4 eggs (optional)
- ✓ 10 cups arugula
- ✓ 1/2 seedless cucumber, chopped
- ✓ 1 cup cooked quinoa, cooled
- ✓ 1 large avocado
- ✓ 1 cup natural almonds, chopped

- ✓ 1/2 cup mixed herbs like mint and dill, chopped
- ✓ 2 cups halved cherry tomatoes and/or heirloom tomatoes cut into wedges
- ✓ Extra virgin olive oil
- ✓ 1 lemon
- ✓ Sea salt, to taste
- ✓ Freshly ground black pepper, to taste

Directions:

- ❖ Cook the eggs by soft-boiling them - Bring a pot of water to a boil, then reduce heat to a simmer. Gently lower all the eggs into water and allow them to simmer for 6 minutes. Remove the eggs from water and run cold water on top to stop the cooking, process set aside and peel when ready to use
- ❖ In a large bowl, combine the arugula, tomatoes, cucumber, and quinoa
- ❖ Divide the salad among 2 containers, store in the fridge for 2 days
- ❖ To Serve: Garnish with the sliced avocado and halved egg, sprinkle herbs

and almonds over top. Drizzle with olive oil, season with salt and pepper, toss to combine. Season with more salt and pepper to taste, a squeeze of lemon juice, and a drizzle of olive oil

Nutrition: Calories:2;Carbs: 18g;Total Fat: 16g;Protein: 10g

125) Mushroom and Spinach Chickpea Omelette

Preparation Time: 25 minutes

Servings: 4

Ingredients:

- ✓ 1 cup chickpea flour
- ✓ ½ tsp onion powder
- ✓ ½ tsp garlic powder
- ✓ ¼ tsp white pepper
- ✓ 1/3 cup nutritional yeast
- ✓ ½ tsp baking soda
- ✓ 1 green bell pepper, chopped
- ✓ 3 scallions, chopped
- ✓ 1 cup sautéed button mushrooms
- ✓ ½ cup chopped fresh spinach
- ✓ 1 cup halved cherry tomatoes
- ✓ 1 tbsp fresh parsley leaves

Directions:

- ❖ In a medium bowl, mix the chickpea flour, onion powder, garlic powder, white pepper, nutritional yeast, and baking soda until well combined. Heat a medium skillet over medium heat and add a quarter of the batter. Swirl the pan to spread the batter across the pan. Scatter a quarter each of the bell pepper, scallions, mushrooms, and spinach on top and cook until the bottom part of the omelet sets, 1-2 minutes.
- ❖ Carefully flip the omelet and cook the other side until set and golden brown. Transfer the omelet to a plate and make the remaining omelets. Serve the omelet with the tomatoes and garnish with the parsley leaves

126) COCONUT-RASPBERRY PANCAKES

Preparation Time: 25 minutes

Servings: 4

Ingredients:

- ✓ 2 tbsp flax seed powder
- ✓ ½ cup coconut milk
- ✓ ¼ cup fresh raspberries, mashed
- ✓ ½ cup oat flour
- ✓ 1 tsp baking soda
- ✓ A pinch salt
- ✓ 1 tbsp coconut sugar
- ✓ 2 tbsp pure date syrup
- ✓ ½ tsp cinnamon powder
- ✓ 2 tbsp unsweetened coconut flakes
- ✓ 2 tsp plant butter
- ✓ Fresh raspberries for garnishing

Directions:

- ❖ In a medium bowl, mix the flax seed powder with the 6 tbsp water and thicken for 5 minutes. Mix in coconut milk and raspberries. Add the oat flour, baking soda, salt, coconut sugar, date syrup, and cinnamon powder. Fold in the coconut flakes until well combined.
- ❖ Working in batches, melt a quarter of the butter in a non-stick skillet and add ¼ cup of the batter. Cook until set beneath and golden brown, 2 minutes. Flip the pancake and cook on the other side until set and golden brown, 2 minutes. Transfer to a plate and make the remaining pancakes using the rest of the ingredients in the same proportions. Garnish the pancakes with some raspberries and serve warm

127) BLUEBERRY-CHIA PUDDING

Preparation Time: 5 minutes + chilling time

Servings: 2

Ingredients:

- ✓ ¾ cup coconut milk
- ✓ ½ tsp vanilla extract
- ✓ ½ cup blueberries
- ✓ 2 tbsp chia seeds
- ✓ Chopped walnuts to garnish

Directions:

- ❖ In a blender, pour the coconut milk, vanilla extract, and half of the blueberries. Process the ingredients at high speed until the blueberries have incorporated into the liquid.
- ❖ Open the blender and mix in the chia seeds. Share the mixture into two breakfast jars, cover, and refrigerate for 4 hours to

allow the mixture to gel. Garnish the pudding with the remaining blueberries and walnuts. Serve immediately

128) POTATO AND CAULIFLOWER BROWNS

Preparation Time: 35 minutes

Servings: 4

Ingredients:

- ✓ 3 tbsp flax seed powder
- ✓ 2 large potatoes, shredded
- ✓ 1 big head cauliflower, riced
- ✓ ½ white onion, grated
- ✓ Salt and black pepper to taste
- ✓ 4 tbsp plant butter

Directions:

- ❖ In a medium bowl, mix the flaxseed powder and 9 tbsp water. Allow thickening for 5 minutes for the vegan "flax egg." Add the potatoes, cauliflower, onion, salt, and black pepper to the vegan "flax egg" and mix until well combined. Allow sitting for 5 minutes to thicken.
- ❖ Working in batches, melt 1 tbsp of plant butter in a non-stick skillet and add 4 scoops of the hashbrown mixture to the skillet. Make sure to have 1 to 2-inch intervals between each scoop.
- ❖ Use the spoon to flatten the batter and cook until compacted and golden brown on the bottom part, 2 minutes. Flip the hashbrowns and cook further for 2 minutes or until the vegetable cook and is golden brown. Transfer to a paper-towel-lined plate to drain grease. Make the remaining hashbrowns using the remaining ingredients. Serve warm

129) Carrot Oatmeal Breakfast

Cooking Time: 10 Minutes

Servings: 2

Ingredients:

- ✓ 1 cup steel-cut oats
- ✓ 1/2 cup raisins
- ✓ 1/2 tsp ground nutmeg
- ✓ 1/2 tsp ground cinnamon
- ✓ 2 carrots, grated
- ✓ 2 cups of water
- ✓ 2 cups unsweetened almond milk
- ✓ 1 tbsp honey

Directions:

- ❖ Spray instant pot from inside with cooking spray.
- ❖ Add all ingredients into the instant pot and stir well.
- ❖ Seal pot with lid and cook on high for 10 minutes.
- ❖ Once done, release pressure using quick release. Remove lid.
- ❖ Stir and serve.

Nutrition: Calories: 3;Fat: 6.6 g;Carbohydrates: 73.8 g;Sugar: 33.7 g;Protein: 8.1 g;Cholesterol: 0 mg

130) ARBORIO RICE RUM-RAISIN PUDDING

Cooking Time: 4 Hours

Servings: 2

Ingredients:

- ✓ ¾ cup Arborio rice
- ✓ 1 can evaporated milk
- ✓ ½ cup raisins
- ✓ ¼ tsp nutmeg, grated
- ✓ 1½ cups water
- ✓ 1/3 cup sugar
- ✓ ¼ cup dark rum
- ✓ sea salt or plain salt

Directions:

- ❖ Start by mixing rum and raisins in a bowl and set aside.
- ❖ Then, heat the evaporated milk and water in a saucepan and then simmer.
- ❖ Now, add sugar and stir until dissolved.
- ❖ Finally, convert this milk mixture into a slow cooker and stir in rice and salt. Cook on low heat for hours.
- ❖ Now, stir in the raisin mixture and nutmeg and let sit for 10 minutes.
- ❖ Serve warm.

Nutrition: Calories: 3, Total Fat: 10.1g, Saturated Fat: 5.9, Cholesterol: 36 mg, Sodium: 161 mg, Total Carbohydrate: 131.5 g, Dietary Fiber: 3.3 g, Total Sugars: 54.8 g, Protein: 14.4 g, Vitamin D: 0 mcg, Calcium: 372 mg, Iron: 2 mg, Potassium: 712 mg

131) SMOOTHIE BOWL OF RASPBERRY AND CHIA

Preparation Time: 10 minutes

Servings: 2

Ingredients:

- ✓ 1 cup coconut milk
- ✓ 2 small-sized bananas, peeled
- ✓ 1 ½ cups raspberries, fresh or frozen
- ✓ 2 dates, pitted
- ✓ 1 tbsp coconut flakes
- ✓ 1 tbsp pepitas
- ✓ 2 tbsp chia seeds

Directions:

- ❖ In your blender or food processor, mix the coconut milk with the bananas, raspberries and dates.
- ❖ Process until creamy and smooth. Divide the smoothie between two bowls.
- ❖ Top each smoothie bowl with the coconut flakes, pepitas and chia seeds. Enjoy

132) BREAKFAST OATS WITH WALNUTS AND CURRANTS

Preparation Time: 10 minutes

Servings: 2

Ingredients:

- ✓ 1 cup water
- ✓ 1 ½ cups oat milk
- ✓ 1 ½ cups rolled oats
- ✓ A pinch of salt
- ✓ A pinch of grated nutmeg
- ✓ 1/4 tsp cardamom
- ✓ 1 handful walnuts, roughly chopped
- ✓ 4 tbsp dried currants

Directions:

- ❖ In a deep saucepan, bring the water and milk to a rolling boil. Add in the oats, cover the saucepan and turn the heat to medium.
- ❖ Add in the salt, nutmeg and cardamom. Continue to cook for about 12 to 13 minutes more, stirring occasionally.
- ❖ Spoon the mixture into serving bowls; top with walnuts and currants. Enjoy

133) APPLESAUCE PANCAKES WITH COCONUT

Preparation Time: 50 minutes

Servings: 8

Ingredients:

- ✓ 1 ¼ cups whole-wheat flour
- ✓ 1 tsp baking powder
- ✓ 1/4 tsp sea salt
- ✓ 1/2 tsp coconut sugar
- ✓ 1/4 tsp ground cloves
- ✓ 1/4 tsp ground cardamom
- ✓ 1/2 tsp ground cinnamon
- ✓ 3/4 cup oat milk
- ✓ 1/2 cup applesauce, unsweetened
- ✓ 2 tbsp coconut oil
- ✓ 8 tbsp coconut, shredded
- ✓ 8 tbsp pure maple syrup

Directions:

- ❖ In a mixing bowl, thoroughly combine the flour, baking powder, salt, sugar and spices. Gradually add in the milk and applesauce.
- ❖ Heat a frying pan over a moderately high flame and add a small amount of the coconut oil.
- ❖ Once hot, pour the batter into the frying pan. Cook for approximately 3 minutes until the bubbles form; flip it and cook on the other side for 3 minutes longer until browned on the underside. Repeat with the remaining oil and batter.
- ❖ Serve with shredded coconut and maple syrup. Enjoy

134) VEGGIE PANINI

Preparation Time: 30 minutes

Servings: 4

Ingredients:

- ✓ 1 tbsp olive oil
- ✓ 1 cup sliced button mushrooms
- ✓ Salt and black pepper to taste
- ✓ 1 ripe avocado, sliced
- ✓ 2 tbsp freshly squeezed lemon juice
- ✓ 1 tbsp chopped parsley
- ✓ ½ tsp pure maple syrup
- ✓ 8 slices whole-wheat ciabatta
- ✓ 4 oz sliced plant-based Parmesan

Directions:

- ❖ Heat the olive oil in a medium skillet over medium heat and sauté the mushrooms until softened, 5 minutes. Season with salt and black pepper. Turn the heat off.
- ❖ Preheat a panini press to medium heat, 3 to 5 minutes. Mash the avocado in a medium bowl and mix in the lemon juice, parsley, and maple syrup. Spread the mixture on 4 bread slices, divide the mushrooms and plant-based Parmesan cheese on top.

❖ Cover with the other bread slices and brush the top with olive oil. Grill the sandwiches one after another in the heated press until golden brown, and the cheese is melted.

❖ Serve

135) CRISPY CORN CAKES

Preparation Time: 35 minutes

Servings: 4

Ingredients:

- ✓ 1 tbsp flaxseed powder
- ✓ 2 cups yellow cornmeal
- ✓ 1 tsp salt
- ✓ 2 tsp baking powder
- ✓ 4 tbsp olive oil
- ✓ 1 cup tofu mayonnaise for serving

Directions:

- ❖ In a bowl, mix the flax seed powder with 3 tbsp water and allow thickening for 5 minutes to form the vegan "flax egg." Mix in 1 cup of water and then whisk in the cornmeal, salt, and baking powder until soup texture forms but not watery.
- ❖ Heat a quarter of the olive oil in a griddle pan and pour in a quarter of the batter. Cook until set and golden brown beneath, 3 minutes. Flip the cake and cook the other side until set and golden brown too. Plate the cake and make three more with the remaining oil and batter.
- ❖ Top the cakes with some tofu mayonnaise before serving

136) CHIA COCONUT PUDDING

Preparation Time: 5 minutes+ cooling time

Servings: 4

Ingredients:

- ✓ 1 cup coconut milk
- ✓ ½ tsp vanilla extract
- ✓ 3 tbsp chia seeds
- ✓ ½ cup granola
- ✓ 2/3 cup chopped sweet nectarine

Directions:

- ❖ In a medium bowl, mix the coconut milk, vanilla, and chia seeds until well combined. Divide the mixture between 4 breakfast cups and refrigerate for at least 4 hours to allow the mixture to gel.
- ❖ Top with the granola and nectarine. Serve

137) CHOCOLATE AND CARROT BREAD WITH RAISINS

Preparation Time: 75 minutes

Servings: 4

Ingredients:

- ✓ 1 ½ cup whole-wheat flour
- ✓ ¼ cup almond flour
- ✓ ¼ tsp salt
- ✓ ¼ tsp cloves powder
- ✓ ¼ tsp cayenne pepper
- ✓ 1 tbsp cinnamon powder
- ✓ ½ tsp nutmeg powder
- ✓ 1 ½ tsp baking powder
- ✓ 2 tbsp flax seed powder
- ✓ ½ cup pure date sugar
- ✓ ¼ cup pure maple syrup
- ✓ ¾ tsp almond extract
- ✓ 1 tbsp grated lemon zest
- ✓ ½ cup unsweetened applesauce
- ✓ ¼ cup olive oil
- ✓ 4 carrots, shredded
- ✓ 3 tbsp unsweetened chocolate chips
- ✓ 2/3 cup black raisins

Directions:

- ❖ Preheat oven to 375 F and line a loaf tin with baking paper. In a bowl, mix all the flours, salt, cloves powder, cayenne pepper, cinnamon powder, nutmeg powder, and baking powder.
- ❖ In another bowl, mix the flax seed powder, 6 tbsp water, and allow thickening for 5 minutes. Mix in the date sugar, maple syrup, almond extract, lemon zest, applesauce, and olive oil. Combine both mixtures until smooth and fold in the carrots, chocolate chips, and raisins.
- ❖ Pour the mixture into a loaf pan and bake in the oven until golden brown on top or a toothpick inserted into the bread comes out clean, 45-50 minutes. Remove from the oven, transfer the bread onto a wire rack to cool, slice, and serve

138) FRENCH TOASTS TROPICAL STYLE

Preparation Time: 55 minutes

Servings: 4

Ingredients:

- 2 tbsp flax seed powder
- 1 ½ cups unsweetened almond milk
- ½ cup almond flour
- 2 tbsp maple syrup + extra for drizzling
- 2 pinches of salt
- ½ tbsp cinnamon powder
- ½ tsp fresh lemon zest
- 1 tbsp fresh pineapple juice
- 8 whole-grain bread slices

Directions:

- Preheat the oven to 400 F and lightly grease a roasting rack with olive oil. Set aside.
- In a medium bowl, mix the flax seed powder with 6 tbsp water and allow thickening for 5 to 10 minutes. Whisk in the almond milk, almond flour, maple syrup, salt, cinnamon powder, lemon zest, and pineapple juice. Soak the bread on both sides in the almond milk mixture and allow sitting on a plate for 2 to 3 minutes.
- Heat a large skillet over medium heat and place the bread in the pan. Cook until golden brown on the bottom side. Flip the bread and cook further until golden brown on the other side, 4 minutes in total. Transfer to a plate, drizzle some maple syrup on top and serve immediately

139)   CREPES WITH MUSHROOM

Preparation Time: 25 minutes   **Servings: 4**

Ingredients:

- 1 cup whole-wheat flour
- 1 tsp onion powder
- ½ tsp baking soda
- ¼ tsp salt
- 1 cup pressed, crumbled tofu
- ⅓ cup plant-based milk
- ¼ cup lemon juice
- 2 tbsp extra-virgin olive oil
- ½ cup finely chopped mushrooms
- ½ cup finely chopped onion
- 2 cups collard greens

Directions:

- Combine the flour, onion powder, baking soda, and salt in a bowl. Blitz the tofu, milk, lemon juice, and oil in a food processor over high speed for 30 seconds. Pour over the flour mixture and mix to combine well. Add in the mushrooms, onion, and collard greens.
- Heat a skillet and grease with cooking spray. Lower the heat and spread a ladleful of the batter across the surface of the skillet. Cook for 4 minutes on both sides or until set. Remove to a plate. Repeat the process until no batter is left, greasing with a little more oil, if needed. Serve

140)   FRENCH TOAST WITH CINNAMON-BANANA

Preparation Time: 25 minutes   **Servings: 3**

Ingredients:

- 1/3 cup coconut milk
- 1/2 cup banana, mashed
- 2 tbsp besan (chickpea flour)
- 1/2 tsp baking powder
- 1/2 tsp vanilla paste
- A pinch of sea salt
- 1 tbsp agave syrup
- 1/2 tsp ground allspice
- A pinch of grated nutmeg
- 6 slices day-old sourdough bread
- 2 bananas, sliced
- 2 tbsp brown sugar
- 1 tsp ground cinnamon

Directions:

- To make the batter, thoroughly combine the coconut milk, mashed banana, besan, baking powder, vanilla, salt, agave syrup, allspice and nutmeg.
- Dredge each slice of bread into the batter until well coated on all sides.
- Preheat an electric griddle to medium heat and lightly oil it with a nonstick cooking spray.
- Cook each slice of bread on the preheated griddle for about 3 minutes per side until golden brown.
- Garnish the French toast with the bananas, brown sugar and cinnamon. Enjoy

141)   INDIAN TRADITIONAL ROTI

Preparation Time: 30 minutes   **Servings: 5**

Ingredients:

- ✓ 2 cups bread flour
- ✓ 1 tsp baking powder
- ✓ 1/2 tsp salt
- ✓ 3/4 warm water
- ✓ 1 cup vegetable oil, for frying

Directions:

- ❖ Thoroughly combine the flour, baking powder and salt in a mixing bowl. Gradually add in the water until the dough comes together.
- ❖ Divide the dough into five balls; flatten each ball to create circles.
- ❖ Heat the olive oil in a frying pan over a moderately high flame. Fry the first bread, turning it over to promote even cooking; fry it for about 10 minutes or until golden brown.
- ❖ Repeat with the remaining dough. Transfer each roti to a paper towel-lined plate to drain the excess oil.
- ❖ Enjoy

142) CHIA CHOCOLATE PUDDING

Preparation Time: 10 minutes + chilling time

Servings: 4

Ingredients:

- ✓ 4 tbsp unsweetened cocoa powder
- ✓ 4 tbsp maple syrup
- ✓ 1 2/3 cups coconut milk
- ✓ A pinch of grated nutmeg
- ✓ A pinch of ground cloves
- ✓ 1/2 tsp ground cinnamon
- ✓ 1/2 cup chia seeds

Directions:

- ❖ Add the cocoa powder, maple syrup, milk and spices to a bowl and stir until everything is well incorporated.
- ❖ Add in the chia seeds and stir again to combine well. Spoon the mixture into four jars, cover and place in your refrigerator overnight.
- ❖ On the actual day, stir with a spoon and serve. Enjoy

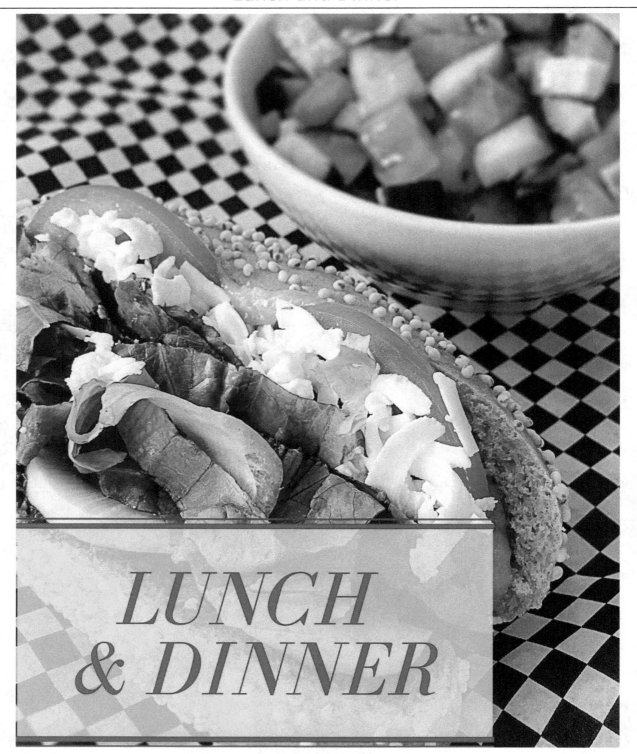

LUNCH & DINNER

143)   TOFU CABBAGE STIR-FRY

Preparation Time: 45 minutes

Servings: 4

Ingredients:

- ✓ 2 ½ cups baby bok choy, quartered
- ✓ 5 oz plant butter
- ✓ 2 cups tofu, cubed
- ✓ 1 tsp garlic powder
- ✓ 1 tsp onion powder
- ✓ 1 tbsp plain vinegar
- ✓ 2 garlic cloves, minced
- ✓ 1 tsp chili flakes
- ✓ 1 tbsp fresh ginger, grated
- ✓ 3 green onions, sliced
- ✓ 1 tbsp sesame oil
- ✓ 1 cup tofu mayonnaise

Directions:

- ❖ Melt half of the butter in a wok over medium heat, add the bok choy, and stir-fry until softened. Season with salt, black pepper, garlic powder, onion powder, and plain vinegar. Sauté for 2 minutes; set aside. Melt the remaining butter in the wok, add and sauté garlic, chili flakes, and ginger until fragrant. Put the tofu in the wok and cook until browned on all sides. Add the green onions and bok choy, heat for 2 minutes, and add the sesame oil. Stir in tofu mayonnaise, cook for 1 minute, and serve

144)   SMOKED TEMPEH WITH BROCCOLI FRITTERS

Preparation Time: 40 minutes

Servings: 4

Ingredients:

- ✓ 4 tbsp flax seed powder
- ✓ 1 tbsp soy sauce
- ✓ 3 tbsp olive oil
- ✓ 1 tbsp grated ginger
- ✓ 3 tbsp fresh lime juice
- ✓ Cayenne pepper to taste
- ✓ 10 oz tempeh slices
- ✓ 1 head broccoli, grated
- ✓ 8 oz tofu, grated
- ✓ 3 tbsp almond flour
- ✓ ½ tsp onion powder
- ✓ 4 ¼ oz plant butter
- ✓ ½ cup mixed salad greens
- ✓ 1 cup tofu mayonnaise
- ✓ Juice of ½ a lemon

Directions:

- ❖ In a bowl, mix the flax seed powder with 12 tbsp water and set aside to soak for 5 minutes. In another bowl, combine soy sauce, olive oil, grated ginger, lime juice, salt, and cayenne pepper. Brush the tempeh slices with the mixture. Heat a grill pan over medium and grill the tempeh on both sides until golden brown and nicely smoked. Remove the slices to a plate.
- ❖ In another bowl, mix the tofu with broccoli. Add in vegan "flax egg," almond flour, onion powder, salt, and black pepper. Mix and form 12 patties out of the mixture. Melt the plant butter in a skillet and fry the patties on both sides until golden brown. Remove to a plate. Add the grilled tempeh with the broccoli fritters and salad greens. Mix the tofu mayonnaise with the lemon juice and drizzle over the salad

145)   CHEESY CAULIFLOWER CASSEROLE

Preparation Time: 35 minutes

Servings: 4

Ingredients:

- ✓ 2 oz plant butter
- ✓ 1 white onion, finely chopped
- ✓ ½ cup celery stalks, finely chopped
- ✓ 1 green bell pepper, chopped
- ✓ Salt and black pepper to taste
- ✓ 1 small head cauliflower, chopped
- ✓ 1 cup tofu mayonnaise
- ✓ 4 oz grated plant-based Parmesan
- ✓ 1 tsp red chili flakes

Directions:

- ❖ Preheat oven to 400 F. Season onion, celery, and bell pepper with salt and black pepper. In a bowl, mix cauliflower, tofu mayonnaise, Parmesan cheese, and red chili flakes. Pour the mixture into a greased baking dish and add the vegetables; mix to distribute. Bake for 20 minutes. Remove and serve warm

146)   SPICY VEGGIE STEAKS WITH GREEN SALAD

Preparation Time: 35 minutes

Servings: 2

Ingredients:

- ✓ 1 eggplant, sliced
- ✓ 1 zucchini, sliced
- ✓ ¼ cup coconut oil
- ✓ Juice of ½ a lemon
- ✓ 5 oz plant-based cheddar, cubed
- ✓ 10 Kalamata olives
- ✓ 2 tbsp pecans
- ✓ 1 oz mixed salad greens
- ✓ ½ cup tofu mayonnaise
- ✓ Salt to taste
- ✓ ½ tsp Cayenne pepper to taste

Directions:

- ❖ Set oven to broil and line a baking sheet with parchment paper. Arrange eggplant and zucchini on the baking sheet. Brush with coconut oil and sprinkle with cayenne pepper. Broil for 15-20 minutes.

- ❖ Remove to a serving platter and drizzle with the lemon juice. Arrange the plant-based cheddar cheese, Kalamata olives, pecans, and mixed greens with the grilled veggies. Top with tofu mayonnaise and serve

147)   BAKED CHEESY SPAGHETTI SQUASH

Preparation Time: 40 minutes

Servings: 4

Ingredients:

- ✓ 2 lb spaghetti squash
- ✓ 1 tbsp coconut oil
- ✓ Salt and black pepper to taste
- ✓ 2 tbsp melted plant butter
- ✓ ½ tbsp garlic powder
- ✓ 1/5 tsp chili powder
- ✓ 1 cup coconut cream
- ✓ 2 oz cashew cream cheese
- ✓ 1 cup plant-based mozzarella
- ✓ 2 oz grated plant-based Parmesan
- ✓ 2 tbsp fresh cilantro, chopped
- ✓ Olive oil for drizzling

Directions:

- ❖ Preheat oven to 350 F.
- ❖ Cut the squash in halves lengthwise and spoon out the seeds and fiber. Place on a baking dish, brush with coconut oil, and season with salt and pepper. Bake for 30 minutes. Remove and use two forks to shred the flesh into strands.
- ❖ Empty the spaghetti strands into a bowl and mix with plant butter, garlic and chili powders, coconut cream, cream cheese, half of the plant-based mozzarella and plant-based Parmesan cheeses. Spoon the mixture into the squash cups and sprinkle with the remaining mozzarella cheese. Bake further for 5 minutes. Sprinkle with cilantro and drizzle with some oil. Serve

148)   KALE AND MUSHROOM PIEROGIS

Preparation Time: 45 minutes

Servings: 4

Ingredients:

- ✓ Stuffing:
- ✓ 2 tbsp plant butter
- ✓ 2 garlic cloves, finely chopped
- ✓ 1 small red onion, finely chopped
- ✓ 3 oz baby Bella mushrooms, sliced
- ✓ 2 oz fresh kale
- ✓ ½ tsp salt
- ✓ ¼ tsp freshly ground black pepper
- ✓ ½ cup dairy-free cream cheese
- ✓ 2 oz plant-based Parmesan, grated
- ✓ Pierogi:
- ✓ 1 tbsp flax seed powder
- ✓ ½ cup almond flour
- ✓ 4 tbsp coconut flour
- ✓ ½ tsp salt
- ✓ 1 tsp baking powder
- ✓ 1 ½ cups grated plant-based Parmesan
- ✓ 5 tbsp plant butter
- ✓ Olive oil for brushing

Directions:

- ❖ Put the plant butter in a skillet and melt over medium heat, then add and sauté the garlic, red onion, mushrooms, and kale until the mushrooms brown. Season the mixture with salt and black pepper and reduce the heat to low. Stir in the cream cheese and plant-based Parmesan cheese and simmer for 1 minute. Turn the heat off and set the filling aside to cool.
- ❖ Make the pierogis: In a small bowl, mix the flax seed powder with 3 tbsp water and allow sitting for 5 minutes. In a bowl, combine almond flour, coconut flour, salt, and baking powder. Put a small pan over low heat, add, and melt the plant-based Parmesan cheese and plant butter while stirring continuously until smooth batter forms. Turn the heat off.
- ❖ Pour the vegan "flax egg" into the cream mixture, continue stirring while adding the flour mixture until a firm dough forms. Mold the dough into four balls, place on a chopping board, and use a rolling pin to flatten each into ½ inch thin round pieces. Spread a generous amount of stuffing on one-half of each dough, then fold over the filling, and seal the dough with your fingers. Brush with olive oil, place on a baking sheet, and bake for 20 minutes at 380 F. Serve with salad

149)   VEGAN MUSHROOM PIZZA

Preparation Time: 35 minutes

Servings: 4

Ingredients:

- ✓ 2 tsp plant butter
- ✓ 1 cup chopped button mushrooms
- ✓ ½ cup sliced mixed bell peppers
- ✓ Salt and black pepper to taste
- ✓ 1 pizza crust
- ✓ 1 cup tomato sauce
- ✓ 1 cup plant-based Parmesan cheese
- ✓ 5-6 basil leaves

Directions:

- ❖ Melt plant butter in a skillet and sauté mushrooms and bell peppers for 10 minutes until softened. Season with salt and black pepper. Put the pizza crust on a pizza pan, spread the tomato sauce all over, and scatter vegetables evenly on top. Sprinkle with plant-based Parmesan cheese. Bake for 20 minutes until the cheese has melted. Garnish with basil and serve

150) MUSHROOM LETTUCE WRAPS

Preparation Time: 25 minutes

Servings: 4

Ingredients:

- ✓ 2 tbsp plant butter
- ✓ 4 oz baby Bella mushrooms, sliced
- ✓ 1 ½ lb tofu, crumbled
- ✓ 1 iceberg lettuce, leaves extracted
- ✓ 1 cup grated plant-based cheddar
- ✓ 1 large tomato, sliced

Directions:

- ❖ Melt the plant butter in a skillet, add in mushrooms and sauté until browned and tender, about 6 minutes. Transfer to a plate. Add the tofu to the skillet and cook until brown, about 10 minutes. Spoon the tofu and mushrooms into the lettuce leaves, sprinkle with the plant-based cheddar cheese, and share the tomato slices on top. Serve the burger immediately

151) CLASSIC GARLICKY RICE

Preparation Time: 20 minutes

Servings: 4

Ingredients:

- ✓ 4 tbsp olive oil
- ✓ 4 cloves garlic, chopped
- ✓ 1 ½ cups white rice
- ✓ 2 ½ cups vegetable broth

Directions:

- ❖ In a saucepan, heat the olive oil over a moderately high flame. Add in the garlic and sauté for about 1 minute or until aromatic.
- ❖ Add in the rice and broth. Bring to a boil; immediately turn the heat to a gentle simmer.
- ❖ Cook for about 15 minutes or until all the liquid has absorbed. Fluff the rice with a fork, season with salt and pepper and serve hot

152) BROWN RICE WITH VEGETABLES AND TOFU

Preparation Time: 45 minutes

Servings: 4

Ingredients:

- ✓ 4 tsp sesame seeds
- ✓ 2 spring garlic stalks, minced
- ✓ 1 cup spring onions, chopped
- ✓ 1 carrot, trimmed and sliced
- ✓ 1 celery rib, sliced
- ✓ 1/4 cup dry white wine
- ✓ 10 ounces tofu, cubed
- ✓ 1 ½ cups long-grain brown rice, rinsed thoroughly
- ✓ 2 tbsp soy sauce
- ✓ 2 tbsp tahini
- ✓ 1 tbsp lemon juice

Directions:

- ❖ In a wok or large saucepan, heat 2 tsp of the sesame oil over medium-high heat. Now, cook the garlic, onion, carrot and celery for about 3 minutes, stirring periodically to ensure even cooking.
- ❖ Add the wine to deglaze the pan and push the vegetables to one side of the wok. Add in the remaining sesame oil and fry the tofu for 8 minutes, stirring occasionally.
- ❖ Bring 2 ½ cups of water to a boil over medium-high heat. Bring to a simmer and cook the rice for about 30 minutes or until it is tender; fluff the rice and stir it with the soy sauce and tahini.
- ❖ Stir the vegetables and tofu into the hot rice; add a few drizzles of the fresh lemon juice and serve warm. Enjoy

153) AMARANTH PORRIDGE

Preparation Time: 35 minutes

Servings: 4

Ingredients:

- ✓ 3 cups water
- ✓ 1 cup amaranth
- ✓ 1/2 cup coconut milk
- ✓ 4 tbsp agave syrup
- ✓ A pinch of kosher salt
- ✓ A pinch of grated nutmeg

Directions:

- ❖ Bring the water to a boil over medium-high heat; add in the amaranth and turn the heat to a simmer.
- ❖ Let it cook for about 30 minutes, stirring periodically to prevent the amaranth from sticking to the bottom of the pan.
- ❖ Stir in the remaining ingredients and continue to cook for 1 to 2

minutes more until cooked through. Enjoy

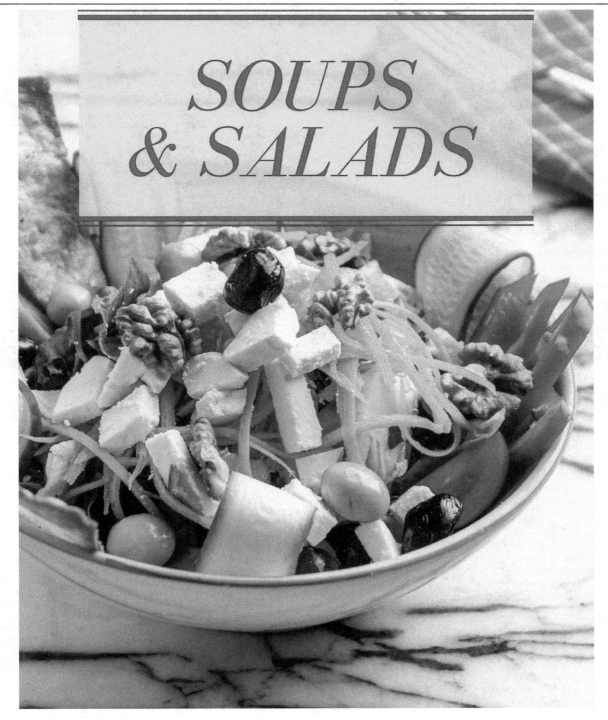

SOUPS
& SALADS

154) SPINACH AND KALE SOUP WITH FRIED COLLARDS

Preparation Time: 16 minutes

Servings: 4

Ingredients:

- ✓ 4 tbsp plant butter
- ✓ 1 cup fresh spinach, chopped
- ✓ 1 cup fresh kale, chopped
- ✓ 1 large avocado
- ✓ 3 ½ cups coconut cream
- ✓ 4 cups vegetable broth
- ✓ 3 tbsp chopped fresh mint leaves
- ✓ Salt and black pepper to taste
- ✓ Juice from 1 lime
- ✓ 1 cup collard greens, chopped
- ✓ 2 garlic cloves, minced
- ✓ 1 pinch of green cardamom powder

Directions:

- ❖ Melt 2 tbsp of plant butter in a saucepan over medium heat and sauté spinach and kale for 5 minutes. Turn the heat off. Add the avocado, coconut cream, vegetable broth, salt, and pepper. Puree the ingredients with an immersion blender until smooth. Pour in the lime juice and set aside.
- ❖ Melt the remaining plant butter in a pan and add the collard greens, garlic, and cardamom; sauté until the garlic is fragrant and has achieved a golden brown color, about 4 minutes. Fetch the soup into serving bowls and garnish with fried collards and mint. Serve warm

155) GOULASH TOFU SOUP

Preparation Time: 25 minutes

Servings: 4

Ingredients:

- ✓ 1 ½ cups extra-firm tofu, crumbled
- ✓ 3 tbsp plant butter
- ✓ 1 white onion
- ✓ 2 garlic cloves
- ✓ 8 oz chopped butternut squash
- ✓ 1 red bell pepper
- ✓ 1 tbsp paprika powder
- ✓ ¼ tsp red chili flakes
- ✓ 1 tbsp dried basil
- ✓ ½ tbsp crushed cardamom seeds
- ✓ Salt and black pepper to taste
- ✓ 1 ½ cups crushed tomatoes
- ✓ 4 cups vegetable broth
- ✓ 1 ½ tsp red wine vinegar
- ✓ Chopped cilantro to serve

Directions:

- ❖ Melt plant butter in a pot over medium heat and sauté onion and garlic for 3 minutes. Stir in tofu and cook for 3 minutes; add the butternut squash, bell pepper, paprika, red chili flakes, basil, cardamom seeds, salt, and pepper. Cook for 2 minutes. Pour in tomatoes and vegetable broth. Bring to a boil, reduce the heat and simmer for 10 minutes. Mix in red wine vinegar. Garnish with cilantro and serve

156) PUMPKIN CREAM COCONUT SOUP

Preparation Time: 55 minutes

Servings: 4

Ingredients:

- ✓ 2 small red onions, cut into wedges
- ✓ 2 garlic cloves, skinned
- ✓ 10 oz pumpkin, cubed
- ✓ 10 oz butternut squash
- ✓ 2 tbsp olive oil
- ✓ 4 tbsp plant butter
- ✓ Juice of 1 lime
- ✓ ¾ cup tofu mayonnaise
- ✓ Toasted pumpkin seeds for garnish

Directions:

- ❖ Preheat oven to 400 F.
- ❖ Place onions, garlic, and pumpkin in a baking sheet and drizzle with olive oil. Season with salt and pepper. Roast for 30 minutes or until the vegetables are golden brown and fragrant. Remove the vegetables from the oven and transfer to a pot. Add 2 cups of water, bring the ingredients to boil over medium heat for 15 minutes. Turn the heat off. Add in plant butter and puree until smooth. Stir in lime juice and tofu mayonnaise. Spoon into serving bowls and garnish with pumpkin seeds to serve

157) CELERY AND POTATO SOUP

Preparation Time: 55 minutes

Servings: 6

Ingredients:

- ✓ 2 tbsp olive oil
- ✓ 1 onion, chopped
- ✓ 1 carrot, chopped
- ✓ 1 celery stalk, chopped
- ✓ 2 garlic cloves, minced
- ✓ 1 golden beet, peeled and diced
- ✓ 1 yellow bell pepper, chopped
- ✓ 1 Yukon Gold potato, diced
- ✓ 6 cups vegetable broth
- ✓ 1 tsp dried thyme
- ✓ Salt and black pepper to taste
- ✓ 1 tbsp lemon juice

Directions:

❖ Heat the oil in a pot over medium heat. Place the onion, carrot, celery, and garlic. Cook for 5 minutes or until softened. Stir in beet, bell pepper, and potato, cook uncovered for 1 minute. Pour in the broth and thyme. Season with salt and pepper. Cook for 45 minutes until the vegetables are tender. Serve sprinkled with lemon juice

158) SPINACH AND POTATO SOUP

Preparation Time: 55 minutes

Servings: 4

Ingredients:

- 2 tbsp olive oil
- 1 onion, chopped
- 2 garlic cloves, minced
- 4 cups vegetable broth
- 2 russet potatoes, cubed
- ½ tsp dried oregano
- ¼ tsp crushed red pepper
- 1 bay leaf
- Salt to taste
- 4 cups chopped spinach
- 1 cup green lentils, rinsed

Directions:

❖ Warm the oil in a pot over medium heat. Place the onion and garlic and cook covered for 5 minutes. Stir in broth, potatoes, oregano, red pepper, bay leaf, lentils, and salt. Bring to a boil, then lower the heat and simmer uncovered for 30 minutes. Add in spinach and cook for another 5 minutes. Discard the bay leaf and serve immediately

159) BEAN TURMERIC SOUP

Preparation Time: 50 minutes

Servings: 6

Ingredients:

- 3 tbsp olive oil
- 1 onion, chopped
- 2 carrots, chopped
- 1 sweet potato, chopped
- 1 yellow bell pepper, chopped
- 2 garlic cloves, minced
- 4 tomatoes, chopped
- 6 cups vegetable broth
- 1 bay leaf
- Salt to taste
- 1 tsp ground cayenne pepper
- 1 (15.5-oz) can white beans, drained
- ⅓ cup whole-wheat pasta
- ¼ tsp turmeric

Directions:

❖ Heat the oil in a pot over medium heat. Place onion, carrots, sweet potato, bell pepper, and garlic. Cook for 5 minutes. Add in tomatoes, broth, bay leaf, salt, and cayenne pepper. Stir and bring to a boil. Lower the heat and simmer for 10 minutes. Put in white beans and simmer for 15 more minutes.

❖ Cook the pasta in a pot with boiling salted water and turmeric for 8-10 minutes, until pasta is al dente. Strain and transfer to the soup. Discard the bay leaf. Spoon into a bowl and serve

160) COCONUT ARUGULA SOUP

Preparation Time: 30 minutes

Servings: 4

Ingredients:

- 1 tsp coconut oil
- 1 onion, diced
- 2 cups green beans
- 4 cups water
- 1 cup arugula, chopped
- 1 tbsp fresh mint, chopped
- Sea salt and black pepper to taste
- ¾ cup coconut milk

Directions:

❖ Place a pot over medium heat and heat the coconut oil. Add in the onion and sauté for 5 minutes. Pour in green beans and water. Bring to a boil, lower the heat and stir in arugula, mint, salt, and pepper. Simmer for 10 minutes. Stir in coconut milk. Transfer to a food processor and blitz the soup until smooth. Serve

161) ORIGINAL LENTIL SOUP WITH SWISS CHARD

Preparation Time: 25 minutes

Servings: 5

Ingredients:

- 2 tbsp olive oil
- 1 white onion, chopped
- 1 tsp garlic, minced
- 2 large carrots, chopped
- 1 parsnip, chopped
- 1/2 tsp dried thyme
- 1/4 tsp ground cumin
- 5 cups roasted vegetable broth
- 1 ¼ cups brown lentils, soaked overnight and rinsed
- 2 cups Swiss chard, torn into pieces

Directions:

❖ In a heavy-bottomed pot, heat the olive oil over a moderate heat. Now, sauté the vegetables along with the spices for about 3 minutes until they are just tender.

❖ Add in the vegetable broth and lentils, bringing it to a boil. Immediately turn the heat to a simmer and add in the bay leaves. Let it cook for about 15 minutes or until lentils are tender.

- ✓ 2 stalks celery, chopped
- ✓ 2 bay leaves

- ❖ Add in the Swiss chard, cover and let it simmer for 5 minutes more or until the chard wilts.
- ❖ Serve in individual bowls and enjoy

162) POMODORO SOUP

Cooking Time: 30 Minutes   **Servings:** 8

Ingredients:

- 4 tbsp olive oil
- 2 medium yellow onions, thinly sliced
- 1 tsp salt (extra for taste if needed)
- 2 tsp curry powder
- 1 tsp red curry powder
- 1 tsp ground coriander
- 1 tsp ground cumin
- ¼-½ tsp red pepper flakes
- 1 15-ounce can diced tomatoes, undrained
- 1 28-ounce can diced or plum tomatoes, undrained
- 5½ cups water (vegetable broth or chicken broth also usable)
- 1 14-ounce can coconut milk optional add-ins: cooked brown rice, lemon wedges, fresh thyme, etc.

Directions:

- ❖ Heat oil in a medium-sized pot over medium heat.
- ❖ Add onions and salt and cook for about 10-1minutes until browned.
- ❖ Stir in curry powder, coriander, red pepper flakes, cumin, and cook for seconds, being sure to keep stirring well.
- ❖ Add tomatoes and water (or broth if you prefer).
- ❖ Simmer the mixture for 1minutes.
- ❖ Take an immersion blender and puree the mixture until a soupy consistency is achieved.
- ❖ Enjoy as it is, or add some extra add-ins for a more flavorful experience

Nutrition: Calories: 217, Total Fat: 19.3 g, Saturated Fat: 11.5 g, Cholesterol: 0 mg, Sodium: 40 mg, Total Carbohydrate: 12.1 g, Dietary Fiber: 3.g, Total Sugars: 7.1 g, Protein: 3 g, Vitamin D: 0 mcg, Calcium: 58 mg, Iron: 2 mg, Potassium: 570 mg

163) ONION CHEESE SOUP

Cooking Time: 25 Minutes   **Servings:** 4

Ingredients:

- 2 large onions, finely sliced
- 2 cups vegetable stock
- 1 tsp brown sugar
- 1 cup red wine
- 1 measure of brandy
- 1 tsp herbs de Provence
- 4 slices stale bread
- 4 ounces grated strong cheese
- 1-ounce grated parmesan
- 1 tbsp plain flour
- 2 tbsp olive oil
- 1-ounce butter
- salt
- pepper

Directions:

- ❖ Heat oil and butter in a pan over medium-high heat.
- ❖ Add onions and brown sugar.
- ❖ Cook until the onions are golden brown.
- ❖ Pour brandy and flambé, making sure to keep stirring until the flames are out.
- ❖ Add plain flour and herbs de Provence and keep stirring well.
- ❖ Slowly add the stock and red wine.
- ❖ Season well and simmer for 20 minutes, making sure to add water if the soup becomes too thick.
- ❖ Ladle the soup into jars.
- ❖ Before serving, place rounds of stale bread on top.
- ❖ Add strong cheese.
- ❖ Garnish with some parmesan.
- ❖ Place the bowls under a hot grill or in an oven until the cheese has melted.

Nutrition: Calories: 403, Total Fat: 22.4 g, Saturated Fat: 10.9 g, Cholesterol: 41 mg, Sodium: 886 mg, Total Carbohydrate: 24.9 g, Dietary Fiber: 3.6 g, Total Sugars: 7 g, Protein: 16.2 g, Vitamin D: 4 mcg, Calcium: 371 mg, Iron: 1 mg, Potassium: 242 mg

164) Herbal Lamb Cutlets and Roasted Veggies

Cooking Time: 45 Minutes   **Servings:** 6

Ingredients:

- ✓ 2 deseeded peppers, cut up into chunks
- ✓ 1 large sweet potato, peeled and chopped
- ✓ 2 sliced courgettes
- ✓ 1 red onion, cut into wedges
- ✓ 1 tbsp olive oil
- ✓ 8 lean lamb cutlets
- ✓ 1 tbsp thyme leaf, chopped
- ✓ 2 tbsp mint leaves, chopped

Directions:

- ❖ Preheat oven to 390degrees F.
- ❖ In a large baking dish, place peppers, courgettes, sweet potatoes, and onion.
- ❖ Drizzle all with oil and season with ground pepper.
- ❖ Roast for about 25 minutes
- ❖ Trim as much fat off the lamb as possible.
- ❖ Mix in herbs with a few twists of ground black pepper.
- ❖ Take the veggies out of the oven and push to one side of a baking dish.
- ❖ Place lamb cutlets on another side, return to oven, and roast for another 10 minutes.
- ❖ Turn the cutlets over, cook for another 10 minutes, and until the veggies are ready (lightly charred and tender).
- ❖ Mix everything on the tray and spread over containers.

Nutrition: Calories: 268, Total Fat: 9.2 g, Saturated Fat: 3 g, Cholesterol: 100 mg, Sodium: mg, Total Carbohydrate: 10.7 g, Dietary Fiber: 2.4 g, Total Sugars: 4.1 g, Protein: 32.4 g, Vitamin D: 0 mcg, Calcium: 20 mg, Iron: 4 mg, Potassium: 365 mg

165) **Mediterranean-Style Potato Salad**

Cooking Time: 30 Minutes   **Servings: 6**

Ingredients:

- ✓ 3 tbsp extra virgin olive oil
- ✓ ½ cup of sliced olives
- ✓ 1 tbsp olive juice
- ✓ 3 tbsp lemon juice, freshly squeezed is best
- ✓ 2 tbsp of mint, fresh and torn
- ✓ ¼ tsp sea salt
- ✓ 2 stalks of sliced celery
- ✓ 2 pounds baby potatoes
- ✓ 2 tbsp of chopped oregano, fresh is best

Directions:

- ❖ Cut the potatoes into inch cubes.
- ❖ Toss the potatoes into a medium saucepan and cover them with water.
- ❖ Place the saucepan on the stove over high heat.
- ❖ Once the potatoes start to boil, bring the heat down to medium-low.
- ❖ Let the potatoes simmer for 13 to 1minutes. When you poke the potatoes with a fork and they feel tender, they are done.
- ❖ As the potatoes are simmering, grab a small bowl and mix the oil, olive juice, lemon juice, and salt. Whisk the ingredients together well.
- ❖ Once the potatoes are done, drain them and pour the potatoes into a bowl.
- ❖ Take the juice mixture and pour 3 tbsp over the potatoes right away.
- ❖ Combine the potatoes with the celery and olives.
- ❖ Prior to serving, sprinkle the potatoes with the mint, oregano, and rest of the dressing.

Nutrition: calories: 175, fats: 7 grams, carbohydrates: 27 grams, protein: 3 grams.

166) **MEDITERRANEAN-STYLE ZUCCHINI NOODLES**

Cooking Time: 10 Minutes   **Servings: 2**

Ingredients:

- ✓ 2 large zucchini or 1 package of store-bought zucchini noodles
- ✓ 1 tsp olive oil
- ✓ 4 cloves garlic diced
- ✓ 10 oz cherry tomatoes cut in half
- ✓ 2-4 oz plain hummus
- ✓ 1 tsp oregano
- ✓ 1/2 tsp red wine vinegar plus more to taste
- ✓ 1/2 cup jarred artichoke hearts, drained and chopped
- ✓ 1/4 cup sun-dried tomatoes, drained and chopped
- ✓ Salt, to taste
- ✓ Pepper to taste
- ✓ Parmesan and fresh basil for topping

Directions:

- ❖ Prepare the zucchini by cutting of the ends off zucchini and spiralize, set aside
- ❖ In a pan over medium heat, add in olive oil
- ❖ Then add in the garlic and cherry tomatoes to the pan, sauté until tomatoes begin to burst, about 4 minutes
- ❖ Add in the zucchini noodles, sun-dried tomatoes, hummus, oregano, artichoke hearts and red wine vinegar to the pan, sauté for 1-2 minutes, or until zucchini is tender-crisp and heated through
- ❖ Season to taste with salt and pepper as needed
- ❖ Allow the zoodle to cool
- ❖ Distribute among the containers, store in the fridge for 2-3 days

❖ To Serve: Reheat in the microwave for 30 seconds or until heated through, serve immediately with parmesan and fresh basil. Enjoy

Nutrition: Calories:241;Carbs: 8g;Total Fat: 37g;Protein: 10g

167)   **Italian-style Baked Beans**

Cooking Time: 15 To 20 Minutes.   **Servings: 6**

Ingredients:

- ✓ ½ cup chopped onion
- ✓ ¼ cup red wine vinegar
- ✓ ¼ tbsp ground cinnamon
- ✓ 15 ounces or 2 cans of great northern beans, do not drain
- ✓ 2 tsp extra virgin olive oil
- ✓ 12 ounces tomato paste, low sodium
- ✓ ½ cup water

Directions:

- ❖ Turn a burner to medium heat and add oil to a saucepan.
- ❖ Add the onion and cook for 4 to 5 minutes. Stir well.
- ❖ Combine the vinegar, tomato paste, cinnamon, and water. Mix until all the ingredients are well combined.
- ❖ Switch the heat to a low setting.
- ❖ Using a colander, drain one can of beans and pour into the pan.
- ❖ Open the second can of beans and pour all of it, including the liquid, into the saucepan and stir.
- ❖ Continue to cook the beans for 10 minutes while stirring frequently.
- ❖ Serve and enjoy!

Nutrition: calories: 236, fats: 3 grams, carbohydrates: 42 grams, protein: 10 grams

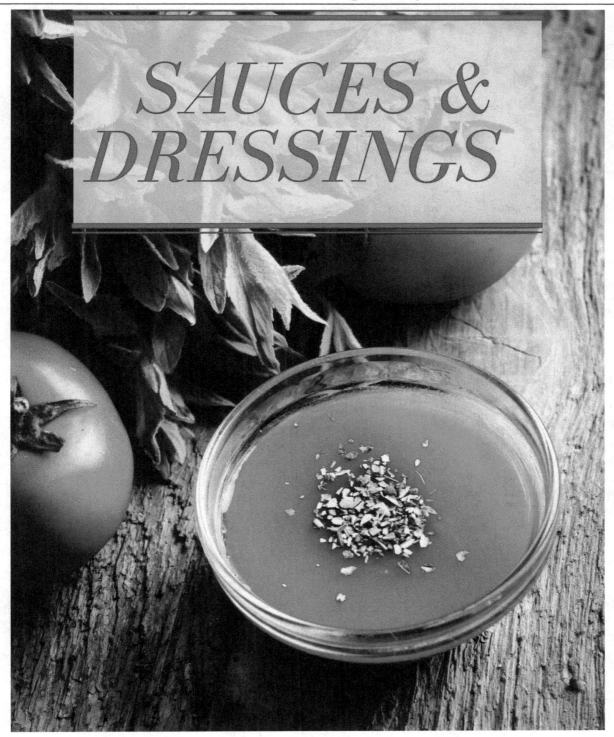

168) MEXICAN-STYLE TORTILLA SOUP

Cooking Time: 40 Minutes   **Servings: 4**

Ingredients:

- ✓ 1-pound chicken breasts, boneless and skinless
- ✓ 1 can (15 ounces whole peeled tomatoes
- ✓ 1 can (10 ounces red enchilada sauce
- ✓ 1 and 1/2 tsp minced garlic
- ✓ 1 yellow onion, diced
- ✓ 1 can (4 ounces fire-roasted diced green chile
- ✓ 1 can (15 ounces black beans, drained and rinsed

- ✓ 1 can (15 ounces fire-roasted corn, undrained
- ✓ 1 container (32 ounces chicken stock or broth
- ✓ 1 tsp ground cumin
- ✓ 2 tsp chili powder
- ✓ 3/4 tsp paprika
- ✓ 1 bay leaf
- ✓ Salt and freshly cracked pepper, to taste
- ✓ 1 tbsp chopped cilantro Tortilla strips, Freshly squeezed lime juice, freshly grated cheddar cheese,

Directions:

- ❖ Set your Instant Pot on Sauté mode.
- ❖ Toss olive oil, onion and garlic into the insert of the Instant Pot.
- ❖ Sauté for 4 minutes then add chicken and remaining ingredients.
- ❖ Mix well gently then seal and lock the lid.
- ❖ Select Manual mode for 7 minutes at high pressure.
- ❖ Once done, release the pressure completely then remove the lid.
- ❖ Adjust seasoning as needed.
- ❖ Garnish with desired toppings.
- ❖ Enjoy.

Nutrition: Calories: 390;Carbohydrate: 5.6g;Protein: 29.5g;Fat: 26.5g;Sugar: 2.1g;Sodium: 620mg

169) Special Cheesy Broccoli Soup

Cooking Time: 30 Minutes   **Servings: 4**

Ingredients:

- ✓ ½ cup heavy whipping cream
- ✓ 1 cup broccoli

- ✓ 1 cup cheddar cheese
- ✓ Salt, to taste
- ✓ 1½ cups chicken broth

Directions:

- ❖ Heat chicken broth in a large pot and add broccoli.
- ❖ Bring to a boil and stir in the rest of the ingredients.
- ❖ Allow the soup to simmer on low heat for about 20 minutes.
- ❖ Ladle out into a bowl and serve hot.

Nutrition: Calories: 188;Carbs: 2.6g;Fats: 15g;Proteins: 9.8g;Sodium: 514mg;Sugar: 0.8g

170) DELICIOUS RICH POTATO SOUP

Cooking Time: 30 Minutes   **Servings: 4**

Ingredients:

- ✓ 1 tbsp butter
- ✓ 1 medium onion, diced
- ✓ 3 cloves garlic, minced
- ✓ 3 cups chicken broth
- ✓ 1 can/box cream of chicken soup
- ✓ 7-8 medium-sized russet potatoes, peeled and chopped
- ✓ 1 1/2 tsp salt

- ✓ Black pepper to taste
- ✓ 1 cup milk
- ✓ 1 tbsp flour
- ✓ 2 cups shredded cheddar cheese Garnish:
- ✓ 5-6 slices bacon, chopped
- ✓ Sliced green onions
- ✓ Shredded cheddar cheese

Directions:

- ❖ Heat butter in the insert of the Instant Pot on sauté mode.
- ❖ Add onions and sauté for 4 minutes until soft.
- ❖ Stir in garlic and sauté it for 1 minute.
- ❖ Add potatoes, cream of chicken, broth, salt, and pepper to the insert.
- ❖ Mix well then seal and lock the lid.
- ❖ Cook this mixture for 10 minutes at Manual Mode with high pressure.
- ❖ Meanwhile, mix flour with milk in a bowl and set it aside.
- ❖ Once the instant pot beeps, release the pressure completely.
- ❖ Remove the Instant Pot lid and switch the instant pot to Sauté mode.
- ❖ Pour in flour slurry and stir cook the mixture for 5 minutes until it thickens.
- ❖ Add 2 cups of cheddar cheese and let it melt.
- ❖ Garnish it as desired.
- ❖ Serve.

Nutrition: Calories: 784;Carbohydrate: 54.8g;Protein: 34g;Fat: 46.5g;Sugar: 7.5g;Sodium: 849mg

171) MEDITERRANEAN-STYLE LENTIL SOUP

Cooking Time: 20 Minutes   **Servings: 4**

Ingredients:

- ✓ 1 tbsp olive oil
- ✓ 1/2 cup red lentils
- ✓ 1 medium yellow or red onion
- ✓ 2 garlic cloves, chopped
- ✓ 1/2 tsp ground cumin
- ✓ 1/2 tsp ground coriander
- ✓ 1/2 tsp ground sumac
- ✓ 1/2 tsp red chili flakes
- ✓ 1/2 tsp dried parsley
- ✓ 3/4 tsp dried mint flakes
- ✓ pinch of sugar
- ✓ 2.5 cups water
- ✓ salt, to taste
- ✓ black pepper, to taste
- ✓ juice of 1/2 lime
- ✓ parsley or cilantro, to garnish

Directions:

- ❖ Preheat oil in the insert of your Instant Pot on Sauté mode.
- ❖ Add onion and sauté until it turns golden brown.
- ❖ Toss in the garlic, parsley sugar, mint flakes, red chili flakes, sumac, coriander, and cumin.
- ❖ Stir cook this mixture for 2 minutes.
- ❖ Add water, lentils, salt, and pepper. Stir gently.
- ❖ Seal and lock the Instant Pot lid and select Manual mode for 8 minutes at high pressure.
- ❖ Once done, release the pressure completely then remove the lid.
- ❖ Stir well then add lime juice.
- ❖ Serve warm.

Nutrition: Calories: 525;Carbohydrate: 59.8g;Protein: 30.1g;Fat: 19.3g;Sugar: 17.3g;Sodium: 897mg

172) Delicious Creamy Keto Cucumber Salad

Cooking Time: 5 Minutes   **Servings: 2**

Ingredients:

- ✓ 2 tbsp mayonnaise
- ✓ Salt and black pepper, to taste
- ✓ 1 cucumber, sliced and quartered
- ✓ 2 tbsp lemon juice

Directions:

- ❖ Mix together the mayonnaise, cucumber slices, and lemon juice in a large bowl.
- ❖ Season with salt and black pepper and combine well.
- ❖ Dish out in a glass bowl and serve while it is cold.

Nutrition: Calories: 8Carbs: 9.3g;Fats: 5.2g;Proteins: 1.2g;Sodium: 111mg;Sugar: 3.8g

173) Classic Minestrone Soup

Cooking Time: 25 Minutes   **Servings:** 6

Ingredients:

- ✓ 2 tbsp olive oil
- ✓ 3 cloves garlic, minced
- ✓ 1 onion, diced
- ✓ 2 carrots, peeled and diced
- ✓ 2 stalks celery, diced
- ✓ 1 1/2 tsp dried basil
- ✓ 1 tsp dried oregano
- ✓ 1/2 tsp fennel seed
- ✓ 6 cups low sodium chicken broth
- ✓ 1 (28-ounce can diced tomatoes

- ✓ 1 (16-ounce can kidney beans, drained and rinsed
- ✓ 1 zucchini, chopped
- ✓ 1 (3-inch Parmesan rind
- ✓ 1 bay leaf
- ✓ 1 bunch kale leaves, chopped
- ✓ 2 tsp red wine vinegar
- ✓ Kosher salt and black pepper, to taste
- ✓ 1/3 cup freshly grated Parmesan
- ✓ 2 tbsp chopped fresh parsley leaves

Directions:

- ❖ Preheat olive oil in the insert of the Instant Pot on Sauté mode.
- ❖ Add carrots, celery, and onion, sauté for 3 minutes.
- ❖ Stir in fennel seeds, oregano, and basil. Stir cook for 1 minute.
- ❖ Add stock, beans, tomatoes, parmesan, bay leaf, and zucchini.
- ❖ Secure and seal the Instant Pot lid then select Manual mode to cook for minutes at high pressure.
- ❖ Once done, release the pressure completely then remove the lid.
- ❖ Add kale and let it sit for 2 minutes in the hot soup.
- ❖ Stir in red wine, vinegar, pepper, and salt.
- ❖ Garnish with parsley and parmesan.
- ❖ Enjoy.

Nutrition: Calories: 805;Carbohydrate: 2.5g;Protein: 124.1g;Fat: 34g;Sugar: 1.4g;Sodium: 634mg

174) SPECIAL KOMBU SEAWEED SALAD

Cooking Time: 40 Minutes   **Servings:** 6

Ingredients:

- ✓ 4 garlic cloves, crushed
- ✓ 1 pound fresh kombu seaweed, boiled and cut into strips

- ✓ 2 tbsp apple cider vinegar
- ✓ Salt, to taste
- ✓ 2 tbsp coconut aminos

Directions:

- ❖ Mix together the kombu, garlic, apple cider vinegar, and coconut aminos in a large bowl.
- ❖ Season with salt and combine well.
- ❖ Dish out in a glass bowl and serve immediately.

Nutrition: Calories: 257;Carbs: 16.9g;Fats: 19.;Proteins: 6.5g;Sodium: 294mg;Sugar: 2.7g

175) LOVELY MINT AVOCADO CHILLED SOUP

Cooking Time: 5 Minutes   **Servings: 2**

Ingredients:

- ✓ Salt, to taste
- ✓ 20 fresh mint leaves

- ✓ 1 cup coconut milk, chilled
- ✓ 1 medium ripe avocado
- ✓ 1 tbsp lime juice

Directions:

- ❖ Put all the ingredients into an immersion blender and blend until a thick mixture is formed.
- ❖ Allow to cool in the fridge for about 10 minutes and serve chilled.

Nutrition: Calories: 286;Carbs: 12.6g;Fats: 26.9g;Proteins: 4.2g;Sodium: 70mg;Sugar: 4.6g

176) CLASSIC SPLIT PEA SOUP

Cooking Time: 30 Minutes   **Servings: 6**

Ingredients:

- ✓ 1 lb. dry split peas sorted and rinsed
- ✓ 6 cups chicken stock
- ✓ 2 bay leaves
- ✓ kosher salt and black pepper

- ✓ 3 tbsp butter
- ✓ 1 onion diced
- ✓ 2 ribs celery diced
- ✓ 2 carrots diced
- ✓ 6 oz. diced ham

Directions:

- ❖ Set your Instant Pot on Sauté mode and melt butter in it.
- ❖ Stir in celery, onion, carrots, salt, and pepper.
- ❖ Sauté them for 5 minutes then stir in split peas, ham bone, chicken stock, and bay leaves.
- ❖ Seal and lock the Instant Pot lid then select Manual mode for 15 minutes at high pressure.
- ❖ Once done, release the pressure completely then remove the lid.
- ❖ Remove the ham bone and separate meat from the bone.
- ❖ Shred or dice the meat and return it to the soup.
- ❖ Adjust seasoning as needed then serve warm.
- ❖ Enjoy.

Nutrition: Calories: 190;Carbohydrate: 30.5g;Protein: 8g;Fat: 3.5g;Sugar: 4.2g;Sodium: 461mg

177) Wine and Lemon Braised Artichokes

Preparation Time: 35 minutes   **Servings: 4**

Ingredients:

- ✓ 2 tbsp basil leaves, finely chopped
- ✓ 2 cloves garlic, minced
- ✓ 1/4 cup dry white wine
- ✓ 1/4 cup extra-virgin olive oil, plus more for drizzling
- ✓ Sea salt and freshly ground black pepper, to taste

- ✓ 1 large lemon, freshly squeezed
- ✓ 1 ½ pounds artichokes, trimmed, tough outer leaves and chokes removed
- ✓ 2 tbsp mint leaves, finely chopped
- ✓ 2 tbsp cilantro leaves, finely chopped

Directions:

- ❖ Fill a bowl with water and add in the lemon juice. Place the cleaned artichokes in the bowl, keeping them completely submerged.
- ❖ In another small bowl, thoroughly combine the herbs and garlic. Rub your artichokes with the herb mixture.
- ❖ Pour the wine and olive oil in a saucepan; add the artichokes to the saucepan. Turn the heat to a simmer and continue to cook, covered, for about 30 minutes until the artichokes are crisp-tender.
- ❖ To serve, drizzle the artichokes with the cooking juices, season them with the salt and black pepper and enjoy

178) ROASTED CARROTS WITH HERBS

Preparation Time: 25 minute   **Servings: 4**

Ingredients:

- ✓ 2 pounds carrots, trimmed and halved lengthwise
- ✓ 4 tbsp olive oil
- ✓ 1 tsp granulated garlic
- ✓ 1 tsp paprika
- ✓ Sea salt and freshly ground black pepper
- ✓ 2 tbsp fresh cilantro, chopped
- ✓ 2 tbsp fresh parsley, chopped
- ✓ 2 tbsp fresh chives, chopped

Directions:

- ❖ Start by preheating your oven to 400 degrees F.
- ❖ Toss the carrots with the olive oil, granulated garlic, paprika, salt and black pepper. Arrange them in a single layer on a parchment-lined roasting sheet.
- ❖ Roast the carrots in the preheated oven for about 20 minutes, until fork-tender.
- ❖ Toss the carrots with the fresh herbs and serve immediately. Enjoy

179) BRAISED GREEN BEANS

Preparation Time: 15 minutes

Servings: 4

Ingredients:

- ✓ 4 tbsp olive oil
- ✓ 1 carrot, cut into matchsticks
- ✓ 1 ½ pounds green beans, trimmed
- ✓ 4 garlic cloves, peeled
- ✓ 1 bay laurel
- ✓ 1 ½ cups vegetable broth
- ✓ Sea salt and ground black pepper, to taste
- ✓ 1 lemon, cut into wedges

Directions:

- ❖ Heat the olive oil in a saucepan over medium flame. Once hot, fry the carrots and green beans for about 5 minutes, stirring periodically to promote even cooking.
- ❖ Add in the garlic and bay laurel and continue sautéing an additional 1 minute or until fragrant.
- ❖ Add in the broth, salt and black pepper and continue to simmer, covered, for about 9 minutes or until the green beans are tender.
- ❖ Taste, adjust the seasonings and serve with lemon wedges. Enjoy

180) BRAISED KALE WITH SESAME SEEDS

Preparation Time: 10 minutes

Servings: 4

Ingredients:

- ✓ 1 cup vegetable broth
- ✓ 1 pound kale, cleaned, tough stems removed, torn into pieces
- ✓ 4 tbsp olive oil
- ✓ 6 garlic cloves, chopped
- ✓ 1 tsp paprika
- ✓ Kosher salt and ground black pepper, to taste
- ✓ 4 tbsp sesame seeds, lightly toasted

Directions:

- ❖ In a saucepan, bring the vegetable broth to a boil; add in the kale leaves and turn the heat to a simmer. Cook for about 5 minutes until kale has softened; reserve.
- ❖ Heat the oil in the same saucepan over medium heat. Once hot, sauté the garlic for about 30 seconds or until aromatic.
- ❖ Add in the reserved kale, paprika, salt and black pepper and let it cook for a few minutes more or until heated through.
- ❖ Garnish with lightly toasted sesame seeds and serve immediately. Enjoy

181) CHINESE CABBAGE STIR-FRY

Preparation Time: 10 minutes

Servings: 3

Ingredients:

3 tbsp sesame oil

1 pound Chinese cabbage, sliced

1/2 tsp Chinese five-spice powder

Kosher salt, to taste

1/2 tsp Szechuan pepper

2 tbsp soy sauce

3 tbsp sesame seeds, lightly toasted

Directions:

❖ In a wok, heat the sesame oil until sizzling. Stir fry the cabbage for about 5 minutes.

❖ Stir in the spices and soy sauce and continue to cook, stirring frequently, for about 5 minutes more, until the cabbage is crisp-tender and aromatic.

❖ Sprinkle sesame seeds over the top and serve immediately

182) SAUTÉED CAULIFLOWER WITH SESAME SEEDS

Preparation Time: 15 minutes

Servings: 4

Ingredients:

1 cup vegetable broth

1 ½ pounds cauliflower florets

4 tbsp olive oil

2 scallion stalks, chopped

4 garlic cloves, minced

Sea salt and freshly ground black pepper, to taste

2 tbsp sesame seeds, lightly toasted

Directions:

❖ In a large saucepan, bring the vegetable broth to a boil; then, add in the cauliflower and cook for about 6 minutes or until fork-tender; reserve.

❖ Then, heat the olive oil until sizzling; now, sauté the scallions and garlic for about 1 minute or until tender and aromatic.

❖ Add in the reserved cauliflower, followed by salt and black pepper; continue to simmer for about 5 minutes or until heated through

❖ Garnish with toasted sesame seeds and serve immediately. Enjoy

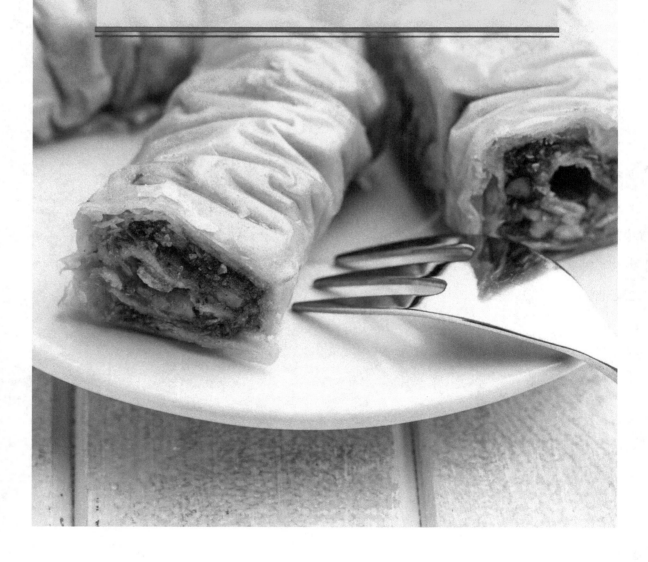

DESSERTS & SNACKS

183) SPECIAL CHUNKY MONKEY TRAIL MIX

Cooking Time: 1 Hour 30 Minutes   **Servings: 6**

Ingredients:

- ✓ 1 cup cashews, halved
- ✓ 2 cups raw walnuts, chopped or halved
- ✓ ⅓ cup coconut sugar
- ✓ ½ cup of chocolate chips
- ✓ 1 tsp vanilla extract
- ✓ 1 cup coconut flakes, unsweetened and make sure you have big flakes and not shredded
- ✓ 6 ounces dried banana slices
- ✓ 1 ½ tsp coconut oil at room temperature

Directions:

- ❖ Turn your crockpot to high and add the cashews, walnuts, vanilla, coconut oil, and sugar. Combine until the ingredients are well mixed and then cook for 45 minutes.
- ❖ Reduce the temperature on your crockpot to low.
- ❖ Continue to cook the mixture for another 20 minutes.
- ❖ Place a piece of parchment paper on your counter.
- ❖ Once the mix is done cooking, remove it from the crockpot and set on top of the parchment paper.
- ❖ Let the mixture sit and cool for 20 minutes.
- ❖ Pour the contents into a bowl and add the dried bananas and chocolate chips. Gently mix the ingredients together. You can store the mixture in Ziplock bags for a quick and easy snack.

Nutrition: calories: 250, fats: 6 grams, carbohydrates: 1grams, protein: 4 grams

184) DELICIOUS FIG-PECAN ENERGY BITES

Cooking Time: 20 Minutes   **Servings: 6**

Ingredients:

- ✓ ½ cup chopped pecans
- ✓ 2 tbsp honey
- ✓ ¾ cup dried figs, about 6 to 8, diced
- ✓ 2 tbsp wheat flaxseed
- ✓ ¼ cup quick oats
- ✓ 2 tbsp regular or powdered peanut butter

Directions:

- ❖ Combine the figs, quick oats, pecans, peanut butter, and flaxseed into a bowl. Stir the ingredients well.
- ❖ Drizzle honey onto the ingredients and mix everything with a wooden spoon. Do your best to press all the ingredients into the honey as you are stirring. If you start to struggle because the mixture is too sticky, set it in the freezer for 3 to 5 minutes.
- ❖ Divide the mixture into four sections.
- ❖ Take a wet rag and get your hands damp. You don't want them too wet or they won't work well with the mixture.
- ❖ Divide each of the four sections into 3 separate sections.
- ❖ Take one of the three sections and roll them up. Repeat with each section so you have a dozen energy bites once you are done.
- ❖ If you want to firm them up, you can place them into the freezer for a few minutes. Otherwise, you can enjoy them as soon as they are little energy balls.
- ❖ To store them, you'll want to keep them in a sealed container and set them in the fridge. They can be stored for about a week.

Nutrition: calories: 157, fats: 6 grams, carbohydrates: 26 grams, protein: 3 grams

185) MEDITERRANEAN STYLE BAKED APPLES

Cooking Time: 25 Minutes   **Servings: 4**

- ✓ ¼ tsp cinnamon

Ingredients:

- ✓ ½ lemon, squeezed for juice
- ✓ 1 ½ pounds of peeled and sliced apples

Directions:

- ❖ Set the temperature of your oven to 350 degrees Fahrenheit so it can preheat.
- ❖ Take a piece of parchment paper and lay on top of a baking pan.
- ❖ Combine your lemon juice, cinnamon, and apples into a medium bowl and mix well.
- ❖ Pour the apples onto the baking pan and arrange them so they are not

doubled up.

❖ Place the pan in the oven and set your timer to 2minutes. The apples should be tender but not mushy.

❖ Remove from the oven, plate and enjoy!

Nutrition: calories: 90, fats: 0.3 grams, carbohydrates: 24 grams, protein: 0.5 grams

186) BREAD PUDDING WITH RAISINS

Preparation Time: 1 hour

Servings: 4

Ingredients:

- 4 cups day-old bread, cubed
- 1 cup brown sugar
- 4 cups coconut milk
- 1/2 tsp vanilla extract
- 1 tsp ground cinnamon
- 2 tbsp rum
- 1/2 cup raisins

Directions:

- Start by preheating your oven to 360 degrees F. Lightly oil a casserole dish with a nonstick cooking spray.
- Place the cubed bread in the prepared casserole dish.
- In a mixing bowl, thoroughly combine the sugar, milk, vanilla, cinnamon, rum and raisins. Pour the custard evenly over the bread cubes.
- Let it soak for about 15 minutes.
- Bake in the preheated oven for about 45 minutes or until the top is golden and set. Enjoy

187) BULGUR WHEAT SALAD

Preparation Time: 25 minutes

Servings: 4

Ingredients:

- 1 cup bulgur wheat
- 1 ½ cups vegetable broth
- 1 tsp sea salt
- 1 tsp fresh ginger, minced
- 4 tbsp olive oil
- 1 onion, chopped
- 8 ounces canned garbanzo beans, drained
- 2 large roasted peppers, sliced
- 2 tbsp fresh parsley, roughly chopped

Directions:

- In a deep saucepan, bring the bulgur wheat and vegetable broth to a simmer; let it cook, covered, for 12 to 13 minutes.
- Let it stand for about 10 minutes and fluff with a fork.
- Add the remaining ingredients to the cooked bulgur wheat; serve at room temperature or well-chilled. Enjoy

188) RYE PORRIDGE WITH BLUEBERRY TOPPING

Preparation Time: 15 minutes

Servings: 3

Ingredients:

- 1 cup rye flakes
- 1 cup water
- 1 cup coconut milk
- 1 cup fresh blueberries
- 1 tbsp coconut oil
- 6 dates, pitted

Directions:

- Add the rye flakes, water and coconut milk to a deep saucepan; bring to a boil over medium-high. Turn the heat to a simmer and let it cook for 5 to 6 minutes.
- In a blender or food processor, puree the blueberries with the coconut oil and dates.
- Ladle into three bowls and garnish with the blueberry topping.
- Enjoy

189) COCONUT SORGHUM PORRIDGE

Preparation Time: 15 minutes

Servings: 2

Ingredients:

- 1/2 cup sorghum
- 1 cup water
- 1/2 cup coconut milk
- 1/4 tsp grated nutmeg
- 1/2 tsp ground cinnamon
- Kosher salt, to taste
- 2 tbsp agave syrup
- 2 tbsp coconut flakes

Directions:

- Place the sorghum, water, milk, nutmeg, cloves, cinnamon and kosher salt in a saucepan; simmer gently for about 15 minutes.
- Spoon the porridge into serving bowls. Top with agave syrup and coconut flakes. Enjoy

- [✓] 1/4 tsp ground cloves

190) LOVELY STRAWBERRY POPSICLE

Cooking Time: 10 Minutes   **Servings: 5**

✓   1 ½ cups fresh strawberries

Ingredients:

✓   ½ cup almond milk

Directions:

❖ Using a blender or hand mixer, combine the almond milk and strawberries thoroughly in a bowl.

❖ Using popsicle molds, pour the mixture into the molds and place the sticks into the mixture.

❖ Set in the freezer for at least 4 hours.

❖ Serve and enjoy—especially on a hot day!

Nutrition: calories: 3 fats: 0.5 grams, carbohydrates: 7 grams, protein: 0.6 grams.

191) SPECIAL FROZEN BLUEBERRY YOGURT

Cooking Time: 30 Minutes   **Servings: 6**

✓   1 juiced and zested lime or lemon. You can even substitute an orange if your tastes prefer.

Ingredients:

✓   ⅔ cup honey
✓   2 cups chilled yogurt
✓   1 pint fresh blueberries

Directions:

❖ With a saucepan on your burner set to medium heat, add the honey, juiced fruit, zest, and blueberries.

❖ Stir the mixture continuously as it begins to simmer for 15 minutes.

❖ When the liquid is nearly gone, pour the contents into a bowl and place in the fridge for several minutes. You will want to stir the ingredients and check to see if they are chilled.

❖ Once the fruit is chilled, combine with the yogurt.

❖ Mix until the ingredients are well incorporated and enjoy.

Nutrition: calories: 233, fats: 3 grams, carbohydrates: 52 grams, protein: 3.5 grams

192) Mum's Aromatic Rice

Preparation Time: 20 minutes   **Servings: 4**

✓   1 bay leaf
✓   1 ½ cups white rice
✓   2 ½ cups vegetable broth
✓   Sea salt and cayenne pepper, to taste

Ingredients:

✓   3 tbsp olive oil
✓   1 tsp garlic, minced
✓   1 tsp dried oregano
✓   1 tsp dried rosemary

Directions:

❖ In a saucepan, heat the olive oil over a moderately high flame. Add in the garlic, oregano, rosemary and bay leaf; sauté for about 1 minute or until aromatic.

❖ Add in the rice and broth. Bring to a boil; immediately turn the heat to a gentle simmer.

❖ Cook for about 15 minutes or until all the liquid has absorbed. Fluff the rice with a fork, season with salt and pepper and serve immediately.

❖ Enjoy

193) EVERYDAY SAVORY GRITS

Preparation Time: 35 minutes   **Servings: 4**

Ingredients:

- ✓ 2 tbsp vegan butter
- ✓ 1 sweet onion, chopped
- ✓ 1 tsp garlic, minced
- ✓ 4 cups water
- ✓ 1 cup stone-ground grits
- ✓ Sea salt and cayenne pepper, to taste

Directions:

- ❖ In a saucepan, melt the vegan butter over medium-high heat. Once hot, cook the onion for about 3 minutes or until tender.
- ❖ Add in the garlic and continue to sauté for 30 seconds more or until aromatic; reserve.
- ❖ Bring the water to a boil over a moderately high heat. Stir in the grits, salt and pepper. Turn the heat to a simmer, cover and continue to cook, for about 30 minutes or until cooked through.
- ❖ Stir in the sautéed mixture and serve warm. Enjoy

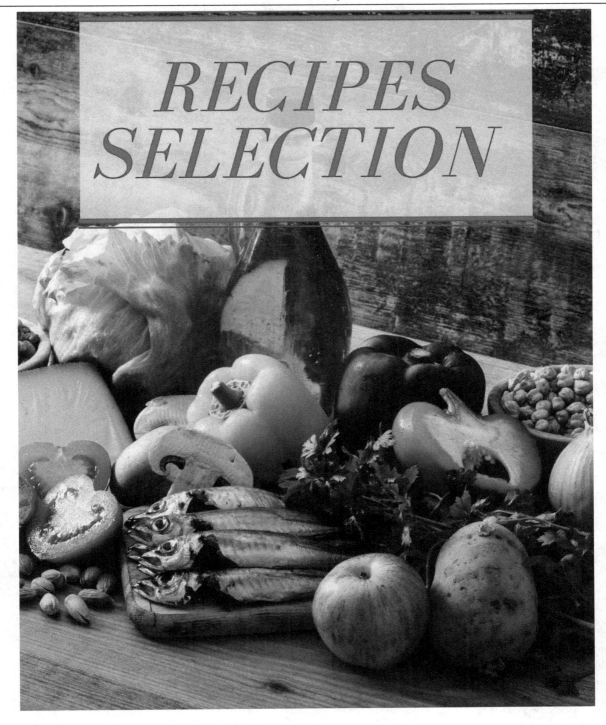

RECIPES
SELECTION

194)   BLACK-EYED PEA OAT BAKE

Preparation Time: 25 minutes

Servings: 4

Ingredients:

- ✓ 1 carrot, shredded
- ✓ 1 onion, chopped
- ✓ 2 garlic cloves, minced
- ✓ 1 (15.5-oz) can black-eyed peas
- ✓ ¾ cup whole-wheat flour
- ✓ ¾ cup quick-cooking oats
- ✓ ½ cup breadcrumbs
- ✓ ¼ cup minced fresh parsley
- ✓ 1 tbsp soy sauce
- ✓ ½ tsp dried sage
- ✓ Salt and black pepper to taste

Directions:

- ❖ Preheat oven to 360 F.
- ❖ Combine the carrot, onion, garlic, and peas and pulse until creamy and smooth in a blender. Add in flour, oats, breadcrumbs, parsley, soy sauce, sage, salt, and pepper. Blend until ingredients are evenly mixed. Spoon the mixture into a greased loaf pan. Bake for 40 minutes until golden. Allow it to cool down for a few minutes before slicing. Serve immediately

195)   PAPRIKA FAVA BEAN PATTIES

Preparation Time: 15 minutes

Servings: 4

Ingredients:

- ✓ 4 tbsp olive oil
- ✓ 1 minced onion
- ✓ 1 garlic clove, minced
- ✓ 1 (15.5-oz) can fava beans
- ✓ 1 tbsp minced fresh parsley
- ✓ ½ cup breadcrumbs
- ✓ ¼ cup almond flour
- ✓ 1 tsp smoked paprika
- ✓ ½ tsp dried thyme
- ✓ 4 burger buns, toasted
- ✓ 4 lettuce leaves
- ✓ 1 ripe tomato, sliced

Directions:

- ❖ In a blender, add onion, garlic, beans, parsley, breadcrumbs, flour, paprika, thyme, salt, and pepper. Pulse until uniform but not smooth. Shape 4 patties out of the mixture. Refrigerate for 15 minutes.
- ❖ Heat olive oil in a skillet over medium heat. Fry the patties for 10 minutes on both sides until golden brown. Serve in toasted buns with lettuce and tomato slices

196)   WALNUT LENTIL BURGERS

Preparation Time: 70 minutes

Servings: 4

Ingredients:

- ✓ 2 tbsp olive oil
- ✓ 1 cup dry lentils, rinsed
- ✓ 2 carrots, grated
- ✓ 1 onion, diced
- ✓ ½ cup walnuts
- ✓ 1 tbsp tomato puree
- ✓ ¾ cup almond flour
- ✓ 2 tsp curry powder
- ✓ 4 whole-grain buns

Directions:

- ❖ Place lentils in a pot and cover with water. Bring to a boil and simmer for 15-20 minutes.
- ❖ Meanwhile, combine the carrots, walnuts, onion, tomato puree, flour, curry powder, salt, and pepper in a bowl. Toss to coat. Once the lentils are ready, drain and transfer into the veggie bowl. Mash the mixture until sticky. Shape the mixture into balls; flatten to make patties.
- ❖ Heat the oil in a skillet over medium heat. Brown the patties for 8 minutes on both sides. To assemble, put the cakes on the buns and top with your desired toppings

197)   COUSCOUS ANDQUINOA BURGERS

Preparation Time: 20 minutes

Servings: 4

Ingredients:

- ✓ 2 tbsp olive oil
- ✓ ¼ cup couscous
- ✓ ¼ cup boiling water
- ✓ 2 cups cooked quinoa
- ✓ 3 tbsp chopped olives
- ✓ ½ tsp garlic powder
- ✓ Salt to taste
- ✓ 4 burger buns
- ✓ Lettuce leaves, for serving
- ✓ Tomato slices, for serving

Directions:

- ❖ Preheat oven to 350 F.
- ❖ In a bowl, place the couscous with boiling water. Let sit covered for 5 minutes. Once the liquid is absorbed, fluff with a fork. Add in quinoa and mash them to form a chunky texture. Stir in vinegar, olive oil, olives, garlic powder, and salt.

✓   2 tbsp balsamic vinegar

❖   Shape the mixture into 4 patties. Arrange them on a greased tray and bake for 25-30 minutes. To assemble, place the patties on the buns and top with lettuce and tomato slices. Serve

198)   FARRO AND BLACK BEAN LOAF

Preparation Time: 50 minutes

Servings: 6

Ingredients:

- ✓ 3 tbsp olive oil
- ✓ 1 onion, minced
- ✓ 1 cup faro
- ✓ 2 (15.5-oz) cans black beans, mashed
- ✓ ½ cup quick-cooking oats
- ✓ 1/3 cup whole-wheat flour
- ✓ 2 tbsp nutritional yeast
- ✓ 1 ½ tsp dried thyme
- ✓ ½ tsp dried oregano

Directions:

- ❖ Heat the oil in a pot over medium heat. Place in onion and sauté for 3 minutes. Add in faro, 2 cups of water, salt, and pepper. Bring to a boil, lower the heat and simmer for 20 minutes. Remove to a bowl.
- ❖ Preheat oven to 350 F.
- ❖ Add the mashed beans, oats, flour, yeast, thyme, and oregano to the faro bowl. Toss to combine. Taste and adjust the seasoning. Shape the mixture into a greased loaf. Bake for 20 minutes. Let cool for a few minutes. Slice and serve

199)   CUBAN-STYLE MILLET

Preparation Time: 40 minutes

Servings: 4

Ingredients:

- ✓ 2 tbsp olive oil
- ✓ 1 onion, chopped
- ✓ 2 zucchinis, chopped
- ✓ 2 garlic cloves, minced
- ✓ 1 tsp dried thyme
- ✓ ½ tsp ground cumin
- ✓ 1 (15.5-oz) can black-eyed peas
- ✓ 1 cup millet
- ✓ 2 tbsp chopped fresh cilantro

Directions:

- ❖ Heat the oil in a pot over medium heat. Place in onion and sauté for 3 minutes until translucent. Add in zucchinis, garlic, thyme, and cumin and cook for 10 minutes. Put in peas, millet, and 2 ½ cups of hot water. Bring to a boil, then lower the heat and simmer for 20 minutes. Fluff the millet using a fork. Serve garnished with cilantro

200)   TRADITIONAL CILANTRO PILAF

Preparation Time: 30 minutes

Servings: 6

Ingredients:

- ✓ 3 tbsp olive oil
- ✓ 1 onion, minced
- ✓ 1 carrot, chopped
- ✓ 2 garlic cloves, minced
- ✓ 1 cup wild rice
- ✓ 1 ½ tsp ground fennel seeds
- ✓ ½ tsp ground cumin
- ✓ Salt and black pepper to taste
- ✓ 3 tbsp minced fresh cilantro

Directions:

- ❖ Heat the oil in a pot over medium heat. Place in onion, carrot, and garlic and sauté for 5 minutes. Stir in rice, fennel seeds, cumin, and 2 cups water. Bring to a boil, then lower the heat and simmer for 20 minutes. Remove to a bowl and fluff using a fork. Serve topped with cilantro and black pepper

201)   ORIENTAL BULGUR ANDWHITE BEANS

Preparation Time: 55 minutes

Servings: 4

Ingredients:

- ✓ 2 tbsp olive oil
- ✓ 3 green onions, chopped
- ✓ 1 cup bulgur
- ✓ 1 cups water
- ✓ 1 tbsp soy sauce
- ✓ Salt to taste
- ✓ 1 ½ cups cooked white beans
- ✓ 1 tbsp nutritional yeast
- ✓ 1 tbsp dried parsley

Directions:

- ❖ Heat the oil in a pot over medium heat. Place in green onions and sauté for 3 minutes. Stir in bulgur, water, soy sauce, and salt. Bring to a boil, then lower the heat and simmer for 20-22 minutes. Mix in beans and yeast. Cook for 5 minutes. Serve topped with parsley

202) RED LENTILS WITH MUSHROOMS

Preparation Time: 25 minutes

Servings: 4

Ingredients:

- ✓ 2 tsp olive oil
- ✓ 2 cloves garlic, minced
- ✓ 2 tsp grated fresh ginger
- ✓ ½ tsp ground cumin
- ✓ ½ tsp fennel seeds
- ✓ 1 cup mushrooms, chopped
- ✓ 1 large tomato, chopped
- ✓ 1 cup dried red lentils
- ✓ 2 tbsp lemon juice

Directions:

- ❖ Heat the oil in a pot over medium heat. Place in the garlic and ginger and cook for 3 minutes. Stir in cumin, fennel, mushrooms, tomato, lentils, and 2 ¼ cups of water. Bring to a boil, then lower the heat and simmer for 15 minutes. Mix in lemon juice and serve

203) COLORFUL RISOTTO WITH VEGETABLES

Preparation Time: 35 minutes

Servings: 5

Ingredients:

- ✓ 2 tbsp sesame oil
- ✓ 1 onion, chopped
- ✓ 2 bell peppers, chopped
- ✓ 1 parsnip, trimmed and chopped
- ✓ 1 carrot, trimmed and chopped
- ✓ 1 cup broccoli florets
- ✓ 2 garlic cloves, finely chopped
- ✓ 1/2 tsp ground cumin
- ✓ 2 cups brown rice
- ✓ Sea salt and black pepper, to taste
- ✓ 1/2 tsp ground turmeric
- ✓ 2 tbsp fresh cilantro, finely chopped

Directions:

- ❖ Heat the sesame oil in a saucepan over medium-high heat.
- ❖ Once hot, cook the onion, peppers, parsnip, carrot and broccoli for about 3 minutes until aromatic.
- ❖ Add in the garlic and ground cumin; continue to cook for 30 seconds more until aromatic.
- ❖ Place the brown rice in a saucepan and cover with cold water by 2 inches. Bring to a boil. Turn the heat to a simmer and continue to cook for about 30 minutes or until tender.
- ❖ Stir the rice into the vegetable mixture; season with salt, black pepper and ground turmeric; garnish with fresh cilantro and serve immediately. Enjoy

204) AMARANT GRITS WITH WALNUTS

Preparation Time: 35 minutes

Servings: 4

Ingredients:

- ✓ 2 cups water
- ✓ 2 cups coconut milk
- ✓ 1 cup amaranth
- ✓ 1 cinnamon stick
- ✓ 1 vanilla bean
- ✓ 4 tbsp maple syrup
- ✓ 4 tbsp walnuts, chopped

Directions:

- ❖ Bring the water and coconut milk to a boil over medium-high heat; add in the amaranth, cinnamon and vanilla and turn the heat to a simmer.
- ❖ Let it cook for about 30 minutes, stirring periodically to prevent the amaranth from sticking to the bottom of the pan.
- ❖ Top with maple syrup and walnuts. Enjoy

205) BARLEY PILAF WITH WILD MUSHROOMS

Preparation Time: 45 minutes

Servings: 4

Ingredients:

- ✓ 2 tbsp vegan butter
- ✓ 1 small onion, chopped
- ✓ 1 tsp garlic, minced
- ✓ 1 jalapeno pepper, seeded and minced
- ✓ 1 pound wild mushrooms, sliced
- ✓ 1 cup medium pearl barley, rinsed
- ✓ 2 ¾ cups vegetable broth

Directions:

- ❖ Melt the vegan butter in a saucepan over medium-high heat.
- ❖ Once hot, cook the onion for about 3 minutes until just tender.
- ❖ Add in the garlic, jalapeno pepper, mushrooms; continue to sauté for 2 minutes or until aromatic.
- ❖ Add in the barley and broth, cover and continue to simmer for about 30

minutes. Once all the liquid has absorbed, allow the barley to rest for about 10 minutes fluff with a fork.

❖ Taste and adjust the seasonings. Enjoy

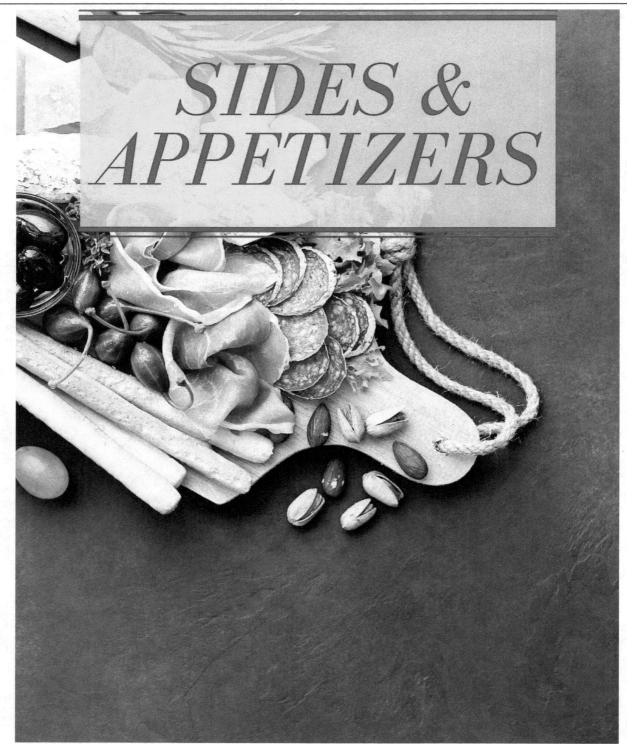

SIDES & APPETIZERS

206)   Artichokes Braised in Lemon and Olive Oil

Preparation Time: 35 minutes

Servings: 4

Ingredients:

- ✓ 1 ½ cups water
- ✓ 2 lemons, freshly squeezed
- ✓ 2 pounds artichokes, trimmed, tough outer leaves and chokes removed
- ✓ 1 handful fresh Italian parsley
- ✓ 2 thyme sprigs
- ✓ 2 rosemary sprigs
- ✓ 2 bay leaves
- ✓ 2 garlic cloves, chopped
- ✓ 1/3 cup olive oil
- ✓ Sea salt and ground black pepper, to taste
- ✓ 1/2 tsp red pepper flakes

Directions:

- ❖ Fill a bowl with water and add in the lemon juice. Place the cleaned artichokes in the bowl, keeping them completely submerged.
- ❖ In another small bowl, thoroughly combine the herbs and garlic. Rub your artichokes with the herb mixture.
- ❖ Pour the lemon water and olive oil in a saucepan; add the artichokes to the saucepan. Turn the heat to a simmer and continue to cook, covered, for about 30 minutes until the artichokes are crisp-tender.
- ❖ To serve, drizzle the artichokes with cooking juices, season them with the salt, black pepper and red pepper flakes. Enjoy

207)   ROSEMARY AND GARLIC ROASTED CARROTS

Preparation Time: 25 minutes

Servings: 4

Ingredients:

- ✓ 2 pounds carrots, trimmed and halved lengthwise
- ✓ 4 tbsp olive oil
- ✓ 2 tbsp champagne vinegar
- ✓ 4 cloves garlic, minced
- ✓ 2 sprigs rosemary, chopped
- ✓ Sea salt and ground black pepper, to taste
- ✓ 4 tbsp pine nuts, chopped

Directions:

- ❖ Begin by preheating your oven to 400 degrees F.
- ❖ Toss the carrots with the olive oil, vinegar, garlic, rosemary, salt and black pepper. Arrange them in a single layer on a parchment-lined roasting sheet.
- ❖ Roast the carrots in the preheated oven for about 20 minutes, until fork-tender.
- ❖ Garnish the carrots with the pine nuts and serve immediately. Enjoy

208)   MEDITERRANEAN-STYLE GREEN BEANS

Preparation Time: 20 minutes

Servings: 4

Ingredients:

- ✓ 2 tbsp olive oil
- ✓ 1 red bell pepper, seeded and diced
- ✓ 1 ½ pounds green beans
- ✓ 4 garlic cloves, minced
- ✓ 1/2 tsp mustard seeds
- ✓ 1/2 tsp fennel seeds
- ✓ 1 tsp dried dill weed
- ✓ 2 tomatoes, pureed
- ✓ 1 cup cream of celery soup
- ✓ 1 tsp Italian herb mix
- ✓ 1 tsp cayenne pepper
- ✓ Salt and freshly ground black pepper

Directions:

- ❖ Heat the olive oil in a saucepan over medium flame. Once hot, fry the peppers and green beans for about 5 minutes, stirring periodically to promote even cooking.
- ❖ Add in the garlic, mustard seeds, fennel seeds and dill and continue sautéing an additional 1 minute or until fragrant.
- ❖ Add in the pureed tomatoes, cream of celery soup, Italian herb mix, cayenne pepper, salt and black pepper. Continue to simmer, covered, for about 9 minutes or until the green beans are tender.
- ❖ Taste, adjust the seasonings and serve warm. Enjoy

209)   ROASTED GARDEN VEGETABLES

Preparation Time: 45 minutes

Servings: 4

Ingredients:

- 1 pound butternut squash, peeled and cut into 1-inch pieces
- 4 sweet potatoes, peeled and cut into 1-inch pieces
- 1/2 cup carrots, peeled and cut into 1-inch pieces
- 2 medium onions, cut into wedges
- 4 tbsp olive oil
- 1 tsp granulated garlic
- 1 tsp paprika
- 1 tsp dried rosemary
- 1 tsp mustard seeds
- Kosher salt and freshly ground black pepper, to taste

Directions:

- Start by preheating your oven to 420 degrees F.
- Toss the vegetables with the olive oil and spices. Arrange them on a parchment-lined roasting pan.
- Roast for about 25 minutes. Stir the vegetables and continue to cook for 20 minutes more.
- Enjoy

210) ROASTED KOHLRABI

Preparation Time: 30 minutes

Servings: 4

Ingredients:

- ✓ 1 pound kohlrabi bulbs, peeled and sliced
- ✓ 4 tbsp olive oil
- ✓ 1/2 tsp mustard seeds
- ✓ 1 tsp celery seeds
- ✓ 1 tsp dried marjoram
- ✓ 1 tsp granulated garlic, minced
- ✓ Sea salt and ground black pepper, to taste
- ✓ 2 tbsp nutritional yeast

Directions:

- ❖ Start by preheating your oven to 450 degrees F.
- ❖ Toss the kohlrabi with the olive oil and spices until well coated. Arrange the kohlrabi in a single layer on a parchment-lined roasting pan.
- ❖ Bake the kohlrabi in the preheated oven for about 15 minutes; stir them and continue to cook an additional 15 minutes.
- ❖ Sprinkle nutritional yeast over the warm kohlrabi and serve immediately. Enjoy

211) CAULIFLOWER WITH TAHINI SAUCE

Preparation Time: 10 minutes

Servings: 4

Ingredients:

- ✓ 1 cup water
- ✓ 2 pounds cauliflower florets
- ✓ Sea salt and ground black pepper, to taste
- ✓ 3 tbsp soy sauce
- ✓ 5 tbsp tahini
- ✓ 2 cloves garlic, minced
- ✓ 2 tbsp lemon juice

Directions:

- ❖ In a large saucepan, bring the water to a boil; then, add in the cauliflower and cook for about 6 minutes or until fork-tender; drain, season with salt and pepper and reserve.
- ❖ In a mixing bowl, thoroughly combine the soy sauce, tahini, garlic and lemon juice. Spoon the sauce over the cauliflower florets and serve.
- ❖ Enjoy

212) HERB CAULIFLOWER MASH

Preparation Time: 25 minutes

Servings: 4

Ingredients:

- ✓ 1 ½ pounds cauliflower florets
- ✓ 4 tbsp vegan butter
- ✓ 4 cloves garlic, sliced
- ✓ Sea salt and ground black pepper, to taste
- ✓ 1/4 cup plain oat milk, unsweetened
- ✓ 2 tbsp fresh parsley, roughly chopped

Directions:

- ❖ Steam the cauliflower florets for about 20 minutes; set it aside to cool.
- ❖ In a saucepan, melt the vegan butter over a moderately high heat; now, sauté the garlic for about 1 minute or until aromatic.
- ❖ Add the cauliflower florets to your food processor followed by the sautéed garlic, salt, black pepper and oat milk. Puree until everything is well incorporated.
- ❖ Garnish with fresh parsley leaves and serve hot. Enjoy

213) GARLIC AND HERB MUSHROOM SKILLET

Preparation Time: 10 minutes

Servings: 4

Ingredients:

- ✓ 4 tbsp vegan butter
- ✓ 1 ½ pounds oyster mushrooms halved
- ✓ 3 cloves garlic, minced
- ✓ 1 tsp dried oregano
- ✓ 1 tsp dried rosemary
- ✓ 1 tsp dried parsley flakes
- ✓ 1 tsp dried marjoram
- ✓ 1/2 cup dry white wine
- ✓ Kosher salt and ground black pepper, to taste

Directions:

- ❖ In a sauté pan, heat the olive oil over a moderately high heat.
- ❖ Now, sauté the mushrooms for 3 minutes or until they release the liquid. Add in the garlic and continue to cook for 30 seconds more or until aromatic.
- ❖ Stir in the spices and continue sautéing an additional 6 minutes, until your mushrooms are lightly browned.
- ❖ Enjoy

214) PAN-FRIED ASPARAGUS

Preparation Time: 10 minutes

Servings: 4

Ingredients:

- ✓ 4 tbsp vegan butter
- ✓ 1 ½ pounds asparagus spears, trimmed
- ✓ 1/2 tsp cumin seeds, ground
- ✓ 1/4 tsp bay leaf, ground
- ✓ Sea salt and ground black pepper, to taste
- ✓ 1 tsp fresh lime juice

Directions:

- ❖ Melt the vegan butter in a saucepan over medium-high heat.
- ❖ Sauté the asparagus for about 3 to 4 minutes, stirring periodically to promote even cooking.
- ❖ Add in the cumin seeds, bay leaf, salt and black pepper and continue to cook the asparagus for 2 minutes more until crisp-tender.
- ❖ Drizzle lime juice over the asparagus and serve warm. Enjoy

215) GINGERY CARROT MASH

Preparation Time: 25 minutes

Servings: 4

Ingredients:

- ✓ 2 pounds carrots, cut into rounds
- ✓ 2 tbsp olive oil
- ✓ 1 tsp ground cumin
- ✓ Salt ground black pepper, to taste
- ✓ 1/2 tsp cayenne pepper
- ✓ 1/2 tsp ginger, peeled and minced
- ✓ 1/2 cup whole milk

Directions:

- ❖ Begin by preheating your oven to 400 degrees F.
- ❖ Toss the carrots with the olive oil, cumin, salt, black pepper and cayenne pepper. Arrange them in a single layer on a parchment-lined roasting sheet.
- ❖ Roast the carrots in the preheated oven for about 20 minutes, until crisp-tender.
- ❖ Add the roasted carrots, ginger and milk to your food processor; puree the ingredients until everything is well blended.
- ❖ Enjoy

216) MEDITERRANEAN-STYLE ROASTED ARTICHOKES

Preparation Time: 50 minutes

Servings: 4

Ingredients:

- ✓ 4 artichokes, trimmed, tough outer leaves and chokes removed, halved
- ✓ 2 lemons, freshly squeezed
- ✓ 4 tbsp extra-virgin olive oil
- ✓ 4 cloves garlic, chopped
- ✓ 1 tsp fresh rosemary
- ✓ 1 tsp fresh basil
- ✓ 1 tsp fresh parsley
- ✓ 1 tsp fresh oregano
- ✓ Flaky sea salt and ground black pepper, to taste
- ✓ 1 tsp red pepper flakes
- ✓ 1 tsp paprika

Directions:

- ❖ Start by preheating your oven to 395 degrees F. Rub the lemon juice all over the entire surface of your artichokes.
- ❖ In a small mixing bowl, thoroughly combine the garlic with herbs and spices
- ❖ Place the artichoke halves in a parchment-lined baking dish, cut-side-up. Brush the artichokes evenly with the olive oil. Fill the cavities with the garlic/herb mixture.
- ❖ Bake for about 20 minutes. Now, cover them with aluminum foil and bake for a further 30 minutes. Serve warm and enjoy

217) THAI-STYLE BRAISED KALE

Preparation Time: 10 minutes

Servings: 4

Ingredients:

- ✓ 1 cup water
- ✓ 1 ½ pounds kale, tough stems and ribs removed, torn into pieces
- ✓ 2 tbsp sesame oil
- ✓ 1 tsp fresh garlic, pressed
- ✓ 1 tsp ginger, peeled and minced
- ✓ 1 Thai chili, chopped
- ✓ 1/2 tsp turmeric powder
- ✓ 1/2 cup coconut milk
- ✓ Kosher salt and ground black pepper, to taste

Directions:

- ❖ In a large saucepan, bring the water to a rapid boil. Add in the kale and let it cook until bright, about 3 minutes. Drain, rinse and squeeze dry.
- ❖ Wipe the saucepan with paper towels and preheat the sesame oil over a moderate heat. Once hot, cook the garlic, ginger and chili for approximately 1 minute or so, until fragrant.
- ❖ Add in the kale and turmeric powder and continue to cook for a further 1 minute or until heated through.
- ❖ Gradually pour in the coconut milk, salt and black pepper; continue to simmer until the liquid has thickened. Taste, adjust the seasonings and serve hot. Enjoy

The Guide on the Combination of the Mediterranean Diet and the Keto Diet to boost your weight loss and Get Fit and Healthy! Cookbook for Beginners: Master Guidance, and More than 150 Recipes to Get You Started! 4-week Meal Plan Included

By

Alexander Sandler & Elizabeth Roberts

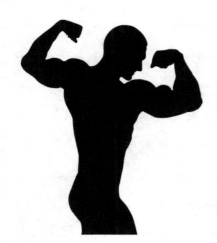
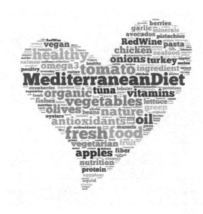

TABLE OF CONTENT

PART III: INTRODUCTION

Today, many people, especially teenagers, fill their plates with pizza, white bread, refined sugar, and processed food with lots of preservatives.

But analysis and research on processed foods such as frozen food, white bread, and carbonated beverages have led to surprising facts. Habitual consumption of these foods can tax the body. Excessive consumption can lead to high insulin production. This can cause diabetes, obesity, and coronary artery malfunction.

The reality of animal fats is not much different. Saturated fats in these foods can hurt our bodies. It causes the accumulation of extra fat in our body and disturbs our body mass index. Saturated fat in animal products like milk and butter increases lousy cholesterol or LDL. In short, it can damage the health of the coronary arteries.

In this technologically advanced society, when we can accomplish our tasks with little effort, physical activities are negligible. Poor health conveniently comes into play. It becomes essential to switch to a healthier diet that meets our body's nutritional needs while keeping us full.

The Mediterranean diet can do this. It is an eating pattern that overflows with whole grains, a plant-based diet in which olive oil is a fat source. This diet has no room for processed foods loaded with sugar or artificial sweeteners. The low amount of fat keeps your heart healthy and provides both essential nutrients and agility. Give it a try, and you won't look back. You will leap into a healthy future.

I wish you all the best in healthy eating.

Scientists have proven that the Mediterranean diet is one of the most effective diets for a healthy body. And more and more people are taking an interest in cooking Mediterranean foods in their homes. But if you are looking for a Mediterranean diet, you will be loaded with tons of recipes that make it almost impossible to find one but don't worry; we are here to make your discoveries more comfortable. We've assembled all the best and most effective Mediterranean recipes for your diet. So, let's start with this one.

START TO GET FAMILIAR WITH THE MEDITERRANEAN DIET

When you read the word "Mediterranean," you tend to think of the sea. This brings to mind seafood. The diet has its roots in the Mediterranean basin, a land that has historically been called a powerhouse of societal evolution. This area of the Nile Valley was good land for the peoples of the East and West. The frequent interaction of people from different regions and cultures had a significant effect on customs, languages, religion, and outlook and positively impacted lifestyles. This integration and cultural clash further influenced eating habits.

Looking at the Mediterranean diet's food content, one can see the reflection of different cultures and classes. Bread, wine, and oil reflect agriculture; lettuce, mushrooms, and mallow further complement this. There is a slight preference for meat but much preference for fish and seafood. This shows the greedy nature of the people of Rome. Here we also have the Germanic flavor of pork with garden vegetables. Beer was made from grains.

The food culture of bread, wine, and oil went beyond the Germanic and Christian Roman culture and entered the borders of the Arabs. The reason was their existence on the southern shore of the Mediterranean. Their food culture was unique because of the variety of leafy vegetables they grew. They had eggplant, spinach, sugarcane, and fruits such as oranges, citrus, lemon, and pomegranate. This influenced the cooking style of the Latinos and influenced their recipes.

The great geographical event that is the discovery of America by Europeans has a great additional impact on the Mediterranean diet. This event added several new foods such as beans, potatoes, tomatoes, chili peppers, and peppers. The tomato, the red plant, was first ornamental and then considered edible. It then became an essential part of the Mediterranean diet.

Historical analysis of the Mediterranean diet shows how the Egyptians' diet at the discovery of America gave us the Mediterranean diet of today. The Mediterranean diet's nutritional model is intimately linked to the Mediterranean people, lifestyle, and history.

Some established health and cultural platforms, such as UNESCO, define the Mediterranean diet, explaining the meaning of the word "diet," which comes from the word "data," meaning lifestyle or way of life. It focuses on food from landscape to table, covering cooking, harvesting, processing, preparation, fishing, cooking, and a specific form of consumption.

There is a variation in the Mediterranean diet in different countries due to ethnic and cultural differences, other religions, and economic disparity. According to the description and recommendation of dieticians and food experts, the Mediterranean diet has the proportion of the following food. In grains, there are whole grains and legumes. For fats, olive oil is the primary source. Onion, garlic, tomatoes, leafy greens, and peppers are the main vegetables. Fresh fruit is the main one in snacks and desserts. Eggs, milk, yogurt, and other dairy products are taken moderately. Foods such as red meat, processed foods, and refined sugar are handled as little as possible.

This diet has a fat ratio of 25% to 35% in calories, and saturated fat never exceeds 8%. As for oil, alternatives are depending on the region. In central and northern Italy, butter and lard are commonly used in cooking. Olive is used primarily for snacks and salad dressing.

This diet reflects Crete's dietary pattern, the rest of Greece, and much of Italy in the early 1960s. It gained widespread recognition in the 1990s. There is an irony to the Mediterranean diet. Although people who live in this region tend to consume a high amount of fat, they enjoy much better cardiovascular health than people in America who consume an equal amount of fat.

The Mediterranean diet tradition offers a cuisine rich in color, taste, flavor, and aroma. Above all, it keeps us closer to nature. It may be simple in appearance, but rich in health and has much to offer that is in no way inferior to any other healthy diet. Some Americans describe the Mediterranean diet as homemade pasta with parmesan sauce and enriched with a few pieces of meat. It includes lots of fresh vegetables with just olive oil drizzled on top. Desserts in this diet include fresh fruit.

An excellent Mediterranean diet does not include soy, canola, or any other refined oil. There is no room for processed meat, refined sugar, white bread, refined grains, white pasta, or pizza dough containing white flour.

This diet features a balanced use of foods with high amounts of fiber, unsaturated fat s, and antioxidants. Besides, there is an approach that prioritizes health by cutting unhealthy animal fats and meat consumption. This way, a balance is achieved between the amount of energy intake and its consumption.

This magical diet is not only a preferred approach to health, with a wide range of magical recipes but also a channel between the most diverse cultures. The inhabitants of this region are children of the earth, and so is their food from the land and soil. It can ensure if consumed rationally, the effectiveness of various bodily functions.

Some well-known health organizations worldwide have designed food pyramids to clarify the most common forms of the Mediterranean region. It has become popular among health activists because people from this region have high life expectancy despite less access to healthcare facilities. It has been stated by the American Heart Association and the American Diabetes Association that the Mediterranean diet lowers the risk of cardiovascular disease and type 2 diabetes. If a Mediterranean diet plan is followed, it can have a lasting effect on health and help reduce and maintain a healthy weight.

THE BENEFITS OF THE MEDITERRANEAN DIET

The Mediterranean diet has gained popularity in medical fields because of its documented benefits for heart health. But, much research has shown that the Mediterranean diet may have a much longer list of health benefits that go beyond the heart. This will review just a few of the many improvements you can experience with your health when you start following the Mediterranean diet.

REDUCES AGE-RELATED MUSCLE AND BONE WEAKNESS

Eating a well-balanced diet that provides a wide range of vitamins and minerals is essential for reducing muscle weakness and bone degradation. This is especially important as you age. Accident-related injuries, such as tripping, falling, or slipping while walking, can cause serious injuries. As you age, this becomes even more concerning because some simple falls can be fatal. Many accidents occur because of weakening muscle mass and loss of bone density. Women, especially those entering the menopausal stage of their lives, are more at risk of severe injuries from accidental falls because estrogen levels decrease significantly during this time—this decrease in estrogen results in a loss of bone muscle mass. Reduced estrogen can also cause bone thinning, which over time develops into osteoporosis.

Maintaining healthy bone mass and muscle agility as you age can be a challenge. When you don't get the proper nutrients to promote healthy bones and muscles, you increase your risk of developing osteoporosis. The Mediterranean diet offers an easy way to meet the dietary needs necessary to improve bone and muscle function.

Antioxidants, vitamins C and K, carotenoids, magnesium, potassium, and phytoestrogens are essential minerals and nutrients for optimal musculoskeletal health. Plant-based foods, unsaturated fats, and whole grains help provide the necessary balance of nutrients that keep bones and muscles healthy. Following a Mediterranean diet can improve and reduce bone loss as you age.

The Mediterranean diet consists of many foods that increase the risk of Alzheimer's, such as processed meats, refined grains like white bread and pasta, and added sugar. Foods that contain dactyl, which is a chemical commonly used in the refining process, increase the buildup of beta-amyloid plaques in the brain. Microwave popcorn, margarine, and butter are some of the most frequently consumed foods that contain this harmful chemical. It's no wonder that Alzheimer's is becoming one of the leading causes of death among Americans.

On the other hand, the Mediterranean diet includes a wide range of foods that have been shown to boost memory and slow cognitive decline. Dark leafy vegetables, fresh berries, extra virgin olive oil, and fresh fish contain vitamins and minerals that can improve brain health. The Mediterranean diet can help you make necessary diet and lifestyle changes that can significantly decrease your risk of Alzheimer's.

The Mediterranean diet encourages improvement in both diet and physical activity. Thanks to these two components are the most important factors that will help you manage the symptoms of diabetes and reduce your risk of developing the condition.

HEART HEALTH AND STROKE RISK REDUCTION

Heart health is strongly influenced by diet. Maintaining healthy cholesterol levels, blood pressure, blood sugar, and staying within a beneficial weight results in optimal heart health. Your diet directly affects each of these components. Those at increased risk are often advised to start on a low-fat diet. A low-fat diet eliminates all fats, including those from oils, nuts, and red meat. Studies have shown that the Mediterranean diet, which includes healthy fats, is more effective at lowering cardiovascular risks than a standard low-fat diet: (that's processed red meat, 2019). This is because the unsaturated fats consumed in the Mediterranean diet lower bad cholesterol levels and increase good cholesterol levels.

The Mediterranean diet emphasizes the importance of daily activity and stress reduction by enjoying quality time with friends and family. Each of these elements, along with eating more plant-based foods, significantly improves heart health and reduces the risk of many heart-related conditions. By increasing your intake of fresh fruits and vegetables and adding regular daily activities, you improve not only your heart health but your overall health.

ADDITIONAL BENEFITS

Aside from the significant benefits to your heart and brain, the Mediterranean diet can significantly improve many other key factors in your life. Since the Mediterranean diet focuses on eating healthy, exercising, and connecting with others, you can see improvements to your mental health, physical health and often feel like you're living a more fulfilling life.

PROTECTS AGAINST CANCER

Many plant-based foods, especially those in the yellow and orange color groups, contain cancer-fighting agents. Increasing the antioxidants consumed by eating fresh fruits and vegetables, and whole grains can protect the body's cells from developing cancer cells. Drinking a glass of red wine also provides cancer-protective compounds.

ENERGY

Following a Mediterranean diet focuses on fueling your body. Other diets focus only on filling your body, and this is often done through empty calories. When your body gets the nutrients it needs, it can function properly, which results in feeling more energized throughout the day. You won't need to rely on sugary drinks, excess caffeine, or sugar-filled energy bars to get you going and keep you moving. You'll feel less weighed down after eating, and that translates into a greater capacity for output.

GET BETTER SLEEP

Sugar and caffeine can cause significant sleep disturbances. Besides, other foods, such as processed foods, can make it harder to get the right amount of sleep. When you eat the right foods, you can see a change in your sleep patterns. Your body will want to rest to recover and properly absorb the vitamins and minerals consumed during the day. Your brain will switch into sleep mode with ease because it has received the vitamins it needs to function correctly. When you get the right amount of sleep, you will, in turn, have more energy the next day, and this can also significantly improve your mood. The Mediterranean diet increases nutrient-dense food consumption and avoids excess sugar and processed foods known to cause sleep problems.

Besides, the Mediterranean diet allows you to maintain a healthy weight, reducing the risk of developing sleep disorders such as sleep apnea. Sleep apnea is common in individuals who are overweight and obese. It causes the airway to become blocked, making it difficult to breathe. This results in not getting enough oxygen when you sleep, which can cause sudden and frequent awakenings during the night.

LONGEVITY

The Mediterranean diet, indeed, helps reduce the risk of many health problems. Its heart, brain, and mood health benefits translate into a longer, more enjoyable life. When you eliminate the risk of developing certain conditions such as cardiovascular disease, diabetes, and dementia, you increase your lifespan. But eliminating these health risks is not the only cause of increased longevity with the Mediterranean diet. Increased physical activity and deep social connection also play a significant role in living a longer life.

CLEAR SKIN

Healthy skin starts on the inside. When you provide your body with healthy foods, it radiates through your skin. The antioxidants in extra virgin olive oil alone are enough to keep your skin young and healthy. But the Mediterranean diet includes many fresh fruits and vegetables that are full of antioxidants. These antioxidants help repair damaged cells in the body and promote the growth of healthy cells. Eating a variety of healthy fats also keeps your skin supple and can protect it from premature aging.

MAINTAINING A HEALTHY WEIGHT

With the Mediterranean diet, you eat mostly whole, fresh foods. Eating more foods rich in vitamins, minerals, and nutrients is essential to maintaining a healthy weight. The diet is easy to stick to, and there are no calorie restrictions to follow strictly. This makes it a highly sustainable plan for those who want to lose weight or maintain a healthy weight. Keep in mind; this is not an option to lose weight fast. This is a lifestyle that will allow you to maintain optimal health for years, not just a few months.

BREAKFAST

218) CAULIFLOWER FRITTERS AND HUMMUS

Cooking Time: 15 Minutes   **Servings:** 4

Ingredients:

- ✓ 2 (15 oz) cans chickpeas, divided
- ✓ 2 1/2 tbsp olive oil, divided, plus more for frying
- ✓ 1 cup onion, chopped, about 1/2 a small onion
- ✓ 2 tbsp garlic, minced
- ✓ 2 cups cauliflower, cut into small pieces, about 1/2 a large head
- ✓ 1/2 tsp salt
- ✓ black pepper
- ✓ Topping:
- ✓ Hummus, of choice
- ✓ Green onion, diced

Directions:

- ❖ Preheat oven to 400°F
- ❖ Rinse and drain 1 can of the chickpeas, place them on a paper towel to dry off well
- ❖ Then place the chickpeas into a large bowl, removing the loose skins that come off, and toss with 1 tbsp of olive oil, spread the chickpeas onto a large pan (being careful not to over-crowd them) and sprinkle with salt and pepper
- ❖ Bake for 20 minutes, then stir, and then bake an additional 5-10 minutes until very crispy
- ❖ Once the chickpeas are roasted, transfer them to a large food processor and process until broken down and crumble - Don't over process them and turn it into flour, as you need to have some texture. Place the mixture into a small bowl, set aside
- ❖ In a large pan over medium-high heat, add the remaining 1 1/2 tbsp of olive oil
- ❖ Once heated, add in the onion and garlic, cook until lightly golden brown, about 2 minutes. Then add in the chopped cauliflower, cook for an additional 2 minutes, until the cauliflower is golden
- ❖ Turn the heat down to low and cover the pan, cook until the cauliflower is fork tender and the onions are golden brown and caramelized, stirring often, about 3-5 minutes
- ❖ Transfer the cauliflower mixture to the food processor, drain and rinse the remaining can of chickpeas and add them into the food processor, along with the salt and a pinch of pepper. Blend until smooth, and the mixture starts to ball, stop to scrape down the sides as needed
- ❖ Transfer the cauliflower mixture into a large bowl and add in 1/2 cup of the roasted chickpea crumbs (you won't use all of the crumbs, but it is easier to break them down when you have a larger amount.), stir until well combined
- ❖ In a large bowl over medium heat, add in enough oil to lightly cover the bottom of a large pan
- ❖ Working in batches, cook the patties until golden brown, about 2-3 minutes, flip and cook again
- ❖ Distribute among the container, placing parchment paper in between the fritters. Store in the fridge for 2-3 days
- ❖ To Serve: Heat through in the oven at 350F for 5-8 minutes. Top with hummus, green onion and enjoy!
- ❖ Recipe Notes: Don't add too much oil while frying the fritter or they will end up soggy. Use only enough to cover the pan. Use a fork while frying and resist the urge to flip them every minute to see if they are golden

Nutrition: Calories:333;Total Carbohydrates: 45g;Total Fat: 13g;Protein: 14g

219) ITALIAN BREAKFAST SAUSAGE AND BABY POTATOES WITH VEGETABLES

Cooking Time: 30 Minutes   **Servings: 4**

Ingredients:

- ✓ 1 lbs sweet Italian sausage links, sliced on the bias (diagonal)
- ✓ 2 cups baby potatoes, halved
- ✓ 2 cups broccoli florets
- ✓ 1 cup onions cut to 1-inch chunks
- ✓ 2 cups small mushrooms -half or quarter the large ones for uniform size
- ✓ 1 cup baby carrots
- ✓ 2 tbsp olive oil
- ✓ 1/2 tsp garlic powder
- ✓ 1/2 tsp Italian seasoning
- ✓ 1 tsp salt
- ✓ 1/2 tsp pepper

Directions:

- ❖ Preheat the oven to 400 degrees F
- ❖ In a large bowl, add the baby potatoes, broccoli florets, onions, small mushrooms, and baby carrots
- ❖ Add in the olive oil, salt, pepper, garlic powder and Italian seasoning and toss to evenly coat
- ❖ Spread the vegetables onto a sheet pan in one even layer
- ❖ Arrange the sausage slices on the pan over the vegetables
- ❖ Bake for 30 minutes – make sure to sake halfway through to prevent sticking
- ❖ Allow to cool
- ❖ Distribute the Italian sausages and vegetables among the containers and store in the fridge for 2-3 days
- ❖ To Serve: Reheat in the microwave for 1-2 minutes, or until heated through and enjoy!
- ❖ Recipe Notes: If you would like crispier potatoes, place them on the pan and bake for 15 minutes before adding the other ingredients to the pan.

Nutrition: Calories:321;Total Fat: 16g;Total Carbs: 23g;Fiber: 4g;Protein: 22g

220) BREAKFAST GREEK QUINOA BOWL

Cooking Time: 20 Minutes   **Servings: 6**

Ingredients:

- ✓ 12 eggs
- ✓ ¼ cup plain Greek yogurt
- ✓ 1 tsp onion powder
- ✓ 1 tsp granulated garlic
- ✓ ½ tsp salt
- ✓ ½ tsp pepper
- ✓ 1 tsp olive oil
- ✓ 1 (5 oz) bag baby spinach
- ✓ 1 pint cherry tomatoes, halved
- ✓ 1 cup feta cheese
- ✓ 2 cups cooked quinoa

Directions:

- ❖ In a large bowl whisk together eggs, Greek yogurt, onion powder, granulated garlic, salt, and pepper, set aside
- ❖ In a large skillet, heat olive oil and add spinach, cook the spinach until it is slightly wilted, about 3-4 minutes
- ❖ Add in cherry tomatoes, cook until tomatoes are softened, 4 minutes
- ❖ Stir in egg mixture and cook until the eggs are set, about 7-9 minutes, stir in the eggs as they cook to scramble
- ❖ Once the eggs have set stir in the feta and quinoa, cook until heated through
- ❖ Distribute evenly among the containers, store for 2-3 days
- ❖ To serve: Reheat in the microwave for 30 seconds to 1 minute or heated through

Nutrition: Calories:357;Total Carbohydrates: ;Total Fat: 20g;Protein: 23g

221)   EGG, HAM WITH CHEESE FREEZER SANDWICHES

Cooking Time: 20 Minutes   **Servings: 6**

Ingredients:

- ✓ Cooking spray or oil to grease the baking dish
- ✓ 7 large eggs
- ✓ ½ cup low-fat (2%) milk
- ✓ ½ tsp garlic powder
- ✓ ½ tsp onion powder
- ✓ 1 tbsp Dijon mustard
- ✓ ½ tsp honey
- ✓ 6 whole-wheat English muffins
- ✓ 6 slices thinly sliced prosciutto
- ✓ 6 slices Swiss cheese

Directions:

- ❖ Preheat the oven to 375°F. Lightly oil or spray an 8-by--inch glass or ceramic baking dish with cooking spray.
- ❖ In a large bowl, whisk together the eggs, milk, garlic powder, and onion powder. Pour the mixture into the baking dish and bake for minutes, until the eggs are set and no longer jiggling. Cool.
- ❖ While the eggs are baking, mix the mustard and honey in a small bowl. Lay out the English muffin halves to start assembly.
- ❖ When the eggs are cool, use a biscuit cutter or drinking glass about the same size as the English muffin diameter to cut 6 egg circles. Divide the leftover egg scraps evenly to be added to each sandwich.
- ❖ Spread ½ tsp of honey mustard on each of the bottom English muffin halves. Top each with 1 slice of prosciutto, 1 egg circle and scraps, 1 slice of cheese, and the top half of the muffin.
- ❖ Wrap each sandwich tightly in foil.
- ❖ STORAGE: Store tightly wrapped sandwiches in the freezer for up to 1 month. To reheat, remove the foil, place the sandwich on a microwave-safe plate, and wrap with a damp paper towel. Microwave on high for 1½ minutes, flip over, and heat again for another 1½ minutes. Because cooking time can vary greatly between microwaves, you may need to experiment with a few sandwiches before you find the perfect amount of time to heat the whole item through.

Nutrition: Total calories: 361; Total fat: 17g; Saturated fat: 7g; Sodium: 953mg; Carbohydrates: 26g; Fiber: 3g; Protein: 24g

222)   HEALTHY SALAD ZUCCHINI KALE TOMATO

Cooking Time: 20 Minutes   **Servings: 4**

Ingredients:

- ✓ 1 lb kale, chopped
- ✓ 2 tbsp fresh parsley, chopped
- ✓ 1 tbsp vinegar
- ✓ 1/2 cup can tomato, crushed
- ✓ 1 tsp paprika
- ✓ 1 cup zucchini, cut into cubes
- ✓ 1 cup grape tomatoes, halved
- ✓ 2 tbsp olive oil
- ✓ 1 onion, chopped
- ✓ 1 leek, sliced
- ✓ Pepper
- ✓ Salt

Directions:

- ❖ Add oil into the inner pot of instant pot and set the pot on sauté mode.
- ❖ Add leek and onion and sauté for 5 minutes.
- ❖ Add kale and remaining ingredients and stir well.
- ❖ Seal pot with lid and cook on high for 15 minutes.
- ❖ Once done, allow to release pressure naturally for 10 minutes then release remaining using quick release. Remove lid.
- ❖ Stir and serve.

Nutrition: Calories: 162;Fat: 3 g;Carbohydrates: 22.2 g;Sugar: 4.8 g;Protein: 5.2 g;Cholesterol: 0 mg

223) CHEESE WITH CAULIFLOWER FRITTATA AND PEPPERS

Cooking Time: 30 Minutes   **Servings: 6**

Ingredients:

- ✓ 10 eggs
- ✓ 1 seeded and chopped bell pepper
- ✓ ½ cup grated Parmigiano-Reggiano
- ✓ ½ cup milk, skim
- ✓ ½ tsp cayenne pepper
- ✓ 1 pound cauliflower, floret
- ✓ ½ tsp saffron
- ✓ 2 tbsp chopped chives
- ✓ Salt and black pepper as desired

Directions:

- ❖ Prepare your oven by setting the temperature to 370 degrees Fahrenheit. You should also grease a skillet suitable for the oven.
- ❖ In a medium-sized bowl, add the milk and eggs. Whisk them until they are frothy.
- ❖ Sprinkle the grated Parmigiano-Reggiano cheese into the frothy mixture and fold the ingredients together.
- ❖ Pour in the salt, saffron, cayenne pepper, and black pepper and gently stir.
- ❖ Add in the chopped bell pepper and gently stir until the ingredients are fully incorporated.
- ❖ Pour the egg mixture into the skillet and cook on medium heat over your stovetop for 4 minutes.
- ❖ Steam the cauliflower florets in a pan. To do this, add ½ inch of water and ½ tsp sea salt. Pour in the cauliflower and cover for 3 to 8 minutes. Drain any extra water.
- ❖ Add the cauliflower into the mixture and gently stir.
- ❖ Set the skillet into the preheated oven and turn your timer to 13 minutes. Once the mixture is golden brown in the middle, remove the frittata from the oven.
- ❖ Set your skillet aside for a couple of minutes so it can cool.
- ❖ Slice and garnish with chives before you serve.

Nutrition: calories: 207, fats: grams, carbohydrates: 8 grams, protein: 17 grams.

224) AVOCADO KALE OMELETTE

Cooking Time: 5 Minutes   **Servings: 1**

Ingredients:

- ✓ 2 eggs
- ✓ 1 tsp milk
- ✓ 2 tsp olive oil
- ✓ 1 cup kale (chopped)
- ✓ 1 tbsp lime juice
- ✓ 1 tbsp cilantro (chopped)
- ✓ 1 tsp sunflower seeds
- ✓ Pinch of red pepper (crushed)
- ✓ ¼ avocado (sliced)
- ✓ sea salt or plain salt
- ✓ freshly ground black pepper

Directions:

- ❖ Toss all the Ingredients: (except eggs and milk) to make the kale salad.
- ❖ Beat the eggs and milk in a bowl.
- ❖ Heat oil in a pan over medium heat. Then pour in the egg mixture and cook it until the bottom settles. Cook for 2 minutes and then flip it over and further cook for 20 seconds.
- ❖ Finally, put the Omelette in containers.
- ❖ Top the Omelette with the kale salad.
- ❖ Serve warm.

Nutrition: Calories: 399, Total Fat: 28.8g, Saturated Fat: 6.2, Cholesterol: 328 mg, Sodium: 162 mg, Total Carbohydrate: 25.2g, Dietary Fiber: 6.3 g, Total Sugars: 9 g, Protein: 15.8 g, Vitamin D: 31 mcg, Calcium: 166 mg, Iron: 4 mg, Potassium: 980 mg

225) BREAKFAST WITH MEDITERRANEAN-STYLE BURRITO

Cooking Time: 5 Minutes   **Servings:** 6

Ingredients:

- ✓ 9 eggs whole
- ✓ 6 tortillas whole 10 inch, regular or sun-dried tomato
- ✓ 3 tbsp sun-dried tomatoes, chopped
- ✓ 1/2 cup feta cheese I use light/low-fat feta
- ✓ 2 cups baby spinach washed and dried
- ✓ 3 tbsp black olives, sliced
- ✓ 3/4 cup refried beans, canned
- ✓ Garnish:
- ✓ Salsa

Directions:

- ❖ Spray a medium frying pan with non- stick spray, add the eggs and scramble and toss for about 5 minutes, or until eggs are no longer liquid
- ❖ Add in the spinach, black olives, sun-dried tomatoes and continue to stir and toss until no longer wet
- ❖ Add in the feta cheese and cover, cook until cheese is melted
- ❖ Add 2 tbsp of refried beans to each tortilla
- ❖ Top with egg mixture, dividing evenly between all burritos, and wrap
- ❖ Frying in a pan until lightly browned
- ❖ Allow to cool completely before slicing
- ❖ Wrap the slices in plastic wrap and then aluminum foil and place in the freezer for up to 2 months or fridge for 2 days
- ❖ To Serve: Remove the aluminum foil and plastic wrap, and microwave for 2 minutes, then allow to rest for 30 seconds, enjoy! Enjoy hot with salsa and fruit

Nutrition: Calories:252;Total Carbohydrates: 21g;Total Fat: 11g;Protein: 14g |

226) SHAKSHUKA AND FETA

Cooking Time: 40 Minutes   **Servings:** 4-6

Ingredients:

- ✓ 6 large eggs
- ✓ 3 tbsp extra-virgin olive oil
- ✓ 1 large onion, halved and thinly sliced
- ✓ 1 large red bell pepper, seeded and thinly sliced
- ✓ 3 garlic cloves, thinly sliced
- ✓ 1 tsp ground cumin
- ✓ 1 tsp sweet paprika
- ✓ ⅛ tsp cayenne, or to taste
- ✓ 1 (28-ounce) can whole plum tomatoes with juices, coarsely chopped
- ✓ ¾ tsp salt, more as needed
- ✓ ¼ tsp black pepper, more as needed
- ✓ 5 oz feta cheese, crumbled, about 1 1/4 cups
- ✓ To Serve:
- ✓ Chopped cilantro
- ✓ Hot sauce

Directions:

- ❖ Preheat oven to 375 degrees F
- ❖ In a large skillet over medium-low heat, add the oil
- ❖ Once heated, add the onion and bell pepper, cook gently until very soft, about 20 minutes
- ❖ Add in the garlic and cook until tender, 1 to 2 minutes, then stir in cumin, paprika and cayenne, and cook 1 minute
- ❖ Pour in tomatoes, season with 3/4 tsp salt and 1/4 tsp pepper, simmer until tomatoes have thickened, about 10 minutes
- ❖ Then stir in crumbled feta
- ❖ Gently crack eggs into skillet over tomatoes, season with salt and pepper
- ❖ Transfer skillet to oven
- ❖ Bake until eggs have just set, 7 to 10 minutes
- ❖ Allow to cool and distribute among the containers, store in the fridge for 2-3 days
- ❖ To Serve: Reheat in the oven at 360 degrees F for 5 minutes or until heated through

Nutrition: Calories:337;Carbs: 17g;Total Fat: 25g;Protein

227)   SPINACH, FETA WITH EGG BREAKFAST QUESADILLAS

Cooking Time: 15 Minutes   **Servings: 5**

Ingredients:

- ✓ 4 handfuls of spinach leaves
- ✓ 1 1/2 cup mozzarella cheese
- ✓ 5 sun-dried tomato tortillas
- ✓ 1/2 cup feta
- ✓ 1/4 tsp salt
- ✓ 1/4 tsp pepper
- ✓ Spray oil

- ✓ 8 eggs (optional)
- ✓ 2 tsp olive oil
- ✓ 1 red bell pepper
- ✓ 1/2 red onion
- ✓ 1/4 cup milk

Directions:

- ❖ In a large non-stick pan over medium heat, add the olive oil
- ❖ Once heated, add the bell pepper and onion, cook for 4-5 minutes until soft
- ❖ In the meantime, whisk together the eggs, milk, salt and pepper in a bowl
- ❖ Add in the egg/milk mixture into the pan with peppers and onions, stirring frequently, until eggs are almost cooked through
- ❖ Add in the spinach and feta, fold into the eggs, stirring until spinach is wilted and eggs are cooked through
- ❖ Remove the eggs from heat and plate
- ❖ Spray a separate large non-stick pan with spray oil, and place over medium heat
- ❖ Add the tortilla, on one half of the tortilla, spread about ½ cup of the egg mixture
- ❖ Top the eggs with around ⅓ cup of shredded mozzarella cheese
- ❖ Fold the second half of the tortilla over, then cook for 2 minutes, or until golden brown
- ❖ Flip and cook for another minute until golden brown
- ❖ Allow the quesadilla to cool completely, divide among the container, store for 2 days or wrap in plastic wrap and foil, and freeze for up to 2 months
- ❖ To Serve: Reheat in oven at 375 for 3-5 minutes or until heated through

Nutrition: (1/2 quesadilla): Calories:213;Total Fat: 11g;Total Carbs: 15g;Protein: 15g

228)   BREAKFAST COBBLER

Cooking Time: 12 Minutes   **Servings: 4**

Ingredients:

- ✓ 1/2 cup dry buckwheat
- ✓ 1/2 cup dates, chopped
- ✓ Pinch of ground ginger

- ✓ 2 lbs apples, cut into chunks
- ✓ 1 1/2 cups water
- ✓ 1/4 tsp nutmeg
- ✓ 1 1/2 tsp cinnamon

Directions:

- ❖ Spray instant pot from inside with cooking spray.
- ❖ Add all ingredients into the instant pot and stir well.
- ❖ Seal pot with a lid and select manual and set timer for 12 minutes.
- ❖ Once done, release pressure using quick release. Remove lid.
- ❖ Stir and serve.

Nutrition: Calories: 195;Fat: 0.9 g;Carbohydrates: 48.3 g;Sugar: 25.8 g;Protein: 3.3 g;Cholesterol: 0 mg

229)

230)   EGG-TOPPED QUINOA BOWL AND KALE

Cooking Time: 5 Minutes   **Servings: 2**

Ingredients:

- ✓ 1 cup cooked quinoa
- ✓ 1 tsp olive oil
- ✓ 2 eggs
- ✓ 1/3 cup avocado, sliced
- sea salt or plain salt
- fresh black pepper

- ✓ 1-ounce pancetta, chopped
- ✓ 1 bunch kale, sliced
- ✓ ½ cup cherry tomatoes, halved
- ✓ 1 tsp red wine vinegar

Directions:

- ❖ Start by heating pancetta in a skillet until golden brown. Add in kale and further cook for 2 minutes.
- ❖ Then, stir in tomatoes, vinegar, and salt and remove from heat.
- ❖ Now, divide this mixture into 2 bowls, add avocado to both, and then set aside.
- ❖ Finally, cook both the eggs and top each bowl with an egg.
- ❖ Serve hot with toppings of your choice.

Nutrition: Calories: 547, Total Fat: 22., Saturated Fat: 5.3, Cholesterol: 179 mg, Sodium: 412 mg, Total Carbohydrate: 62.5 g, Dietary Fiber: 8.6 g, Total Sugars:

1.7 g, Protein: 24.7 g, Vitamin D: 15 mcg, Calcium: 117 mg, Iron: 6 mg, Potassium: 1009 mg

231) STRAWBERRY GREEK COLD YOGURT

Cooking Time: 2-4 Hours   **Servings: 5**

Ingredients:

- ✓ 3 cups plain Greek low-fat yogurt
- ✓ 1 cup sugar
- ✓ ¼ cup lemon juice, freshly squeezed
- ✓ 2 tsp vanilla
- ✓ 1/8 tsp salt
- ✓ 1 cup strawberries, sliced

Directions:

- ❖ In a medium-sized bowl, add yogurt, lemon juice, sugar, vanilla, and salt.
- ❖ Whisk the whole mixture well.
- ❖ Freeze the yogurt mix in a 2-quart ice cream maker according to the given instructions.
- ❖ During the final minute, add the sliced strawberries.
- ❖ Transfer the yogurt to an airtight container.
- ❖ Place in the freezer for 2-4 hours.
- ❖ Remove from the freezer and allow it to stand for 5-15 minutes.
- ❖ Serve and enjoy!

Nutrition: Calories: 251, Total Fat: 0.5 g, Saturated Fat: 0.1 g, Cholesterol: 3 mg, Sodium: 130 mg, Total Carbohydrate: 48.7 g, Dietary Fiber: 0.6 g, Total Sugars: 47.3 g, Protein: 14.7 g, Vitamin D: 1 mcg, Calcium: 426 mg, Iron: 0 mg, Potassium: 62 mg

232) PEACH ALMOND OATMEAL

Cooking Time: 10 Minutes   **Servings: 2**

Ingredients:

- ✓ 1 cup unsweetened almond milk
- ✓ 2 cups of water
- ✓ 1 cup oats
- ✓ 2 peaches, diced
- ✓ Pinch of salt

Directions:

- ❖ Spray instant pot from inside with cooking spray.
- ❖ Add all ingredients into the instant pot and stir well.
- ❖ Seal pot with a lid and select manual and set timer for 10 minutes.
- ❖ Once done, allow to release pressure naturally for 10 minutes then release remaining using quick release. Remove lid.
- ❖ Stir and serve.

Nutrition: Calories: 234;Fat: 4.8 g;Carbohydrates: 42.7 g;Sugar: 9 g;Protein: 7.3 g;Cholesterol: 0 mg

233) BANANA PEANUT BUTTER PUDDING

Cooking Time: 25 Minutes   **Servings: 1**

Ingredients:

- ✓ 2 bananas, halved
- ✓ ¼ cup smooth peanut butter
- ✓ Coconut for garnish, shredded

Directions:

- ❖ Start by blending bananas and peanut butter in a blender and mix until smooth or desired texture obtained.
- ❖ Pour into a bowl and garnish with coconut if desired.
- ❖ Enjoy.

Nutrition: Calories: 589, Total Fat: 33.3g, Saturated Fat: 6.9, Cholesterol: 0 mg, Sodium: 13 mg, Total Carbohydrate: 66.5 g, Dietary Fiber: 10 g, Total Sugars: 38 g, Protein: 18.8 g, Vitamin D: 0 mcg, Calcium: 40 mg, Iron: 2 mg, Potassium: 1264 mg

234) COCONUT BANANA MIX

Cooking Time: 4 Minutes   **Servings: 4**

Ingredients:

- ✓ 3 tbsp chopped raisins
- ✓ ⅛ tsp nutmeg
- ✓ ⅛ tsp cinnamon
- ✓ Salt to taste

- ✓ 1 cup coconut milk
- ✓ 1 banana
- ✓ 1 cup dried coconut
- ✓ 2 tbsp ground flax seed

Directions:

- ❖ Set a large skillet on the stove and set it to low heat.
- ❖ Chop up the banana.
- ❖ Pour the coconut milk, nutmeg, and cinnamon into the skillet.
- ❖ Pour in the ground flaxseed while stirring continuously.
- ❖ Add the dried coconut and banana. Mix the ingredients until combined well.
- ❖ Allow the mixture to simmer for 2 to 3 minutes while stirring occasionally.
- ❖ Set four airtight containers on the counter.
- ❖ Remove the pan from heat and sprinkle enough salt for your taste buds.
- ❖ Divide the mixture into the containers and place them into the fridge overnight. They can remain in the fridge for up to 3 days.
- ❖ Before you set this tasty mixture in the microwave to heat up, you need to let it thaw on the counter for a bit.

Nutrition: calories: 279, fats: 22 grams, carbohydrates: 25 grams, protein: 6.4 grams

235) **OLIVE OIL RASPBERRY-LEMON MUFFINS**

Cooking Time: 20 Minutes   **Servings: 12**

Ingredients:

- ✓ ⅛ tsp kosher salt
- ✓ 1¼ cups buttermilk
- ✓ 1 large egg
- ✓ ¼ cup extra-virgin olive oil
- ✓ 1 tbsp freshly squeezed lemon juice
- ✓ Zest of 2 lemons
- ✓ 1¼ cups frozen raspberries (do not thaw)

- ✓ Cooking spray to grease baking liners
- ✓ 1 cup all-purpose flour
- ✓ 1 cup whole-wheat flour
- ✓ ½ cup tightly packed light brown sugar
- ✓ ½ tsp baking soda
- ✓ ½ tsp aluminum-free baking powder

Directions:

- ❖ Preheat the oven to 400°F and line a muffin tin with baking liners. Spray the liners lightly with cooking spray.
- ❖ In a large mixing bowl, whisk together the all-purpose flour, whole-wheat flour, brown sugar, baking soda, baking powder, and salt.
- ❖ In a medium bowl, whisk together the buttermilk, egg, oil, lemon juice, and lemon zest.
- ❖ Pour the wet ingredients into the dry ingredients and stir just until blended. Do not overmix.
- ❖ Fold in the frozen raspberries.
- ❖ Scoop about ¼ cup of batter into each muffin liner and bake for 20 minutes, or until the tops look browned and a paring knife comes out clean when inserted. Remove the muffins from the tin to cool.
- ❖ STORAGE: Store covered containers at room temperature for up to 4 days. To freeze muffins for up to 3 months, wrap them in foil and place in an airtight resealable bag.

Nutrition: Total calories: 166; Total fat: 5g; Saturated fat: 1g; Sodium: 134mg; Carbohydrates: 30g; Fiber: 3g; Protein: 4g

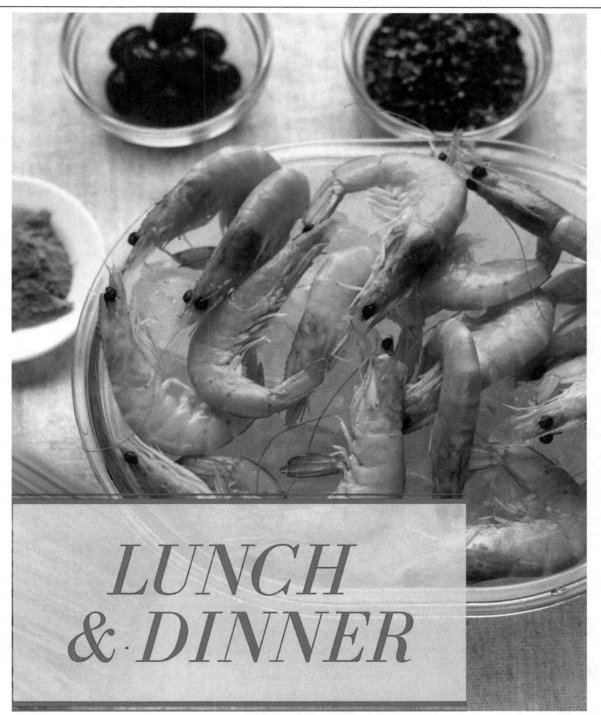

LUNCH
& DINNER

236) MARINATED TUNA STEAK SPECIAL

Cooking Time: 15-20 Minutes   **Servings: 4**

Ingredients:

- ✓ Olive oil (2 tbsp.)
- ✓ Orange juice (.25 cup)
- ✓ Soy sauce (.25 cup)
- ✓ Lemon juice (1 tbsp.)
- ✓ Fresh parsley (2 tbsp.)
- ✓ Garlic clove (1)
- ✓ Ground black pepper (.5 tsp.)
- ✓ Fresh oregano (.5 tsp.)
- ✓ Tuna steaks (4 - 4 oz. Steaks)

Directions:

- ❖ Mince the garlic and chop the oregano and parsley.
- ❖ In a glass container, mix the pepper, oregano, garlic, parsley, lemon juice, soy sauce, olive oil, and orange juice.
- ❖ Warm the grill using the high heat setting. Grease the grate with oil.
- ❖ Add to tuna steaks and cook for five to six minutes. Turn and baste with the marinated sauce.
- ❖ Cook another five minutes or until it's the way you like it. Discard the remaining marinade.

Nutrition: Calories: 200;Protein: 27.4 grams;Fat: 7.9 grams

237) SHRIMP AND GARLIC PASTA

Cooking Time: 15 Minutes   **Servings: 4**

Ingredients:

- ✓ 6 ounces whole wheat spaghetti
- ✓ 12 ounces raw shrimp, peeled and deveined, cut into 1-inch pieces
- ✓ 1 bunch asparagus, trimmed
- ✓ 1 large bell pepper, thinly sliced
- ✓ 1 cup fresh peas
- ✓ 3 garlic cloves, chopped
- ✓ 1 and ¼ tsp kosher salt
- ✓ ½ and ½ cups non-fat plain yogurt
- ✓ 3 tbsp lemon juice
- ✓ 1 tbsp extra-virgin olive oil
- ✓ ½ tsp fresh ground black pepper
- ✓ ¼ cup pine nuts, toasted

Directions:

- ❖ Take a large sized pot and bring water to a boil
- ❖ Add your spaghetti and cook them for about minutes less than the directed package instruction
- ❖ Add shrimp, bell pepper, asparagus and cook for about 2- 4 minutes until the shrimp are tender
- ❖ Drain the pasta and the contents well
- ❖ Take a large bowl and mash garlic until a paste form
- ❖ Whisk in yogurt, parsley, oil, pepper and lemon juice into the garlic paste
- ❖ Add pasta mix and toss well
- ❖ Serve by sprinkling some pine nuts!
- ❖ Enjoy!
- ❖ Meal Prep/Storage Options: Store in airtight containers in your fridge for 1-3 days.

Nutrition: Calories: 406;Fat: 22g;Carbohydrates: 28g;Protein: 26g

238) BUTTER PAPRIKA SHRIMPS

Cooking Time: 30 Minutes   **Servings: 2**

Ingredients:

- ✓ ¼ tbsp smoked paprika
- ✓ 1/8 cup sour cream
- ✓ ½ pound tiger shrimps
- ✓ 1/8 cup butter
- ✓ Salt and black pepper, to taste

Directions:

- ❖ Preheat the oven to 390 degrees F and grease a baking dish.
- ❖ Mix together all the ingredients in a large bowl and transfer into the baking dish.
- ❖ Place in the oven and bake for about 15 minutes.
- ❖ Place paprika shrimp in a dish and set aside to cool for meal prepping. Divide it in 2 containers and cover the lid. Refrigerate for 1-2 days and reheat in microwave before serving.

Nutrition: Calories: 330 ;Carbohydrates: 1.;Protein: 32.6g;Fat: 21.5g;Sugar: 0.2g;Sodium: 458mg

239) MEDITERRANEAN-STYLE SALMON AVOCADO SALAD

Cooking Time: 10 Minutes   **Servings: 4**

Ingredients:

- ✓ 1 lb skinless salmon fillets
- ✓ Marinade/Dressing:
- ✓ 3 tbsp olive oil
- ✓ Salad:
- ✓ 4 cups Romaine (or Cos) lettuce leaves, washed and dried
- ✓ 1 large cucumber, diced
- ✓ 2 Roma tomatoes, diced
- ✓ 1 red onion, sliced
- ✓ 1 avocado, sliced

Directions:

- ❖ In a jug, whisk together the olive oil, lemon juice, red wine vinegar, chopped parsley, garlic minced, oregano, salt and pepper
- ❖ Pour out half of the marinade into a large, shallow dish, refrigerate the

- ✓ 2 tbsp lemon juice fresh, squeezed
- ✓ 1 tbsp red wine vinegar, optional
- ✓ 1 tbsp fresh chopped parsley
- ✓ 2 tsp garlic minced
- ✓ 1 tsp dried oregano
- ✓ 1 tsp salt
- ✓ Cracked pepper, to taste

- ✓ 1/2 cup feta cheese crumbled
- ✓ 1/3 cup pitted Kalamata olives or black olives, sliced
- ✓ Lemon wedges to serve

- ❖ remaining marinade to use as the dressing
- ❖ Coat the salmon in the rest of the marinade
- ❖ Place a skillet pan or grill over medium-high, add 1 tbsp oil and sear salmon on both sides until crispy and cooked through
- ❖ Allow the salmon to cool
- ❖ Distribute the salmon among the containers, store in the fridge for 2-3 days
- ❖ To Serve: Prepare the salad by placing the romaine lettuce, cucumber, roma tomatoes, red onion, avocado, feta cheese, and olives in a large salad bowl. Reheat the salmon in the microwave for 30seconds to 1 minute or until heated through.
- ❖ Slice the salmon and arrange over salad. Drizzle the salad with the remaining untouched dressing, serve with lemon wedges.

Nutrition: Calories:411;Carbs: 12g;Total Fat: 27g;Protein: 28g

240)   KALE BEET SALAD

Cooking Time: 50 Minutes   **Servings: 6**

Ingredients:

- ✓ 1 bunch of kale, washed and dried, ribs removed, chopped
- ✓ 6 pieces washed beets, peeled and dried and cut into ½ inches
- ✓ ½ tsp dried rosemary
- ✓ ½ tsp garlic powder
- ✓ salt
- ✓ pepper
- ✓ olive oil
- ✓ ¼ medium red onion, thinly sliced

- ✓ 1-2 tbsp slivered almonds, toasted
- ✓ ¼ cup olive oil
- ✓ Juice of 1½ lemon
- ✓ ¼ cup honey
- ✓ ¼ tsp garlic powder
- ✓ 1 tsp dried rosemary
- ✓ salt
- ✓ pepper

Directions:

- ❖ Preheat oven to 400 degrees F.
- ❖ Take a bowl and toss the kale with some salt, pepper, and olive oil.
- ❖ Lightly oil a baking sheet and add the kale.
- ❖ Roast in the oven for 5 minutes, and then remove and place to the side.
- ❖ Place beets in a bowl and sprinkle with a bit of rosemary, garlic powder, pepper, and salt; ensure beets are coated well.
- ❖ Spread the beets on the oiled baking sheet, place on the middle rack of your oven, and roast for 45 minutes, turning twice.
- ❖ Make the lemon vinaigrette by whisking all of the listed Ingredients: in a bowl.
- ❖ Once the beets are ready, remove from the oven and allow it to cool.
- ❖ Take a medium-sized salad bowl and add kale, onions, and beets.
- ❖ Dress with lemon honey vinaigrette and toss well.
- ❖ Garnish with toasted almonds.
- ❖ Enjoy!

Nutrition: Calories: 245, Total Fat: 17.6 g, Saturated Fat: 2.6 g, Cholesterol: 0 mg, Sodium: 77 mg, Total Carbohydrate: 22.9 g, Dietary Fiber: 3 g, Total Sugars:

17.7 g, Protein: 2.4 g, Vitamin D: 0 mcg, Calcium: 50 mg, Iron: 1 mg, Potassium: 416 mg

241)   MOROCCAN FISH

Cooking Time: 1 Hour 25 Minutes   **Servings: 12**

Ingredients:

- ✓ Garbanzo beans (15 oz. Can)
- ✓ Red bell peppers (2)
- ✓ Large carrot (1)
- ✓ Vegetable oil (1 tbsp.)
- ✓ Onion (1)
- ✓ Garlic (1 clove)
- ✓ Tomatoes (3 chopped/14.5 oz can)

- ✓ Olives (4 chopped)
- ✓ Chopped fresh parsley (.25 cup)
- ✓ Ground cumin (.25 cup)
- ✓ Paprika (3 tbsp.)
- ✓ Chicken bouillon granules (2 tbsp.)
- ✓ Cayenne pepper (1 tsp.)
- ✓ Salt (to your liking)
- ✓ Tilapia fillets (5 lb.)

Directions:

- ❖ Drain and rinse the beans. Thinly slice the carrot and onion. Mince the garlic and chop the olives. Discard the seeds from the peppers and slice them into strips.
- ❖ Warm the oil in a frying pan using the medium temperature setting. Toss in the onion and garlic. Simmer them for approximately five minutes.
- ❖ Fold in the bell peppers, beans, tomatoes, carrots, and olives.
- ❖ Continue sautéing them for about five additional minutes.
- ❖ Sprinkle the veggies with the cumin, parsley, salt, chicken bouillon, paprika, and cayenne.
- ❖ Stir thoroughly and place the fish on top of the veggies.
- ❖ Pour in water to cover the veggies.
- ❖ Lower the heat setting and cover the pan to slowly cook until the fish is flaky (about 40 min..

Nutrition: Calories: 268;Protein: 42 grams;Fat: 5 grams

242) SARDINES WITH NIÇOISE-INSPIRED SALAD

Cooking Time: 15 Minutes   **Servings:** 4

Ingredients:

- ✓ 4 eggs
- ✓ 12 ounces baby red potatoes (about 12 potatoes)
- ✓ 6 ounces green beans, halved
- ✓ 4 cups baby spinach leaves or mixed greens
- ✓ 1 bunch radishes, quartered (about 1⅓ cups)
- ✓ 1 cup cherry tomatoes
- ✓ 20 kalamata or niçoise olives (about ⅓ cup)
- ✓ 3 (3.75-ounce) cans skinless, boneless sardines packed in olive oil, drained
- ✓ 8 tbsp Dijon Red Wine Vinaigrette

Directions:

- ❖ Place the eggs in a saucepan and cover with water. Bring the water to a boil. As soon as the water starts to boil, place a lid on the pan and turn the heat off. Set a timer for minutes.
- ❖ When the timer goes off, drain the hot water and run cold water over the eggs to cool. Peel the eggs when cool and cut in half.
- ❖ Prick each potato a few times with a fork. Place them on a microwave-safe plate and microwave on high for 4 to 5 minutes, until the potatoes are tender. Let cool and cut in half.
- ❖ Place green beans on a microwave-safe plate and microwave on high for 1½ to 2 minutes, until the beans are crisp-tender. Cool.
- ❖ Place 1 egg, ½ cup of green beans, 6 potato halves, 1 cup of spinach, ⅓ cup of radishes, ¼ cup of tomatoes, olives, and 3 sardines in each of 4 containers. Pour 2 tbsp of vinaigrette into each of 4 sauce containers.
- ❖ STORAGE: Store covered containers in the refrigerator for up to 4 days.

Nutrition: Total calories: 450; Total fat: 32g; Saturated fat: 5g; Sodium: 6mg; Carbohydrates: 22g; Fiber: 5g; Protein: 21g

243) POMODORO LETTUCE SALAD

Cooking Time: 15 Minutes   **Servings:** 6

Ingredients:

- ✓ 1 heart of Romaine lettuce, chopped
- ✓ 3 Roma tomatoes, diced
- ✓ 1 English cucumber, diced
- ✓ 1 small red onion, finely chopped
- ✓ ½ cup curly parsley, finely chopped
- ✓ 2 tbsp virgin olive oil
- ✓ lemon juice, ½ large lemon
- ✓ 1 tsp garlic powder
- ✓ salt
- ✓ pepper

Directions:

- ❖ Add all Ingredients: to a large bowl.
- ❖ Toss well and transfer them to containers.
- ❖ Enjoy!

Nutrition: Calories: 68, Total Fat: 9 g, Saturated Fat: 0.8 g, Cholesterol: 0 mg, Sodium: 7 mg, Total Carbohydrate: 6 g, Dietary Fiber: 1.5 g, Total Sugars: 3.3 g,

Protein: 1.3 g, Vitamin D: 0 mcg, Calcium: 18 mg, Iron: 1 mg, Potassium: 309 mg

244) Mediterranean-Style Chicken Pasta Bake

Cooking Time: 30 Minutes   **Servings:** 4

Ingredients:

- ✓ Marinade:
- ✓ 1½ lbs. boneless, skinless chicken thighs, cut into bite-sized pieces*
- ✓ 2 garlic cloves, thinly sliced
- ✓ 2-3 tbsp. marinade from artichoke hearts
- ✓ 4 sprigs of fresh oregano, leaves stripped
- ✓ Olive oil
- ✓ Red wine vinegar
- ✓ Pasta:
- ✓ ½ cup marinated artichoke hearts, roughly chopped
- ✓ ½ cup white beans, rinsed + drained (I use northern white beans)
- ✓ ½ cup Kalamata olives, roughly chopped
- ✓ ⅓ cup parsley and basil leaves, roughly chopped
- ✓ 2-3 handfuls of part-skim shredded mozzarella cheese
- ✓ Salt, to taste
- ✓ Pepper, to taste
- ✓ Garnish:
- ✓ Parsley

Directions:

- ❖ Create the chicken marinade by drain the artichoke hearts reserving the juice
- ❖ In a large bowl, add the artichoke juice, garlic, chicken, and oregano leaves, drizzle with olive oil, a splash of red wine vinegar, and mix well to coat
- ❖ Marinate for at least 1 hour, maximum hours
- ❖ Cook the pasta in boiling salted water, drain and set aside
- ❖ Preheat your oven to 42degrees F
- ❖ In a casserole dish, add the sliced onions and tomatoes, toss with olive oil, salt and pepper. Then cook, stirring occasionally, until the onions are soft and the tomatoes start to burst, about 15-20 minutes
- ❖ In the meantime, in a large skillet over medium heat, add 1 tsp of olive oil

Ingredients:

- 1 lb whole wheat fusilli pasta
- 1 red onion, thinly sliced
- 1 pint grape or cherry tomatoes, whole
- Basil leaves

Directions:

- Remove the chicken from the marinade, pat dry, and season with salt and pepper
- Working in batches, brown the chicken on both sides, leaving slightly undercooked
- Remove the casserole dish from the oven, add in the cooked pasta, browned chicken, artichoke hearts, beans, olives, and chopped herbs, stir to combine
- Top with grated cheese
- Bake for an additional 5-7 minutes, until the cheese is brown and bubbling
- Remove from the oven and allow the dish to cool completely
- Distribute among the containers, store for 2-3 days
- To Serve: Reheat in the microwave for 1-2 minutes or until heated through.
- Garnish with fresh herbs and serve

Nutrition: Calories:487;Carbs: 95g;Total Fat: 5g;Protein: 22g

245) VEGETABLE FLATBREAD ROAST

Cooking Time: 25 Minutes   **Servings: 12**

Ingredients:

- 16 oz pizza dough, homemade or frozen
- 6 oz soft goat cheese, divided
- ¾ cup grated Parmesan cheese divided
- 3 tbsp chopped fresh dill, divided
- 1 small red onion, sliced thinly
- 1 small zucchini, sliced thinly
- 2 small tomatoes, thinly sliced
- 1 small red pepper, thinly sliced into rings
- Olive oil
- Salt, to taste
- Pepper, to taste

Directions:

- Preheat the oven to 400 degrees F
- Roll the dough into a large rectangle, and then place it on a piece of parchment paper sprayed with non-stick spray
- Take a knife and spread half the goat cheese onto one half of the dough, then sprinkle with half the dill and half the Parmesan cheese
- Carefully fold the other half of the dough on top of the cheese, spread and sprinkle the remaining parmesan and goat cheese
- Layer the thinly sliced vegetables over the top
- Brush the olive oil over the top of the veggies and sprinkle with salt, pepper, and the remaining dill
- Bake for 22-25 minutes, until the edges are medium brown, cut in half, lengthwise
- Then slice the flatbread in long 2-inch slices and allow to cool
- Distribute among the containers, store for 2 days
- To Serve: Reheat in the oven at 375 degrees for 5 minutes or until hot. Enjoy with a fresh salad.

Nutrition: Calories:170;Carbs: 21g;Total Fat: 6g;Protein: 8g

246) COBB SALAD WITH STEAK

Cooking Time: 15 Minutes   **Servings: 4**

Ingredients:

- 6 large eggs
- 2 tbsp unsalted butter
- 1 lb steak
- 2 tbsp olive oil
- 6 cups baby spinach
- 1 cup cherry tomatoes, halved
- 1 cup pecan halves
- 1/2 cup crumbled feta cheese
- Kosher salt, to taste
- Freshly ground black pepper, to taste

Directions:

- In a large skillet over medium high heat, melt butter
- Using paper towels, pat the steak dry, then drizzle with olive oil and season with salt and pepper, to taste
- Once heated, add the steak to the skillet and cook, flipping once, until cooked through to desired doneness, - cook for 4 minutes per side for a medium-rare steak
- Transfer the steak to a plate and allow it to cool before dicing
- Place the eggs in a large saucepan and cover with cold water by 1 inch
- Bring to a boil and cook for 1 minute, cover the eggs with a tight-fitting lid and remove from heat, set aside for 8-10 minutes, then drain well and allow to cool before peeling and dicing
- Assemble the salad in the container by placing the spinach at the bottom of the container, top with arranged rows of steak, eggs, feta, tomatoes, and pecans
- To Serve: Top with the balsamic vinaigrette, or desired dressing
- Recipe Note: You can also use New York, rib-eye or filet mignon for this recipe

Nutrition: Calories:640;Total Fat: 51g;Total Carbs: 9.8g;Fiber: 5g;Protein: 38.8g

247) LAMB CHOPS GRILL

Cooking Time: 10 Minutes   **Servings: 4**

- ✓ 1 tbsp chopped garlic
- ✓ ¼ tsp ground black pepper
- ✓ ½ cup olive oil
- ✓ 2 tbsp fresh basil, shredded

Ingredients:

- ✓ 4 8-ounce lamb shoulder chops
- ✓ 2 tbsp Dijon mustard
- ✓ 2 tbsp balsamic vinegar

Directions:

- ❖ Pat the lamb chops dry and arrange them in a shallow glass-baking dish.
- ❖ Take a bowl and whisk in Dijon mustard, garlic, balsamic vinegar, and pepper.
- ❖ Mix well to make the marinade.
- ❖ Whisk oil slowly into the marinade until it is smooth.
- ❖ Stir in basil.
- ❖ Pour the marinade over the lamb chops, making sure to coat both sides.
- ❖ Cover, refrigerate and allow the chops to marinate for anywhere from 1-4 hours.
- ❖ Remove the chops from the refrigerator and leave out for 30 minutes or until room temperature.
- ❖ Preheat grill to medium heat and oil grate.
- ❖ Grill the lamb chops until the center reads 145 degrees F and they are nicely browned, about 5-minutes per side.
- ❖ Enjoy!

Nutrition: Calories: 1587, Total Fat: 97.5 g, Saturated Fat: 27.6 g, Cholesterol: 600 mg, Sodium: 729 mg, Total Carbohydrate: 1.3 g, Dietary Fiber: 0.4 g, Total

Sugars: 0.1 g, Protein: 176.5 g, Vitamin D: 0 mcg, Calcium: 172 mg, Iron: 15 mg, Potassium: 30 mg

248) CHILI BROILED CALAMARI

Cooking Time: 8 Minutes   **Servings: 4**

- ✓ Dash of sea salt
- ✓ 1 and ½ pounds squid, cleaned and split open, with tentacles cut into ½ inch rounds
- ✓ 2 tbsp cilantro, chopped
- ✓ 2 tbsp red bell pepper, minced

Ingredients:

- ✓ 2 tbsp extra virgin olive oil
- ✓ 1 tsp chili powder
- ✓ ½ tsp ground cumin
- ✓ Zest of 1 lime
- ✓ Juice of 1 lime

Directions:

- ❖ Take a medium bowl and stir in olive oil, chili powder, cumin, lime zest, sea salt, lime juice and pepper
- ❖ Add squid and let it marinade and stir to coat, coat and let it refrigerate for 1 hour
- ❖ Pre-heat your oven to broil
- ❖ Arrange squid on a baking sheet, broil for 8 minutes turn once until tender
- ❖ Garnish the broiled calamari with cilantro and red bell pepper
- ❖ Serve and enjoy!
- ❖ Meal Prep/Storage Options: Store in airtight containers in your fridge for 1-2 days.

Nutrition: Calories:159;Fat: 13g;Carbohydrates: 12g;Protein: 3g

249) SALMON AND CORN PEPPER SALSA

Cooking Time: 12 Minutes   **Servings: 2**

Ingredients:

- ✓ 1 garlic clove, grated
- ✓ ½ tsp mild chili powder
- ✓ ½ tsp ground coriander
- ✓ ¼ tsp ground cumin
- ✓ 2 limes – 1, zest and juice; 1 cut into wedges
- ✓ 2 tsp rapeseed oil

- ✓ 2 wild salmon fillets
- ✓ 1 ear of corn on the cob, husk removed
- ✓ 1 red onion, finely chopped
- ✓ ,1 avocado, cored, peeled, and finely chopped
- ✓ 1 red pepper, deseeded and finely chopped
- ✓ 1 red chili, halved and deseeded
- ✓ ½ a pack of finely chopped coriander

Directions:

- ❖ Boil the corn in water for about 6-8 minutes until tender.
- ❖ Drain and cut off the kernels.
- ❖ In a bowl, combine garlic, spices, 1 tbsp of limejuice, and oil; mix well to prepare spice rub.
- ❖ Coat the salmon with the rub.
- ❖ Add the zest to the corn and give it a gentle stir.
- ❖ Heat a frying pan over medium heat.
- ❖ Add salmon and cook for about 2 minutes per side.
- ❖ Serve the cooked salmon with salsa and lime wedges.
- ❖ Enjoy!

Nutrition: Calories: 949, Total Fat: 57.4 g, Saturated Fat: 9.7 g, Cholesterol: 2mg, Sodium: 180 mg, Total Carbohydrate: 33.5 g, Dietary Fiber: 11.8 g, Total Sugars: 8.3 g, Protein: 76.8 g, Vitamin D: 0 mcg, Calcium: 100 mg, Iron: 3 mg, Potassium: 856 mg

250) ITALIAN-INSPIRED ROTISSERIE CHICKEN WITH BROCCOLI SLAW

Cooking Time: 15 Minutes   **Servings:** 4

Ingredients:

- ✓ 4 cups packaged broccoli slaw
- ✓ 1 cooked rotisserie chicken, meat removed (about 10 to 12 ounces)
- ✓ 1 bunch red radishes, stemmed, halved, and thickly sliced (about 1¼ cups)
- ✓ 1 cup sliced red onion

- ✓ ½ cup pitted kalamata or niçoise olives, roughly chopped
- ✓ ½ cup sliced pepperoncini
- ✓ 8 tbsp Dijon Red Wine Vinaigrette, divided

Directions:

- ❖ Place the broccoli slaw, chicken, radishes, onion, olives, and pepperoncini in a large mixing bowl. Toss to combine.
- ❖ Place cups of salad in each of 4 containers. Pour 2 tbsp of vinaigrette into each of 4 sauce containers.
- ❖ STORAGE: Store covered containers in the refrigerator for up to 5 days.

Nutrition: Total calories: 329; Total fat: 2; Saturated fat: 4g; Sodium: 849mg; Carbohydrates: 10g; Fiber: 3g; Protein: 20g

251) Flatbread and Roasted Vegetables

Cooking Time: 45 Minutes   **Servings:** 12

Ingredients:

- ✓ 5 ounces goat cheese
- ✓ 1 thinly sliced onion
- ✓ 2 thinly sliced tomatoes
- ✓ Olive oil
- ✓ ¼ tsp pepper

- ✓ ⅛ tsp salt
- ✓ 16 ounces homemade or frozen pizza dough
- ✓ ¾ tbsp chopped dill, fresh is better
- ✓ 1 thinly sliced zucchini
- ✓ 1 red pepper, cup into rings

Directions:

- ❖ Set your oven to 400 degrees Fahrenheit.
- ❖ Set the dough on a large piece of parchment paper. Use a rolling pin to roll the dough into a large rectangle.
- ❖ Spread half of the goat cheese on ½ of the pizza dough.
- ❖ Sprinkle half of the dill on the other half of the dough.
- ❖ Fold the dough so the half with the dill is on top of the cheese.
- ❖ Spread the remaining goat cheese on the pizza dough and then sprinkle the rest of the dill over the cheese.
- ❖ Layer the vegetables on top in any arrangement you like.
- ❖ Drizzle olive oil on top of the vegetables.
- ❖ Sprinkle salt and pepper over the olive oil.
- ❖ Set the piece of parchment paper on a pizza pan or baking pan and place it in the oven.
- ❖ Set the timer for 22 minutes. If the edges are not a medium brown, leave the flatbread in the oven for another couple of minutes.
- ❖ Remove the pizza from the oven when it is done and cut the flatbread in half lengthwise.
- ❖ Slice the flatbread into 2-inch long pieces and enjoy!

Nutrition: calories: 170, fats: 5 grams, carbohydrates: 20 grams, protein: 8 grams.

252) SEAFOOD RICE

Cooking Time: 40 Minutes   **Servings: 4-5**

Ingredients:

- ✓ 4 small lobster tails (6-12 oz each)
- ✓ Water
- ✓ 3 tbsp Extra Virgin Olive Oil
- ✓ 1 large yellow onion, chopped
- ✓ 2 cups Spanish rice or short grain rice, soaked in water for 15 minutes and then drained
- ✓ 4 garlic cloves, chopped
- ✓ 2 large pinches of Spanish saffron threads soaked in 1/2 cup water
- ✓ 1 tsp Sweet Spanish paprika
- ✓ 1 tsp cayenne pepper
- ✓ 1/2 tsp aleppo pepper flakes
- ✓ Salt, to taste
- ✓ 2 large Roma tomatoes, finely chopped
- ✓ 6 oz French green beans, trimmed
- ✓ 1 lb prawns or large shrimp or your choice, peeled and deveined
- ✓ 1/4 cup chopped fresh parsley

Directions:

- ❖ In a large pot, add 3 cups of water and bring it to a rolling boil
- ❖ Add in the lobster tails and allow boil briefly, about 1-minutes or until pink, remove from heat
- ❖ Using tongs transfer the lobster tails to a plate and Do not discard the lobster cooking water
- ❖ Allow the lobster is cool, then remove the shell and cut into large chunks.
- ❖ In a large deep pan or skillet over medium-high heat, add 3 tbsp olive oil
- ❖ Add the chopped onions, sauté the onions for 2 minutes and then add the rice, and cook for 3 more minutes, stirring regularly
- ❖ Then add in the lobster cooking water and the chopped garlic and, stir in the saffron and its soaking liquid, cayenne pepper, aleppo pepper, paprika, and salt
- ❖ Gently stir in the chopped tomatoes and green beans, bring to a boil and allow the liquid slightly reduce, then cover (with lid or tightly wrapped foil) and cook over low heat for 20 minutes
- ❖ Once done, uncover and spread the shrimp over the rice, push it into the rice slightly, add in a little water, if needed
- ❖ Cover and cook for another 15 minutes until the shrimp turn pink
- ❖ Then add in the cooked lobster chunks
- ❖ Once the lobster is warmed through, remove from heat allow the dish to cool completely
- ❖ Distribute among the containers, store for 2 days
- ❖ To Serve: Reheat in the microwave for 1-2 minutes or until heated through. Garnish with parsley and enjoy!
- ❖ Recipe Notes: Remember to soak your rice if needed to help with the cooking process

Nutrition: Calories:536;Carbs: 56g;Total Fat: 26g;Protein: 50g

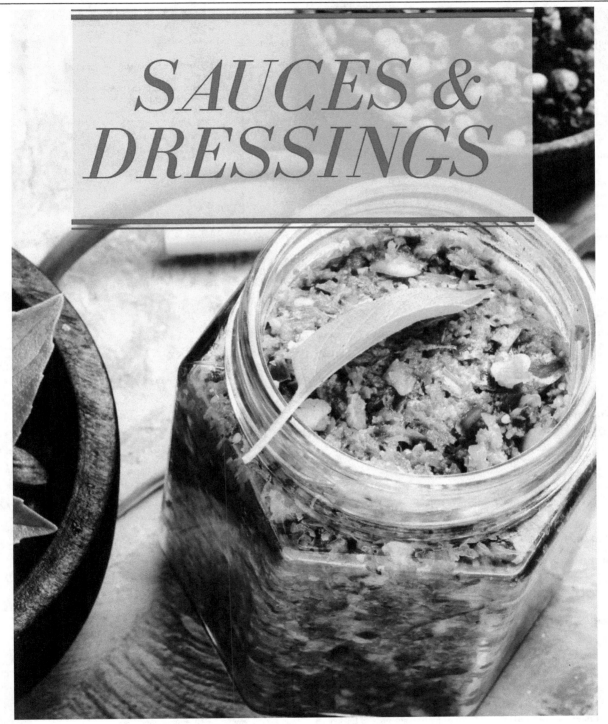

SAUCES & DRESSINGS

253) SPECIAL POMEGRANATE VINAIGRETTE

Cooking Time: 5 Minutes   **Servings:** ½ Cup

✓   ½ tsp dried mint
✓   2 tbsp plus 2 tsp olive oil

Ingredients:

✓   ⅓ cup pomegranate juice
✓   1 tsp Dijon mustard
✓   1 tbsp apple cider vinegar

Directions:

❖   Place the pomegranate juice, mustard, vinegar, and mint in a small bowl and whisk to combine.
❖   Whisk in the oil, pouring it into the bowl in a thin steam.
❖   Pour the vinaigrette into a container and refrigerate.
❖   STORAGE: Store the covered container in the refrigerator for up to 2 weeks. Bring the vinaigrette to room temperature and shake before serving.

Nutrition: (2 tbsp): Total calories: 94; Total fat: 10g; Saturated fat: 2g; Sodium: 30mg; Carbohydrates: 3g; Fiber: 0g; Protein: 0g

254) GREEN OLIVE WITH SPINACH TAPENADE

Cooking Time: 20 Minutes   **Servings:** 1½ Cups

✓   ½ tsp dried oregano
✓   ⅓ cup packed fresh basil
✓   2 tbsp olive oil
✓   2 tsp red wine vinegar

Ingredients:

✓   1 cup pimento-stuffed green olives, drained
✓   3 packed cups baby spinach
✓   1 tsp chopped garlic

Directions:

❖   Place all the ingredients in the bowl of a food processor and pulse until the mixture looks finely chopped but not puréed.
❖   Scoop the tapenade into a container and refrigerate.
❖   STORAGE: Store the covered container in the refrigerator for up to 5 days.

Nutrition: (¼ cup): Total calories: 80; Total fat: 8g; Saturated fat: 1g; Sodium: 6mg; Carbohydrates: 1g; Fiber: 1g; Protein: 1g

255) BULGUR PILAF AND ALMONDS

Cooking Time: 20 Minutes   **Servings:** 4

✓   1 cup small diced red bell pepper
✓   ⅓ cup chopped fresh cilantro
✓   1 tbsp olive oil
✓   ¼ tsp salt

Ingredients:

✓   ⅔ cup uncooked bulgur
✓   1⅓ cups water
✓   ¼ cup sliced almonds

Directions:

❖   Place the bulgur and water in a saucepan and bring the water to a boil. Once the water is at a boil, cover the pot with a lid and turn off the heat. Let the covered pot stand for 20 minutes.
❖   Transfer the cooked bulgur to a large mixing bowl and add the almonds, peppers, cilantro, oil, and salt. Stir to combine.
❖   Place about 1 cup of bulgur in each of 4 containers.
❖   STORAGE: Store covered containers in the refrigerator for up to 5 days. Bulgur can be either reheated or eaten at room temperature.

Nutrition: Total calories: 17 Total fat: 7g; Saturated fat: 1g; Sodium: 152mg; Carbohydrates: 25g; Fiber: 6g; Protein: 4g

256) SPANISH GARLIC YOGURT SAUCE

Cooking Time: 5 Minutes   **Servings:** 1 Cup

✓   1 tbsp olive oil
✓   ¼ tsp kosher salt

Ingredients:

✓   1 cup low-fat (2%) plain Greek yogurt
✓   ½ tsp garlic powder
✓   1 tbsp freshly squeezed lemon juice

Directions:

❖   Mix all the ingredients in a medium bowl until well combined.
❖   Spoon the yogurt sauce into a container and refrigerate.
❖   STORAGE: Store the covered container in the refrigerator for up to 7 days

Nutrition: (¼ cup): Total calories: 75; Total fat: 5g; Saturated fat: 1g; Sodium: 173mg; Carbohydrates: 3g; Fiber: 0g; Protein: 6g.

257) ORANGE WITH CINNAMON–SCENTED WHOLE-WHEAT COUSCOUS

Cooking Time: 10 Minutes   **Servings: 4**

Ingredients:

- ✓ ½ cup water
- ✓ ⅛ tsp ground cinnamon
- ✓ ¼ tsp kosher salt
- ✓ 1 cup whole-wheat couscous

- ✓ 2 tsp olive oil
- ✓ ¼ cup minced shallot
- ✓ ½ cup freshly squeezed orange juice (from 2 oranges)

Directions:

- ❖ Heat the oil in a saucepan over medium heat. Once the oil is shimmering, add the shallot and cook for 2 minutes, stirring frequently. Add the orange juice, water, cinnamon, and salt, and bring to a boil.
- ❖ Once the liquid is boiling, add the couscous, cover the pan, and turn off the heat. Leave the couscous covered for 5 minutes. When the couscous is done, fluff with a fork.
- ❖ Place ¾ cup of couscous in each of 4 containers.
- ❖ STORAGE: Store covered containers in the refrigerator for up to 5 days. Freeze for up to 2 months.

Nutrition: Total calories: 21 Total fat: 4g; Saturated fat: <1g; Sodium: 147mg; Carbohydrates: 41g; Fiber: 5g; Protein: 8g

258) CHUNKY ROASTED CHERRY TOMATO WITH BASIL SAUCE

Cooking Time: 40 Minutes   **Servings: 1⅓ Cups**

Ingredients:

- ✓ ¼ tsp kosher salt
- ✓ ½ tsp chopped garlic
- ✓ ¼ cup fresh basil leaves

- ✓ 2 pints cherry tomatoes (20 ounces total)
- ✓ 2 tsp olive oil, plus 3 tbsp

Directions:

- ❖ Preheat the oven to 350°F. Line a sheet pan with a silicone baking mat or parchment paper.
- ❖ Place the tomatoes on the lined sheet pan and toss with tsp of oil. Roast for 40 minutes, shaking the pan halfway through.
- ❖ While the tomatoes are still warm, place them in a medium mixing bowl and add the salt, the garlic, and the remaining tbsp of oil. Mash the tomatoes with the back of a fork. Stir in the fresh basil.
- ❖ Scoop the sauce into a container and refrigerate.
- ❖ STORAGE: Store the covered container in the refrigerator for up to days.

Nutrition: (⅓ cup): Total calories: 141; Total fat: 13g; Saturated fat: 2g; Sodium: 158mg; Carbohydrates: 7g; Fiber: 2g; Protein: 1g

259) CELERY HEART, BASIL, AND ALMOND PESTO

Cooking Time: 10 Minutes   **Servings: 1 Cup**

Ingredients:

- ✓ ¼ tsp kosher salt
- ✓ 1 tbsp freshly squeezed lemon juice
- ✓ ¼ cup olive oil
- ✓ 3 tbsp water

- ✓ ½ cup raw, unsalted almonds
- ✓ 3 cups fresh basil leaves, (about 1½ ounces)
- ✓ ½ cup chopped celery hearts with leaves

Directions:

- ❖ Place the almonds in the bowl of a food processor and process until they look like coarse sand.
- ❖ Add the basil, celery hearts, salt, lemon juice, oil and water and process until smooth. The sauce will be somewhat thick. If you would like a thinner sauce, add more water, oil, or lemon juice, depending on your taste preference.
- ❖ Scoop the pesto into a container and refrigerate.
- ❖ STORAGE: Store the covered container in the refrigerator for up to 2 weeks. Pesto may be frozen for up to 6 months.

Nutrition: (¼ cup): Total calories: 231; Total fat: 22g; Saturated fat: 3g; Sodium: 178mg; Carbohydrates: 6g; Fiber: 3g; Protein: 4g

260) SAUTÉED KALE AND GARLIC WITH LEMON

Cooking Time: 7 Minutes   **Servings: 4**

Ingredients:

- ✓ 1 tbsp olive oil
- ✓ 3 bunches kale, stemmed and roughly chopped
- ✓ 2 tsp chopped garlic
- ✓ ¼ tsp kosher salt
- ✓ 1 tbsp freshly squeezed lemon juice

Directions:

- ❖ Heat the oil in a -inch skillet over medium-high heat. Once the oil is shimmering, add as much kale as will fit in the pan. You will probably only fit half the leaves into the pan at first. Mix the kale with tongs so that the leaves are coated with oil and start to wilt. As the kale wilts, keep adding more of the raw kale, continuing to use tongs to mix. Once all the kale is in the pan, add the garlic and salt and continue to cook until the kale is tender. Total cooking time from start to finish should be about 7 minutes.
- ❖ Mix the lemon juice into the kale. Add additional salt and/or lemon juice if necessary. Place 1 cup of kale in each of 4 containers and refrigerate.
- ❖ STORAGE: Store covered containers in the refrigerator for up to 5 days

Nutrition: Total calories: 8 Total fat: 1g; Saturated fat: <1g; Sodium: 214mg; Carbohydrates: 17g; Fiber: 6g; Protein: 6g

261) CREAMY POLENTA AND CHIVES WITH PARMESAN

Cooking Time: 15 Minutes   **Servings: 5**

Ingredients:

- ✓ 1 tsp olive oil
- ✓ ¼ cup minced shallot
- ✓ ½ cup white wine
- ✓ 3¼ cups water
- ✓ ¾ cup cornmeal
- ✓ 3 tbsp grated Parmesan cheese
- ✓ ½ tsp kosher salt
- ✓ ¼ cup chopped chives

Directions:

- ❖ Heat the oil in a saucepan over medium heat. Once the oil is shimmering, add the shallot and sauté for 2 minutes. Add the wine and water and bring to a boil.
- ❖ Pour the cornmeal in a thin, even stream into the liquid, stirring continuously until the mixture starts to thicken.
- ❖ Reduce the heat to low and continue to cook for 10 to 12 minutes, whisking every 1 to 2 minutes.
- ❖ Turn the heat off and stir in the cheese, salt, and chives. Cool.
- ❖ Place about ¾ cup of polenta in each of containers.
- ❖ STORAGE: Store covered containers in the refrigerator for up to 5 days.

Nutrition: Total calories: 110; Total fat: 3g; Saturated fat: 1g; Sodium: 29g; Carbohydrates: 16g; Fiber: 1g; Protein: 3g

262) SPECIAL MOCHA-NUT STUFFED DATES

Cooking Time: 10 Minutes   **Servings: 5**

Ingredients:

- ✓ 2 tbsp creamy, unsweetened, unsalted almond butter
- ✓ 1 tsp unsweetened cocoa powder
- ✓ 3 tbsp walnut pieces
- ✓ 2 tbsp water
- ✓ ¼ tsp honey
- ✓ ¾ tsp instant espresso powder
- ✓ 10 Medjool dates, pitted

Directions:

- ❖ In a small bowl, combine the almond butter, cocoa powder, and walnut pieces.
- ❖ Place the water in a small microwaveable mug and heat on high for 30 seconds. Add the honey and espresso powder to the water and stir to dissolve.
- ❖ Add the espresso water to the cocoa bowl and combine thoroughly until a creamy, thick paste forms.
- ❖ Stuff each pitted date with 1 tsp of mocha filling.
- ❖ Place 2 dates in each of small containers.
- ❖ STORAGE: Store covered containers in the refrigerator for up to 5 days.

Nutrition: Total calories: 205; Total fat: ; Saturated fat: 1g; Sodium: 1mg; Carbohydrates: 39g; Fiber: 4g; Protein: 3g

263) EGGPLANT DIP ROAST (BABA GHANOUSH)

Cooking Time: 45 Minutes   **Servings: 2 Cups**

Ingredients:

- ✓ 2 eggplants (close to 1 pound each)
- ✓ 1 tsp chopped garlic
- ✓ 3 tbsp unsalted tahini
- ✓ ¼ cup freshly squeezed lemon juice
- ✓ 1 tbsp olive oil
- ✓ ½ tsp kosher salt

Directions:

- ❖ Preheat the oven to 450°F and line a sheet pan with a silicone baking mat or parchment paper.
- ❖ Prick the eggplants in many places with a fork, place on the sheet pan, and roast in the oven until extremely soft, about 45 minutes. The eggplants should look like they are deflating.
- ❖ When the eggplants are cool, cut them open and scoop the flesh into a

large bowl. You may need to use your hands to pull the flesh away from the skin. Discard the skin. Mash the flesh very well with a fork.

❖ Add the garlic, tahini, lemon juice, oil, and salt. Taste and adjust the seasoning with additional lemon juice, salt, or tahini if needed.

❖ Scoop the dip into a container and refrigerate.

❖ STORAGE: Store the covered container in the refrigerator for up to 5 days.

Nutrition: (¼ cup): Total calories: 8 Total fat: 5g; Saturated fat: 1g; Sodium: 156mg; Carbohydrates: 10g; Fiber: 4g; Protein: 2g

264) DELICIOUS HONEY-LEMON VINAIGRETTE

Cooking Time: 5 Minutes   **Servings:** ½ Cup

Ingredients:

- ✓ 2 tsp Dijon mustard
- ✓ ⅛ tsp kosher salt
- ✓ ¼ cup olive oil

- ✓ ¼ cup freshly squeezed lemon juice
- ✓ 1 tsp honey

Directions:

- ❖ Place the lemon juice, honey, mustard, and salt in a small bowl and whisk to combine.
- ❖ Whisk in the oil, pouring it into the bowl in a thin steam.
- ❖ Pour the vinaigrette into a container and refrigerate.
- ❖ STORAGE: Store the covered container in the refrigerator for up to 2 weeks. Allow the vinaigrette to come to room temperature and shake before serving.

Nutrition: (2 tbsp): Total calories: 131; Total fat: 14g; Saturated fat: 2g; Sodium: 133mg; Carbohydrates: 3g; Fiber: <1g; Protein: <1g

265) SPANISH-STYLE ROMESCO SAUCE

Cooking Time: 10 Minutes   **Servings:** 1⅔ Cups

Ingredients:

- ✓ 1 tsp smoked paprika
- ✓ ½ tsp kosher salt
- ✓ Pinch cayenne pepper
- ✓ 2 tsp red wine vinegar
- ✓ 2 tbsp olive oil

- ✓ ½ cup raw, unsalted almonds
- ✓ 4 medium garlic cloves (do not peel)
- ✓ 1 (12-ounce) jar of roasted red peppers, drained
- ✓ ½ cup canned diced fire-roasted tomatoes, drained

Directions:

- ❖ Preheat the oven to 350°F.
- ❖ Place the almonds and garlic cloves on a sheet pan and toast in the oven for 10 minutes. Remove from the oven and peel the garlic when cool enough to handle.
- ❖ Place the almonds in the bowl of a food processor. Process the almonds until they resemble coarse sand, to 45 seconds. Add the garlic, peppers, tomatoes, paprika, salt, and cayenne. Blend until smooth.
- ❖ Once the mixture is smooth, add the vinegar and oil and blend until well combined. Taste and add more vinegar or salt if needed.
- ❖ Scoop the romesco sauce into a container and refrigerate.
- ❖ STORAGE: Store the covered container in the refrigerator for up to 7 days.

Nutrition: (⅓ cup): Total calories: 158; Total fat: 13g; Saturated fat: 1g; Sodium: 292mg; Carbohydrates: 10g; Fiber: 3g; Protein: 4g

266) CARDAMOM MASCARPONE AND STRAWBERRIES

Cooking Time: 10 Minutes   **Servings:** 4

Ingredients:

- ✓ ¼ tsp ground cardamom
- ✓ 2 tbsp milk
- ✓ 1 pound strawberries (should be 24 strawberries in the pack)

- ✓ 1 (8-ounce) container mascarpone cheese
- ✓ 2 tsp honey

Directions:

- ❖ Combine the mascarpone, honey, cardamom, and milk in a medium mixing bowl.
- ❖ Mix the ingredients with a spoon until super creamy, about 30 seconds.
- ❖ Place 6 strawberries and 2 tbsp of the mascarpone mixture in each of 4 containers.
- ❖ STORAGE: Store covered containers in the refrigerator for up to 5 days.

Nutrition: Total calories: 289; Total fat: 2; Saturated fat: 10g; Sodium: 26mg; Carbohydrates: 11g; Fiber: 3g; Protein: 1g

267) SWEET SPICY GREEN PUMPKIN SEEDS

Cooking Time: 15 Minutes   **Servings:** 2 Cups

Ingredients:

- ✓ 1 tbsp chili powder
- ✓ ¼ tsp cayenne pepper
- ✓ 1 tsp ground cinnamon
- ✓ ¼ tsp kosher salt

- ✓ 2 cups raw green pumpkin seeds (pepitas)
- ✓ 1 egg white, beaten until frothy
- ✓ 3 tbsp honey

Directions:

- ❖ Preheat the oven to 350°F. Line a sheet pan with a silicone baking mat or parchment paper.
- ❖ In a medium bowl, mix all the ingredients until the seeds are well coated. Place on the lined sheet pan in a single, even layer.
- ❖ Bake for 15 minutes. Cool the seeds on the sheet pan, then peel clusters from the baking mat and break apart into small pieces.

- ❖ Place ¼ cup of seeds in each of 8 small containers or resealable sandwich bags.
- ❖ STORAGE: Store covered containers or resealable bags at room temperature for up to days.

Nutrition: (¼ cup): Total calories: 209; Total fat: 15g; Saturated fat: 3g; Sodium: 85mg; Carbohydrates: 11g; Fiber: 2g; Protein: 10g

268) **DELICIOUS RASPBERRY RED WINE SAUCE**

Cooking Time: 20 Minutes | **Servings: 1 Cup**

Ingredients:

- ✓ 2 tsp olive oil
- ✓ 2 tbsp finely chopped shallot
- ✓ 1½ cups frozen raspberries
- ✓ 1 cup dry, fruity red wine
- ✓ 1 tsp thyme leaves, roughly chopped
- ✓ 1 tsp honey
- ✓ ¼ tsp kosher salt
- ✓ ½ tsp unsweetened cocoa powder

Directions:

- ❖ In a -inch skillet, heat the oil over medium heat. Add the shallot and cook until soft, about 2 minutes.
- ❖ Add the raspberries, wine, thyme, and honey and cook on medium heat until reduced, about 15 minutes. Stir in the salt and cocoa powder.
- ❖ Transfer the sauce to a blender and blend until smooth. Depending on how much you can scrape out of your blender, this recipe makes ¾ to 1 cup of sauce.
- ❖ Scoop the sauce into a container and refrigerate.
- ❖ STORAGE: Store the covered container in the refrigerator for up to 7 days.

Nutrition: (¼ cup): Total calories: 107; Total fat: 3g; Saturated fat: <1g; Sodium: 148mg; Carbohydrates: 1g; Fiber: 4g; Protein: 1g

269) **ANTIPASTO SHRIMP SKEWERS**

Cooking Time: 10 Minutes | **Servings: 4**

Ingredients:

- ✓ 16 pitted kalamata or green olives
- ✓ 16 fresh mozzarella balls (ciliegine)
- ✓ 16 cherry tomatoes
- ✓ 16 medium (41 to 50 per pound) precooked peeled, deveined shrimp
- ✓ 8 (8-inch) wooden or metal skewers

Directions:

- ❖ Alternate 2 olives, 2 mozzarella balls, 2 cherry tomatoes, and 2 shrimp on 8 skewers.
- ❖ Place skewers in each of 4 containers.
- ❖ STORAGE: Store covered containers in the refrigerator for up to 4 days.

Nutrition: Total calories: 108; Total fat: 6g; Saturated fat: 1g; Sodium: 328mg; Carbohydrates: ; Fiber: 1g; Protein: 9g

270) **SMOKED PAPRIKA WITH OLIVE OIL–MARINATED CARROTS**

Cooking Time: 5 Minutes | **Servings: 4**

Ingredients:

- ✓ 1 (1-pound) bag baby carrots (not the petite size)
- ✓ 2 tbsp olive oil
- ✓ 2 tbsp red wine vinegar
- ✓ ¼ tsp garlic powder
- ✓ ¼ tsp ground cumin
- ✓ ¼ tsp smoked paprika
- ✓ ⅛ tsp red pepper flakes
- ✓ ¼ cup chopped parsley
- ✓ ¼ tsp kosher salt

Directions:

- ❖ Pour enough water into a saucepan to come ¼ inch up the sides. Turn the heat to high, bring the water to a boil, add the carrots, and cover with a lid. Steam the carrots for 5 minutes, until crisp tender.
- ❖ After the carrots have cooled, mix with the oil, vinegar, garlic powder, cumin, paprika, red pepper, parsley, and salt.
- ❖ Place ¾ cup of carrots in each of 4 containers.
- ❖ STORAGE: Store covered containers in the refrigerator for up to 5 days.

Nutrition: Total calories: 109; Total fat: 7g; Saturated fat: 1g; Sodium: 234mg; Carbohydrates: 11g; Fiber: 3g; Protein: 2g

271) **GREEK TZATZIKI SAUCE**

Cooking Time: 15 Minutes | **Servings: 2½ Cups**

Ingredients:

- ✓ 1 English cucumber
- ✓ 2 cups low-fat (2%) plain Greek yogurt
- ✓ 1 tbsp olive oil
- ✓ 2 tsp freshly squeezed lemon juice
- ✓ ½ tsp chopped garlic
- ✓ ½ tsp kosher salt
- ✓ ⅛ tsp freshly ground black pepper
- ✓ 2 tbsp chopped fresh dill
- ✓ 2 tbsp chopped fresh mint

Directions:

- ❖ Place a sieve over a medium bowl. Grate the cucumber, with the skin, over the sieve. Press the grated cucumber into the sieve with the flat surface of a spatula to press as much liquid out as possible.
- ❖ In a separate medium bowl, place the yogurt, oil, lemon juice, garlic, salt, pepper, dill, and mint and stir to combine.
- ❖ Press on the cucumber one last time, then add it to the yogurt mixture. Stir to combine. Taste and add more salt and lemon juice if necessary.
- ❖ Scoop the sauce into a container and refrigerate.
- ❖ STORAGE: Store the covered container in the refrigerator for up to days.

Nutrition: (¼ cup): Total calories: 51; Total fat: 2g; Saturated fat: 1g; Sodium: 137mg; Carbohydrates: 3g; Fiber: <1g; Protein: 5g

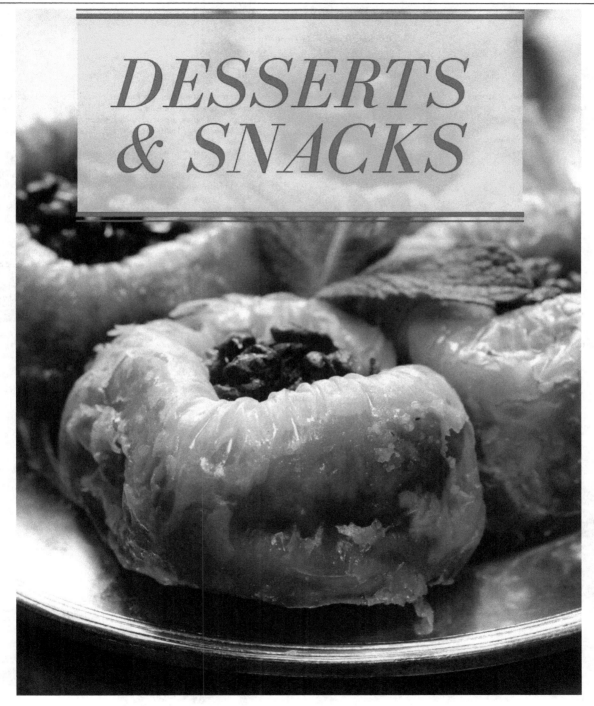

DESSERTS & SNACKS

272) CHERRY BROWNIES AND WALNUTS

Cooking Time: 25 To 30 Minutes **Servings: 9**

Ingredients:

- 9 fresh cherries that are stemmed and pitted or 9 frozen cherries
- ½ cup sugar or sweetener substitute
- ¼ cup extra virgin olive oil
- 1 tsp vanilla extract
- ¼ tsp sea salt
- ½ cup whole-wheat pastry flour
- ¼ tsp baking powder
- ⅓ cup walnuts, chopped
- 2 eggs
- ½ cup plain Greek yogurt
- ⅓ cup cocoa powder, unsweetened

Directions:

- Make sure one of the metal racks in your oven is set in the middle.
- Turn the temperature on your oven to 375 degrees Fahrenheit.
- Using cooking spray, grease a 9-inch square pan.
- Take a large bowl and add the oil and sugar or sweetener substitute. Whisk the ingredients well.
- Add the eggs and use a mixer to beat the ingredients together.
- Pour in the yogurt and continue to beat the mixture until it is smooth.
- Take a medium bowl and combine the cocoa powder, flour, sea salt, and baking powder by whisking them together.
- Combine the powdered ingredients into the wet ingredients and use your electronic mixer to incorporate the ingredients together thoroughly.
- Add in the walnuts and stir.
- Pour the mixture into the pan.
- Sprinkle the cherries on top and push them into the batter. You can use any design, but it is best to make three rows and three columns with the cherries. This ensures that each piece of the brownie will have one cherry.
- Put the batter into the oven and turn your timer to 20 minutes.
- Check that the brownies are done using the toothpick test before removing them from the oven. Push the toothpick into the middle of the brownies and once it comes out clean, remove the brownies.
- Let the brownies cool for 5 to 10 minutes before cutting and serving.

Nutrition: calories: 225, fats: 10 grams, carbohydrates: 30 grams, protein: 5 grams

273) SPECIAL FRUIT DIP

Cooking Time: 10 To 15 Minutes **Servings: 10**

Ingredients:

- ¼ cup coconut milk, full-fat is best
- ¼ cup vanilla yogurt
- ⅓ cup marshmallow creme
- 1 cup cream cheese, set at room temperature
- 2 tbsp maraschino cherry juice

Directions:

- In a large bowl, add the coconut milk, vanilla yogurt, marshmallow creme, cream cheese, and cherry juice.
- Using an electric mixer, set to low speed and blend the ingredients together until the fruit dip is smooth.
- Serve the dip with some of your favorite fruits and enjoy!

Nutrition: calories: 110, fats: 11 grams, carbohydrates: 3 grams, protein: 3 grams

274) DELICIOUS LEMONY TREAT

Cooking Time: 30 Minutes   **Servings:** 4

Ingredients:

- ✓ 1 lemon, medium in size
- ✓ 1 ½ tsp cornstarch
- ✓ 1 cup Greek yogurt, plain is best
- ✓ Fresh fruit
- ✓ ¼ cup cold water
- ✓ ⅔ cup heavy whipped cream
- ✓ 3 tbsp honey
- ✓ Optional: mint leaves

Directions:

- ❖ Take a large glass bowl and your metal, electric mixer and set them in the refrigerator so they can chill.
- ❖ In a separate bowl, add the yogurt and set that in the fridge.
- ❖ Zest the lemon into a medium bowl that is microwavable.
- ❖ Cut the lemon in half and then squeeze 1 tbsp of lemon juice into the bowl.
- ❖ Combine the cornstarch and water. Mix the ingredients thoroughly.
- ❖ Pour in the honey and whisk the ingredients together.
- ❖ Put the mixture into the microwave for 1 minute on high.
- ❖ Once the microwave stops, remove the mixture and stir.
- ❖ Set it back into the microwave for 15 to 30 seconds or until the mixture starts to bubble and thicken.
- ❖ Take the bowl of yogurt from the fridge and pour in the warm mixture while whisking.
- ❖ Put the yogurt mixture back into the fridge.
- ❖ Take the large bowl and beaters out of the fridge.
- ❖ Put your electronic mixer together and pour the whipped cream into the chilled bowl.
- ❖ Beat the cream until soft peaks start to form. This can take up to 3 minutes, depending on how fresh your cream is.
- ❖ Remove the yogurt from the fridge.
- ❖ Fold the yogurt into the cream using a rubber spatula. Remember to lift and turn the mixture so it doesn't deflate.
- ❖ Place back into the fridge until you are serving the dessert or for 15 minutes. The dessert should not be in the fridge for longer than 1 hour.
- ❖ When you serve the lemony goodness, you will spoon it into four dessert dishes and drizzle with extra honey or even melt some chocolate to drizzle on top.
- ❖ Add a little fresh mint and enjoy!

Nutrition: calories: 241, fats: 16 grams, carbohydrates: 21 grams, protein: 7 grams

275) MELON AND GINGER

Cooking Time: 10 To 15 Minutes   **Servings:** 4

Ingredients:

- ✓ ½ cantaloupe, cut into 1-inch chunks
- ✓ 2 cups of watermelon, cut into 1-inch chunks
- ✓ 2 cups honeydew melon, cut into 1-inch chunks
- ✓ 2 tbsp of raw honey
- ✓ Ginger, 2 inches in size, peeled, grated, and preserve the juice

Directions:

- ❖ In a large bowl, combine your cantaloupe, honeydew melon, and watermelon. Gently mix the ingredients.
- ❖ Combine the ginger juice and stir.
- ❖ Drizzle on the honey, serve, and enjoy! You can also chill the mixture for up to an hour before serving.

Nutrition: calories: 91, fats: 0 grams, carbohydrates: 23 grams, protein: 1 gram.

276) DELICIOUS ALMOND SHORTBREAD COOKIES

Cooking Time: 25 Minutes   **Servings: 16**

Ingredients:

- ✓ ½ cup coconut oil
- ✓ 1 tsp vanilla extract
- ✓ 2 egg yolks
- ✓ 1 tbsp brandy
- ✓ 1 cup powdered sugar
- ✓ 1 cup finely ground almonds
- ✓ 3 ½ cups cake flour
- ✓ ½ cup almond butter
- ✓ 1 tbsp water or rose flower water

Directions:

- ❖ In a large bowl, combine the coconut oil, powdered sugar, and butter. If the butter is not soft, you want to wait until it softens up. Use an electric mixer to beat the ingredients together at high speed.
- ❖ In a small bowl, add the egg yolks, brandy, water, and vanilla extract. Whisk well.
- ❖ Fold the egg yolk mixture into the large bowl.
- ❖ Add the flour and almonds. Fold and mix with a wooden spoon.
- ❖ Place the mixture into the fridge for at least 1 hour and 30 minutes.
- ❖ Preheat your oven to 325 degrees Fahrenheit.
- ❖ Take the mixture, which now looks like dough, and divide it into 1-inch balls.
- ❖ With a piece of parchment paper on a baking sheet, arrange the cookies and flatten them with a fork or your fingers.
- ❖ Place the cookies in the oven for 13 minutes, but watch them so they don't burn.
- ❖ Transfer the cookies onto a rack to cool for a couple of minutes before enjoying!

Nutrition: calories: 250, fats: 14 grams, carbohydrates: 30 grams, protein: 3 grams

277) CLASSIC CHOCOLATE FRUIT KEBABS

Cooking Time: 30 Minutes   **Servings: 6**

Ingredients:

- ✓ 24 blueberries
- ✓ 12 strawberries with the green leafy top part removed
- ✓ 12 green or red grapes, seedless
- ✓ 12 pitted cherries
- ✓ 8 ounces chocolate

Directions:

- ❖ Line a baking sheet with a piece of parchment paper and place 6, -inch long wooden skewers on top of the paper.
- ❖ Start by threading a piece of fruit onto the skewers. You can create and follow any pattern that you like with the ingredients. An example pattern is 1 strawberry, 1 cherry, blueberries, 2 grapes. Repeat the pattern until all of the fruit is on the skewers.
- ❖ In a saucepan on medium heat, melt the chocolate. Stir continuously until the chocolate has melted completely.
- ❖ Carefully scoop the chocolate into a plastic sandwich bag and twist the bag closed starting right above the chocolate.
- ❖ Snip the corner of the bag with scissors.
- ❖ Drizzle the chocolate onto the kebabs by squeezing it out of the bag.
- ❖ Put the baking pan into the freezer for 20 minutes.
- ❖ Serve and enjoy!

Nutrition: calories: 254, fats: 15 grams, carbohydrates: 28 grams, protein: 4 grams 278)

279) PEACHES AND BLUE CHEESE CREAM

Cooking Time: 20 Hours 10 Minutes   **Servings: 4**

Ingredients:

- ✓ 4 peaches
- ✓ 1 cinnamon stick
- ✓ 4 ounces sliced blue cheese
- ✓ ⅓ cup orange juice, freshly squeezed is best
- ✓ 3 whole cloves
- ✓ 1 tsp of orange zest, taken from the orange peel
- ✓ ¼ tsp cardamom pods
- ✓ ⅔ cup red wine
- ✓ 2 tbsp honey, raw or your preferred variety
- ✓ 1 vanilla bean
- ✓ 1 tsp allspice berries
- ✓ 4 tbsp dried cherries

Directions:

- ❖ Set a saucepan on top of your stove range and add the cinnamon stick, cloves, orange juice, cardamom, vanilla, allspice, red wine, and orange zest. Whisk the ingredients well. Add your peaches to the mixture and poach them for hours or until they become soft.
- ❖ Take a spoon to remove the peaches and boil the rest of the liquid to make the syrup. You want the liquid to reduce itself by at least half.
- ❖ While the liquid is boiling, combine the dried cherries, blue cheese, and honey into a bowl. Once your peaches are cooled, slice them into halves.
- ❖ Top each peach with the blue cheese mixture and then drizzle the liquid onto the top. Serve and enjoy!

Nutrition: calories: 211, fats: 24 grams, carbohydrates: 15 grams, protein: 6 grams

280)   MEDITERRANEAN-STYLE BLACKBERRY ICE CREAM

Cooking Time: 15 Minutes   **Servings: 6**

Ingredients:

- ✓ 1 tsp arrowroot powder
- ✓ ¼ tsp ground cloves
- ✓ 5 ounces sugar or sweetener substitute
- ✓ 1 pound heavy cream

- ✓ 3 egg yolks
- ✓ 1 container of Greek yogurt
- ✓ 1 pound mashed blackberries
- ✓ ½ tsp vanilla essence

Directions:

- ❖ In a small bowl, add the arrowroot powder and egg yolks. Whisk or beat them with an electronic mixture until they are well combined.
- ❖ Set a saucepan on top of your stove and turn your heat to medium.
- ❖ Add the heavy cream and bring it to a boil.
- ❖ Turn off the heat and add the egg mixture into the cream through folding.
- ❖ Turn the heat back on to medium and pour in the sugar. Cook the mixture for 10 minutes or until it starts to thicken.
- ❖ Remove the mixture from heat and place it in the fridge so it can completely cool. This should take about one hour.
- ❖ Once the mixture is cooled, add in the Greek yogurt, ground cloves, blackberries, and vanilla by folding in the ingredients.
- ❖ Transfer the ice cream into a container and place it in the freezer for at least two hours.
- ❖ Serve and enjoy!

Nutrition: calories: 402, fats: 20 grams, carbohydrates: 52 grams, protein: 8 grams

281)   CLASSIC STUFFED FIGS

Cooking Time: 20 Minutes   **Servings: 6**

Ingredients:

- ✓ 4 ounces goat cheese, divided
- ✓ 2 tbsp of raw honey

- ✓ 10 halved fresh figs
- ✓ 20 chopped almonds

Directions:

- ❖ Turn your oven to broiler mode and set it to a high temperature.
- ❖ Place your figs, cut side up, on a baking sheet. If you like to place a piece of parchment paper on top you can do this, but it is not necessary.
- ❖ Sprinkle each fig with half of the goat cheese.
- ❖ Add a tbsp of chopped almonds to each fig.
- ❖ Broil the figs for 3 to 4 minutes.
- ❖ Take them out of the oven and let them cool for 5 to 7 minutes.
- ❖ Sprinkle with the remaining goat cheese and honey.

Nutrition: calories: 209, fats: 9 grams, carbohydrates: 26 grams, protein: grams.

282)   CHIA PUDDING AND STRAWBERRIES

Cooking Time: 4 Hours 5 Minutes   **Servings: 4**

Ingredients:

- ✓ 2 cups unsweetened almond milk
- ✓ 1 tbsp vanilla extract
- ✓ 2 tbsp raw honey
- ✓ ¼ cup chia seeds
- ✓ 2 cups fresh and sliced strawberries

Directions:

- ❖ In a medium bowl, combine the honey, chia seeds, vanilla, and unsweetened almond milk. Mix well.
- ❖ Set the mixture in the refrigerator for at least 4 hours.
- ❖ When you serve the pudding, top it with strawberries. You can even create a design in a glass serving bowl or dessert dish by adding a little pudding on the bottom, a few strawberries, top the strawberries with some more pudding, and then top the dish with a few strawberries.

Nutrition: calories: 108, fats: grams, carbohydrates: 17 grams, protein: 3 grams

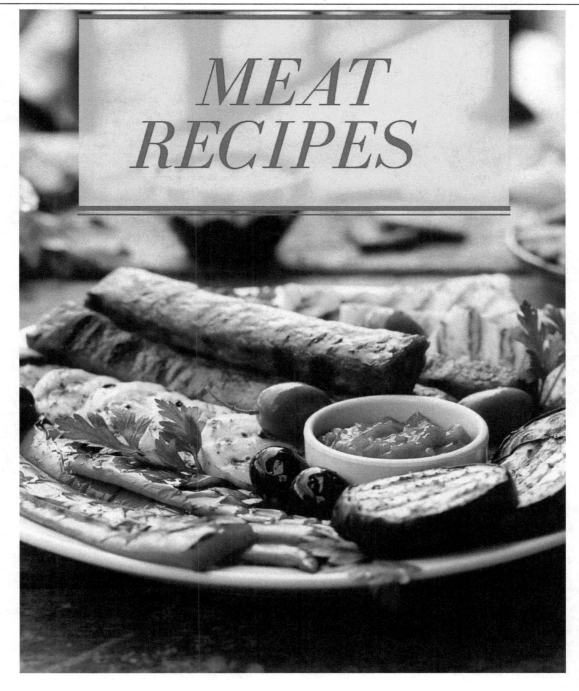

MEAT
RECIPES

283) CLASSIC AIOLI BAKED CHICKEN WINGS

Cooking Time: 35 Minutes   **Servings: 4**

Ingredients:

- ✓ 4 chicken wings
- ✓ 1 cup Halloumi cheese, cubed
- ✓ 1 tbsp garlic, finely minced
- ✓ 1 tbsp fresh lime juice
- ✓ 1 tbsp fresh coriander, chopped
- ✓ 6 black olives, pitted and halved
- ✓ 1 ½ tbsp butter
- ✓ 1 hard-boiled egg yolk
- ✓ 1 tbsp balsamic vinegar
- ✓ 1/2 cup extra-virgin olive oil
- ✓ 1/4 tsp flaky sea salt
- ✓ Sea salt and pepper, to season

Directions:

- ❖ In a saucepan, melt the butter until sizzling. Sear the chicken wings for 5 minutes per side. Season with salt and pepper to taste.
- ❖ Place the chicken wings on a parchment-lined baking pan
- ❖ Mix the egg yolk, garlic, lime juice, balsamic vinegar, olive oil, and salt in your blender until creamy, uniform and smooth.
- ❖ Spread the Aioli over the fried chicken. Now, scatter the coriander and black olives on top of the chicken wings.
- ❖ Bake in the preheated oven at 380 degrees F for 20 to 2minutes. Top with the cheese and bake an additional 5 minutes until hot and bubbly.
- ❖ Storing
- ❖ Place the chicken wings in airtight containers or Ziploc bags; keep in your refrigerator for up to 3 to 4 days.
- ❖ For freezing, place the chicken wings in airtight containers or heavy-duty freezer bags. Freeze up to 3 months. Once thawed in the refrigerator, heat in the preheated oven at 375 degrees F for 20 to 25 minutes or until heated through. Enjoy!

Nutrition: 562 Calories; 43.8g Fat; 2.1g Carbs; 40.8g Protein; 0.4g Fiber

284) SPECIAL SMOKED PORK SAUSAGE KETO BOMBS

Cooking Time: 15 Minutes   **Servings: 6**

Ingredients:

- ✓ 3/4 pound smoked pork sausage, ground
- ✓ 1 tsp ginger-garlic paste
- ✓ 2 tbsp scallions, minced
- ✓ 1 tbsp butter, room temperature
- ✓ 1 tomato, pureed
- ✓ 4 ounces mozzarella cheese, crumbled
- ✓ 2 tbsp flaxseed meal
- ✓ 8 ounces cream cheese, room temperature
- ✓ Sea salt and ground black pepper, to taste

Directions:

- ❖ Melt the butter in a frying pan over medium-high heat. Cook the sausage for about 4 minutes, crumbling with a spatula.
- ❖ Add in the ginger-garlic paste, scallions, and tomato; continue to cook over medium-low heat for a further 6 minutes. Stir in the remaining ingredients.
- ❖ Place the mixture in your refrigerator for 1 to 2 hours until firm. Roll the mixture into bite-sized balls.
- ❖ Storing
- ❖ Transfer the balls to the airtight containers and place in your refrigerator for up to 3 days.
- ❖ For freezing, place in a freezer safe containers and freeze up to 1 month. Enjoy!

Nutrition: 383 Calories; 32. Fat; 5.1g Carbs; 16.7g Protein; 1.7g Fiber

285) TURKEY MEATBALLS AND TANGY BASIL CHUTNEY

Cooking Time: 30 Minutes   **Servings: 6**

Ingredients:

- ✓ 2 tbsp sesame oil
- ✓ For the Meatballs:
- ✓ 1/2 cup Romano cheese, grated
- ✓ 1 tsp garlic, minced
- ✓ 1/2 tsp shallot powder
- ✓ 1/4 tsp dried thyme
- ✓ 1/2 tsp mustard seeds
- ✓ 2 small-sized eggs, lightly beaten
- ✓ 1 ½ pounds ground turkey
- ✓ 1/2 tsp sea salt
- ✓ 1/4 tsp ground black pepper, or more to taste
- ✓ 3 tbsp almond meal
- ✓ For the Basil Chutney:
- ✓ 2 tbsp fresh lime juice
- ✓ 1/4 cup fresh basil leaves
- ✓ 1/4 cup fresh parsley
- ✓ 1/2 cup cilantro leaves
- ✓ 1 tsp fresh ginger root, grated
- ✓ 2 tbsp olive oil
- ✓ 2 tbsp water
- ✓ 1 tbsp habanero chili pepper, deveined and minced

Directions:

- ❖ In a mixing bowl, combine all ingredients for the meatballs. Roll the mixture into meatballs and reserve.
- ❖ Heat the sesame oil in a frying pan over a moderate flame. Sear the meatballs for about 8 minutes until browned on all sides.
- ❖ Make the chutney by mixing all the ingredients in your blender or food processor.
- ❖ Storing
- ❖ Place the meatballs in airtight containers or Ziploc bags; keep in your refrigerator for up to 3 to 4 days.
- ❖ Freeze the meatballs in airtight containers or heavy-duty freezer bags. Freeze up to 3 to 4 months. To defrost, slowly reheat in a frying pan.
- ❖ Store the basil chutney in the refrigerator for up to a week. Bon appétit!

Nutrition: 390 Calories; 27.2g Fat; 1. Carbs; 37.4g Protein; 0.3g Fiber

286)   ROASTED CHICKEN AND CASHEW PESTO

Cooking Time: 35 Minutes   **Servings: 4**

Ingredients:

- ✓ 1 cup leeks, chopped
- ✓ 1 pound chicken legs, skinless
- ✓ Salt and ground black pepper, to taste
- ✓ 1/2 tsp red pepper flakes
- ✓ For the Cashew-Basil Pesto:

- ✓ 1/2 cup cashews
- ✓ 2 garlic cloves, minced
- ✓ 1/2 cup fresh basil leaves
- ✓ 1/2 cup Parmigiano-Reggiano cheese, preferably freshly grated
- ✓ 1/2 cup olive oil

Directions:

- ❖ Place the chicken legs in a parchment-lined baking pan. Season with salt and pepper, Then, scatter the leeks around the chicken legs.
- ❖ Roast in the preheated oven at 390 degrees F for 30 to 35 minutes, rotating the pan occasionally.
- ❖ Pulse the cashews, basil, garlic, and cheese in your blender until pieces are small. Continue blending while adding olive oil to the mixture. Mix until the desired consistency is reached.
- ❖ Storing
- ❖ Place the chicken in airtight containers or Ziploc bags; keep in your refrigerator for up 3 to 4 days.
- ❖ To freeze the chicken legs, place them in airtight containers or heavy-duty freezer bags. Freeze up to 3 months. Once thawed in the refrigerator, heat in the preheated oven at 375 degrees F for 20 to 25 minutes.
- ❖ Store your pesto in the refrigerator for up to a week. Bon appétit!

Nutrition: 5 Calories; 44.8g Fat; 5g Carbs; 38.7g Protein; 1g Fiber

287)   SPECIAL DUCK BREASTS IN BOOZY SAUCE

Cooking Time: 20 Minutes   **Servings: 4**

Ingredients:

- ✓ 1 ½ pounds duck breasts, butterflied
- ✓ 1 tbsp tallow, room temperature
- ✓ 1 ½ cups chicken consommé
- ✓ 3 tbsp soy sauce

- ✓ 2 ounces vodka
- ✓ 1/2 cup sour cream
- ✓ 4 scallion stalks, chopped
- ✓ Salt and pepper, to taste

Directions:

- ❖ Melt the tallow in a frying pan over medium-high flame. Sear the duck breasts for about 5 minutes, flipping them over occasionally to ensure even cooking.
- ❖ Add in the scallions, salt, pepper, chicken consommé, and soy sauce. Partially cover and continue to cook for a further 8 minutes.
- ❖ Add in the vodka and sour cream; remove from the heat and stir to combine well.
- ❖ Storing
- ❖ Place the duck breasts in airtight containers or Ziploc bags; keep in your refrigerator for up to 3 to 4 days.
- ❖ For freezing, place duck breasts in airtight containers or heavy-duty freezer bags. Freeze up to 2 to 3 months. Once thawed in the refrigerator, reheat in a saucepan. Bon appétit!

Nutrition: 351 Calories; 24. Fat; 6.6g Carbs; 22.1g Protein; 0.6g Fiber

288) WHITE CAULIFLOWER WITH CHICKEN CHOWDER

Cooking Time: 30 Minutes   **Servings: 6**

Ingredients:

- ✓ 1 cup leftover roast chicken breasts
- ✓ 1 head cauliflower, broken into small-sized florets
- ✓ Sea salt and ground white pepper, to taste
- ✓ 2 ½ cups water
- ✓ 3 cups chicken consommé
- ✓ 1 ¼ cups sour cream
- ✓ 1/2 stick butter
- ✓ 1/2 cup white onion, finely chopped
- ✓ 1 tsp fresh garlic, finely minced
- ✓ 1 celery, chopped

Directions:

- ❖ In a heavy bottomed pot, melt the butter over a moderate heat. Cook the onion, garlic and celery for about 5 minutes or until they've softened.
- ❖ Add in the salt, white pepper, water, chicken consommé, chicken, and cauliflower florets; bring to a boil. Reduce the temperature to simmer and continue to cook for 30 minutes.
- ❖ Puree the soup with an immersion blender. Fold in sour cream and stir to combine well.
- ❖ Storing
- ❖ Spoon your chowder into airtight containers or Ziploc bags; keep in your refrigerator for up to 3 to 4 days.
- ❖ For freezing, place your chowder in airtight containers. It will maintain the best quality for about 4 to months. Defrost in the refrigerator. Bon appétit!

Nutrition: 231 Calories; 18.2g Fat; 5.9g Carbs; 11.9g Protein; 1.4g Fiber

289) Taro Leaf with Chicken Soup

Cooking Time: 45 Minutes   **Servings: 4**

Ingredients:

- ✓ 1 pound whole chicken, boneless and chopped into small chunks
- ✓ 1/2 cup onions, chopped
- ✓ 1/2 cup rutabaga, cubed
- ✓ 2 carrots, peeled
- ✓ 2 celery stalks
- ✓ Salt and black pepper, to taste
- ✓ 1 cup chicken bone broth
- ✓ 1/2 tsp ginger-garlic paste
- ✓ 1/2 cup taro leaves, roughly chopped
- ✓ 1 tbsp fresh coriander, chopped
- ✓ 3 cups water
- ✓ 1 tsp paprika

Directions:

- ❖ Place all ingredients in a heavy-bottomed pot. Bring to a boil over the highest heat.
- ❖ Turn the heat to simmer. Continue to cook, partially covered, an additional 40 minutes.
- ❖ Storing
- ❖ Spoon the soup into four airtight containers or Ziploc bags; keep in your refrigerator for up to 3 to days.
- ❖ For freezing, place the soup in airtight containers. It will maintain the best quality for about to 6 months. Defrost in the refrigerator. Bon appétit!

Nutrition: 25Calories; 12.9g Fat; 3.2g Carbs; 35.1g Protein; 2.2g Fiber

290) CREAMY GREEK-STYLE SOUP

Cooking Time: 30 Minutes   **Servings: 4**

Ingredients:

- ✓ 1/2 stick butter
- ✓ 1/2 cup zucchini, diced
- ✓ 2 garlic cloves, minced
- ✓ 4 ½ cups roasted vegetable broth
- ✓ Sea salt and ground black pepper, to season
- ✓ 1 ½ cups leftover turkey, shredded
- ✓ 1/3 cup double cream
- ✓ 1/2 cup Greek-style yogurt

Directions:

- ❖ In a heavy-bottomed pot, melt the butter over medium-high heat. Once hot, cook the zucchini and garlic for 2 minutes until they are fragrant.
- ❖ Add in the broth, salt, black pepper, and leftover turkey. Cover and cook for minutes, stirring periodically.
- ❖ Then, fold in the cream and yogurt. Continue to cook for 5 minutes more or until thoroughly warmed.
- ❖ Storing
- ❖ Spoon the soup into four airtight containers or Ziploc bags; keep in your refrigerator for up to 3 to 4 days.
- ❖ For freezing, place the soup in airtight containers. It will maintain the best quality for about 4 to months. Defrost in the refrigerator. Enjoy!

Nutrition: 256 Calories; 18.8g Fat; 5.4g Carbs; 15.8g Protein; 0.2g Fiber

291) LOW-CARB PORK WRAPS

Cooking Time: 15 Minutes   **Servings: 4**

Ingredients:

- ✓ 1 pound ground pork
- ✓ 2 garlic cloves, finely minced
- ✓ 1 chili pepper, deveined and finely minced
- ✓ 1 tsp mustard powder
- ✓ 1 tbsp sunflower seeds
- ✓ 2 tbsp champagne vinegar
- ✓ 1 tbsp coconut aminos
- ✓ Celery salt and ground black pepper, to taste
- ✓ 2 scallion stalks, sliced
- ✓ 1 head lettuce

Directions:

- ❖ Sear the ground pork in the preheated pan for about 8 minutes. Stir in the garlic, chili pepper, mustard seeds, and sunflower seeds; continue to sauté for minute longer or until aromatic.
- ❖ Add in the vinegar, coconut aminos, salt, black pepper, and scallions. Stir to combine well.
- ❖ Storing
- ❖ Place the ground pork mixture in airtight containers or Ziploc bags; keep in your refrigerator for up to 3 to days.
- ❖ For freezing, place the ground pork mixture it in airtight containers or heavy-duty freezer bags. Freeze up to 2 to 3 months. Defrost in the refrigerator and reheat in the skillet.
- ❖ Add spoonfuls of the pork mixture to the lettuce leaves, wrap them and serve.

Nutrition: 281 Calories; 19.4g Fat; 5.1g Carbs; 22.1g Protein; 1.3g Fiber

292) MISSISSIPPI-STYLE PULLED PORK

Cooking Time: 6 Hours   **Servings:** 4

Ingredients:

- ✓ 1 ½ pounds pork shoulder
- ✓ 1 tbsp liquid smoke sauce
- ✓ 1 tsp chipotle powder
- ✓ Au Jus gravy seasoning packet
- ✓ 2 onions, cut into wedges
- ✓ Kosher salt and freshly ground black pepper, taste

Directions:

- ❖ Mix the liquid smoke sauce, chipotle powder, Au Jus gravy seasoning packet, salt and pepper. Rub the spice mixture into the pork on all sides.
- ❖ Wrap in plastic wrap and let it marinate in your refrigerator for 3 hours.
- ❖ Prepare your grill for indirect heat. Place the pork butt roast on the grate over a drip pan and top with onions; cover the grill and cook for about 6 hours.
- ❖ Transfer the pork to a cutting board. Now, shred the meat into bite-sized pieces using two forks.
- ❖ Storing
- ❖ Divide the pork between four airtight containers or Ziploc bags; keep in your refrigerator for up to 3 to 5 days.
- ❖ For freezing, place the pork in airtight containers or heavy-duty freezer bags. Freeze up to 4 months. Defrost in the refrigerator. Bon appétit!

Nutrition: 350 Calories; 11g Fat; 5g Carbs; 53.6g Protein; 2.2g Fiber

293) SPICY WITH CHEESY TURKEY DIP

Cooking Time: 25 Minutes   **Servings:** 4

Ingredients:

- ✓ 1 Fresno chili pepper, deveined and minced
- ✓ 1 ½ cups Ricotta cheese, creamed, 4% fat, softened
- ✓ 1/4 cup sour cream
- ✓ 1 tbsp butter, room temperature
- ✓ 1 shallot, chopped
- ✓ 1 tsp garlic, pressed
- ✓ 1 pound ground turkey
- ✓ 1/2 cup goat cheese, shredded
- ✓ Salt and black pepper, to taste
- ✓ 1 ½ cups Gruyère, shredded

Directions:

- ❖ Melt the butter in a frying pan over a moderately high flame. Now, sauté the onion and garlic until they have softened.
- ❖ Stir in the ground turkey and continue to cook until it is no longer pink.
- ❖ Transfer the sautéed mixture to a lightly greased baking dish. Add in Ricotta, sour cream, goat cheese, salt, pepper, and chili pepper.
- ❖ Top with the shredded Gruyère cheese. Bake in the preheated oven at 350 degrees F for about 20 minutes or until hot and bubbly in top.
- ❖ Storing
- ❖ Place your dip in an airtight container; keep in your refrigerator for up 3 to 4 days. Enjoy!

Nutrition: 284 Calories; 19g Fat; 3.2g Carbs; 26. Protein; 1.6g Fiber

294) TURKEY CHORIZO AND BOK CHOY

Cooking Time: 50 Minutes   **Servings:** 4

Ingredients:

- ✓ 4 mild turkey Chorizo, sliced
- ✓ 1/2 cup full-fat milk
- ✓ 6 ounces Gruyère cheese, preferably freshly grated
- ✓ 1 yellow onion, chopped
- ✓ Coarse salt and ground black pepper, to taste
- ✓ 1 pound Bok choy, tough stem ends trimmed
- ✓ 1 cup cream of mushroom soup
- ✓ 1 tbsp lard, room temperature

Directions:

- ❖ Melt the lard in a nonstick skillet over a moderate flame; cook the Chorizo sausage for about 5 minutes, stirring occasionally to ensure even cooking; reserve.
- ❖ Add in the onion, salt, pepper, Bok choy, and cream of mushroom soup. Continue to cook for 4 minutes longer or until the vegetables have softened.
- ❖ Spoon the mixture into a lightly oiled casserole dish. Top with the reserved Chorizo.
- ❖ In a mixing bowl, thoroughly combine the milk and cheese. Pour the cheese mixture over the sausage.
- ❖ Cover with foil and bake at 36degrees F for about 35 minutes.

- ❖ Storing
- ❖ Cut your casserole into four portions. Place each portion in an airtight container; keep in your refrigerator for 3 to 4 days.
- ❖ For freezing, wrap your portions tightly with heavy-duty aluminum foil or freezer wrap. Freeze up to 1 to 2 months. Defrost in the refrigerator. Enjoy!

Nutrition: 18Calories; 12g Fat; 2.6g Carbs; 9.4g Protein; 1g Fiber

295) FLATBREAD AND CHICKEN LIVER PÂTÉ

Cooking Time: 2 Hours 15 Minutes   **Servings:** 4

Ingredients:

- ✓ 1 yellow onion, finely chopped
- ✓ 10 ounces chicken livers
- ✓ 1/2 tsp Mediterranean seasoning blend
- ✓ 4 tbsp olive oil
- ✓ 1 garlic clove, minced

- ✓ For Flatbread:
- ✓ 1 cup lukewarm water
- ✓ 1/2 stick butter
- ✓ 1/2 cup flax meal
- ✓ 1 ½ tbsp psyllium husks
- ✓ 1 ¼ cups almond flour

Directions:

- ❖ Pulse the chicken livers along with the seasoning blend, olive oil, onion and garlic in your food processor; reserve.
- ❖ Mix the dry ingredients for the flatbread. Mix in all the wet ingredients. Whisk to combine well.
- ❖ Let it stand at room temperature for 2 hours. Divide the dough into 8 balls and roll them out on a flat surface.
- ❖ In a lightly greased pan, cook your flatbread for 1 minute on each side or until golden.
- ❖ Storing
- ❖ Wrap the chicken liver pate in foil before packing it into airtight containers; keep in your refrigerator for up to 7 days.
- ❖ For freezing, place the chicken liver pate in airtight containers or heavy-duty freezer bags. Freeze up to 2 months. Defrost overnight in the refrigerator.
- ❖ As for the keto flatbread, wrap them in foil before packing them into airtight containers; keep in your refrigerator for up to 4 days.
- ❖ Bon appétit!

Nutrition: 395 Calories; 30.2g Fat; 3.6g Carbs; 17.9g Protein; 0.5g Fiber

296) SATURDAY CHICKEN WITH CAULIFLOWER SALAD

Cooking Time: 20 Minutes   **Servings:** 2

Ingredients:

- ✓ 1 tsp hot paprika
- ✓ 2 tbsp fresh basil, snipped
- ✓ 1/2 cup mayonnaise
- ✓ 1 tsp mustard
- ✓ 2 tsp butter
- ✓ 2 chicken wings

- ✓ 1/2 cup cheddar cheese, shredded
- ✓ Sea salt and ground black pepper, to taste
- ✓ 2 tbsp dry sherry
- ✓ 1 shallot, finely minced
- ✓ 1/2 head of cauliflower

Directions:

- ❖ Boil the cauliflower in a pot of salted water until it has softened; cut into small florets and place in a salad bowl.
- ❖ Melt the butter in a saucepan over medium-high heat. Cook the chicken for about 8 minutes or until the skin is crisp and browned. Season with hot paprika salt, and black pepper.
- ❖ Whisk the mayonnaise, mustard, dry sherry, and shallot and dress your salad. Top with cheddar cheese and fresh basil.
- ❖ Storing
- ❖ Place the chicken wings in airtight containers or Ziploc bags; keep in your refrigerator for up 3 to 4 days.
- ❖ Keep the cauliflower salad in your refrigerator for up 3 days.
- ❖ For freezing, place the chicken wings in airtight containers or heavy-duty freezer bags. Freeze up to 3 months. Once thawed in the refrigerator, reheat in a saucepan until thoroughly warmed.

Nutrition: 444 Calories; 36g Fat; 5.7g Carbs; 20.6g Protein; 4.3g Fiber

297) SPECIAL KANSAS-STYLE MEATLOAF

Cooking Time: 1 Hour 10 Minutes   **Servings:** 8

Ingredients:

- ✓ 2 pounds ground pork
- ✓ 2 eggs, beaten
- ✓ 1/2 cup onions, chopped
- ✓ 1/2 cup marinara sauce, bottled
- ✓ 8 ounces Colby cheese, shredded
- ✓ 1 tsp granulated garlic

- ✓ Sea salt and freshly ground black pepper, to taste
- ✓ 1 tsp lime zest
- ✓ 1 tsp mustard seeds
- ✓ 1/2 cup tomato puree
- ✓ 1 tbsp Erythritol

Directions:

- ❖ Mix the ground pork with the eggs, onions, marinara salsa, cheese, granulated garlic, salt, pepper, lime zest, and mustard seeds; mix to combine.
- ❖ Press the mixture into a lightly-greased loaf pan. Mix the tomato paste with the Erythritol and spread the mixture over the top of your meatloaf.
- ❖ Bake in the preheated oven at 5 degrees F for about 1 hour 10 minutes, rotating the pan halfway through the cook time. Storing Wrap your meatloaf tightly with heavy-duty aluminum foil or plastic wrap. Then, keep in your refrigerator for up to 3 to 4 days.
- ❖ For freezing, wrap your meatloaf tightly to prevent freezer burn. Freeze up to 3 to 4 months. Defrost in the refrigerator. Bon appétit!

Nutrition: 318 Calories; 14. Fat; 6.2g Carbs; 39.3g Protein; 0.3g Fiber

298) ORIGINAL TURKEY KEBABS

Cooking Time: 30 Minutes   **Servings: 6**

Ingredients:

- ✓ 1 ½ pounds turkey breast, cubed
- ✓ 3 Spanish peppers, sliced
- ✓ 2 zucchinis, cut into thick slices

- ✓ 1 onion, cut into wedges
- ✓ 2 tbsp olive oil, room temperature
- ✓ 1 tbsp dry ranch seasoning

Directions:

- ❖ Thread the turkey pieces and vegetables onto bamboo skewers. Sprinkle the skewers with dry ranch seasoning and olive oil.
- ❖ Grill your kebabs for about 10 minutes, turning them periodically to ensure even cooking.
- ❖ Storing
- ❖ Wrap your kebabs in foil before packing them into airtight containers; keep in your refrigerator for up to 3 to days.
- ❖ For freezing, place your kebabs in airtight containers or heavy-duty freezer bags. Freeze up to 2-3 months. Defrost in the refrigerator. Bon appétit!

Nutrition: 2 Calories; 13.8g Fat; 6.7g Carbs; 25.8g Protein; 1.2g Fiber

299) ORIGINAL MEXICAN-STYLE TURKEY BACON BITES

Cooking Time: 5 Minutes   **Servings: 4**

Ingredients:

- ✓ 4 ounces turkey bacon, chopped
- ✓ 4 ounces Neufchatel cheese
- ✓ 1 tbsp butter, cold

- ✓ 1 jalapeno pepper, deveined and minced
- ✓ 1 tsp Mexican oregano
- ✓ 2 tbsp scallions, finely chopped

Directions:

- ❖ Thoroughly combine all ingredients in a mixing bowl.
- ❖ Roll the mixture into 8 balls.
- ❖ Storing
- ❖ Divide the turkey bacon bites between two airtight containers or Ziploc bags; keep in your refrigerator for up 3 to days.

Nutrition: 19Calories; 16.7g Fat; 2.2g Carbs; 8.8g Protein; 0.3g Fiber

300) ORIGINAL MUFFINS WITH GROUND PORK

Cooking Time: 25 Minutes   **Servings: 6**

Ingredients:

- ✓ 1 stick butter
- ✓ 3 large eggs, lightly beaten
- ✓ 2 tbsp full-fat milk
- ✓ 1/2 tsp ground cardamom
- ✓ 3 ½ cups almond flour
- ✓ 2 tbsp flaxseed meal
- ✓ 1 tsp baking powder
- ✓ 2 cups ground pork
- ✓ Salt and pepper, to your liking
- ✓ 1/2 tsp dried basil

Directions:

- ❖ In the preheated frying pan, cook the ground pork until the juices run clear, approximately 5 minutes.
- ❖ Add in the remaining ingredients and stir until well combined.
- ❖ Spoon the mixture into lightly greased muffin cups. Bake in the preheated oven at 5 degrees F for about 17 minutes.
- ❖ Allow your muffins to cool down before unmolding and storing.
- ❖ Storing
- ❖ Place your muffins in the airtight containers or Ziploc bags; keep in the refrigerator for a week.
- ❖ For freezing, divide your muffins among Ziploc bags and freeze up to 3 months. Defrost in your microwave for a couple of minutes. Bon appétit!

Nutrition: 330 Calories; 30.3g Fat; 2.3g Carbs; 19g Protein; 1.2g Fiber

301) CLASSIC TURKEY WINGS WITH GRAVY SAUCE

Cooking Time: 6 Hours **Servings:** 6

Ingredients:

- 2 pounds turkey wings
- 1/2 tsp cayenne pepper
- 4 garlic cloves, sliced
- 1 large onion, chopped
- Salt and pepper, to taste
- 1 tsp dried marjoram
- 1 tbsp butter, room temperature
- 1 tbsp Dijon mustard
- For the Gravy:
- 1 cup double cream
- Salt and black pepper, to taste
- 1/2 stick butter
- 3/4 tsp guar gum

Directions:

- ❖ Rub the turkey wings with the Dijon mustard and tbsp of butter. Preheat a grill pan over medium-high heat.
- ❖ Sear the turkey wings for 10 minutes on all sides.
- ❖ Transfer the turkey to your Crock pot; add in the garlic, onion, salt, pepper, marjoram, and cayenne pepper. Cover and cook on low setting for 6 hours.
- ❖ Melt 1/2 stick of the butter in a frying pan. Add in the cream and whisk until cooked through.
- ❖ Next, stir in the guar gum, salt, and black pepper along with cooking juices. Let it cook until the sauce has reduced by half.
- ❖ Storing
- ❖ Wrap the turkey wings in foil before packing them into airtight containers; keep in your refrigerator for up to 3 to 4 days.
- ❖ For freezing, place the turkey wings in airtight containers or heavy-duty freezer bags. Freeze up to 2 to 3 months. Defrost in the refrigerator.
- ❖ Keep your gravy in refrigerator for up to 2 days.

Nutrition: 280 Calories; 22.2g Fat; 4.3g Carbs; 15.8g Protein; 0.8g Fiber

302) AUTHENTIC PORK CHOPS WITH HERBS

Cooking Time: 20 Minutes **Servings:** 4

Ingredients:

- 1 tbsp butter
- 1 pound pork chops
- 2 rosemary sprigs, minced
- 1 tsp dried marjoram
- 1 tsp dried parsley
- A bunch of spring onions, roughly chopped
- 1 thyme sprig, minced
- 1/2 tsp granulated garlic
- 1/2 tsp paprika, crushed
- Coarse salt and ground black pepper, to taste

Directions:

- ❖ Season the pork chops with the granulated garlic, paprika, salt, and black pepper.
- ❖ Melt the butter in a frying pan over a moderate flame. Cook the pork chops for 6 to 8 minutes, turning them occasionally to ensure even cooking.
- ❖ Add in the remaining ingredients and cook an additional 4 minutes.
- ❖ Storing
- ❖ Divide the pork chops into four portions; place each portion in a separate airtight container or Ziploc bag; keep in your refrigerator for 3 to 4 days.
- ❖ Freeze the pork chops in airtight containers or heavy-duty freezer bags. Freeze up to 4 months. Defrost in the refrigerator. Bon appétit!

Nutrition: 192 Calories; 6.9g Fat; 0.9g Carbs; 29.8g Protein; 0.4g Fiber

303) ORIGINAL GROUND PORK STUFFED PEPPERS

Cooking Time: 40 Minutes **Servings:** 4

Ingredients:

- 6 bell peppers, deveined
- 1 tbsp vegetable oil
- 1 shallot, chopped
- 1 garlic clove, minced
- 1/2 pound ground pork
- 1/3 pound ground veal
- 1 ripe tomato, chopped
- 1/2 tsp mustard seeds
- Sea salt and ground black pepper, to taste

Directions:

- ❖ Parboil the peppers for 5 minutes.
- ❖ Heat the vegetable oil in a frying pan that is preheated over a moderate heat. Cook the shallot and garlic for 3 to 4 minutes until they've softened.
- ❖ Stir in the ground meat and cook, breaking apart with a fork, for about 6 minutes. Add the chopped tomatoes, mustard seeds, salt, and pepper.
- ❖ Continue to cook for 5 minutes or until heated through. Divide the filling between the peppers and transfer them to a baking pan.

- ❖ Bake in the preheated oven at 36degrees F approximately 25 minutes.
- ❖ Storing
- ❖ Place the peppers in airtight containers or Ziploc bags; keep in your refrigerator for up to 3 to 4 days.
- ❖ For freezing, place the peppers in airtight containers or heavy-duty freezer bags. Freeze up to 2 to 3 months. Defrost in the refrigerator. Bon appétit!

Nutrition: 2 Calories; 20.5g Fat; 8.2g Carbs; 18.2g Protein; 1.5g Fiber

304) GRILL-STYLE CHICKEN SALAD WITH AVOCADO

Cooking Time: 20 Minutes   **Servings: 4**

Ingredients:

- ✓ 1/3 cup olive oil
- ✓ 2 chicken breasts
- ✓ Sea salt and crushed red pepper flakes
- ✓ 2 egg yolks
- ✓ 1 tbsp fresh lemon juice
- ✓ 1/2 tsp celery seeds
- ✓ 1 tbsp coconut aminos
- ✓ 1 large-sized avocado, pitted and sliced

Directions:

- ❖ Grill the chicken breasts for about 4 minutes per side. Season with salt and pepper, to taste.
- ❖ Slice the grilled chicken into bite-sized strips.
- ❖ To make the dressing, whisk the egg yolks, lemon juice, celery seeds, olive oil and coconut aminos in a measuring cup.
- ❖ Storing
- ❖ Place the chicken breasts in airtight containers or Ziploc bags; keep in your refrigerator for 3 to 4 days.
- ❖ For freezing, place the chicken breasts in airtight containers or heavy-duty freezer bags. It will maintain the best quality for about 4 months. Defrost in the refrigerator.
- ❖ Store dressing in your refrigerator for 3 to 4 days. Dress the salad and garnish with fresh avocado. Bon appétit!

Nutrition: 40Calories; 34.2g Fat; 4.8g Carbs; 22.7g Protein; 3.1g Fiber

305) EASY-COOKING FALL-OFF-THE-BONE RIBS

Cooking Time: 8 Hours   **Servings: 4**

Ingredients:

- ✓ 1 pound baby back ribs
- ✓ 4 tbsp coconut aminos
- ✓ 1/4 cup dry red wine
- ✓ 1/2 tsp cayenne pepper
- ✓ 1 garlic clove, crushed
- ✓ 1 tsp Italian herb mix
- ✓ 1 tbsp butter
- ✓ 1 tsp Serrano pepper, minced
- ✓ 1 Italian pepper, thinly sliced
- ✓ 1 tsp grated lemon zest

Directions:

- ❖ Butter the sides and bottom of your Crock pot. Place the pork and peppers on the bottom.
- ❖ Add in the remaining ingredients.
- ❖ Slow cook for 9 hours on Low heat setting.
- ❖ Storing
- ❖ Divide the baby back ribs into four portions. Place each portion of the ribs along with the peppers in an airtight container; keep in your refrigerator for 3 to days.
- ❖ For freezing, place the ribs in airtight containers or heavy-duty freezer bags. Freeze up to 4 to months. Defrost in the refrigerator. Reheat in your oven at 250 degrees F until heated through.

Nutrition: 192 Calories; 6.9g Fat; 0.9g Carbs; 29.8g Protein; 0.5g Fiber

306) CLASSIC BRIE-STUFFED MEATBALLS

Cooking Time: 25 Minutes   **Servings: 5**

Ingredients:

- ✓ 2 eggs, beaten
- ✓ 1 pound ground pork
- ✓ 1/3 cup double cream
- ✓ 1 tbsp fresh parsley
- ✓ Kosher salt and ground black pepper
- ✓ 1 tsp dried rosemary
- ✓ 10 (1-inch cubes of brie cheese
- ✓ 2 tbsp scallions, minced
- ✓ 2 cloves garlic, minced

Directions:

- ❖ Mix all ingredients, except for the brie cheese, until everything is well incorporated.
- ❖ Roll the mixture into 10 patties; place a piece of cheese in the center of each patty and roll into a ball.
- ❖ Roast in the preheated oven at 0 degrees F for about 20 minutes.
- ❖ Storing
- ❖ Place the meatballs in airtight containers or Ziploc bags; keep in your refrigerator for up to 3 to 4 days.
- ❖ Freeze the meatballs in airtight containers or heavy-duty freezer bags. Freeze up to 3 to 4 months. To defrost, slowly reheat in a saucepan. Bon

appétit!

Nutrition: 302 Calories; 13g Fat; 1.9g Carbs; 33.4g Protein; 0.3g Fiber

307) SPECIAL SPICY AND TANGY CHICKEN DRUMSTICKS

Cooking Time: 55 Minutes   **Servings: 6**

Ingredients:

- ✓ 3 chicken drumsticks, cut into chunks
- ✓ 1/2 stick butter
- ✓ 2 eggs
- ✓ 1/4 cup hemp seeds, ground
- ✓ Salt and cayenne pepper, to taste
- ✓ 2 tbsp coconut aminos
- ✓ 3 tsp red wine vinegar
- ✓ 2 tbsp salsa
- ✓ 2 cloves garlic, minced

Directions:

- ❖ Rub the chicken with the butter, salt, and cayenne pepper.
- ❖ Drizzle the chicken with the coconut aminos, vinegar, salsa, and garlic. Allow it to stand for 30 minutes in your refrigerator.
- ❖ Whisk the eggs with the hemp seeds. Dip each chicken strip in the egg mixture. Place the chicken chunks in a parchment-lined baking pan.
- ❖ Roast in the preheated oven at 390 degrees F for 25 minutes.
- ❖ Storing
- ❖ Divide the roasted chicken between airtight containers; keep in your refrigerator for up 3 to 4 days.
- ❖ For freezing, place the roasted chicken in airtight containers or heavy-duty freezer bags. Freeze up to 3 months. Defrost in the refrigerator and reheat in a pan. Enjoy!

Nutrition: 420 Calories; 22g Fat; 5g Carbs; 35.3g Protein; 0.8g Fiber

308) ORIGINAL ITALIAN-STYLE CHICKEN MEATBALLS WITH PARMESAN

Cooking Time: 20 Minutes   **Servings: 6**

Ingredients:

- ✓ For the Meatballs:
- ✓ 1 ¼ pounds chicken, ground
- ✓ 1 tbsp sage leaves, chopped
- ✓ 1 tsp shallot powder
- ✓ 1 tsp porcini powder
- ✓ 2 garlic cloves, finely minced
- ✓ 1/3 tsp dried basil
- ✓ 3/4 cup Parmesan cheese, grated
- ✓ 2 eggs, lightly beaten
- ✓ Salt and ground black pepper, to your liking
- ✓ 1/2 tsp cayenne pepper
- ✓ For the sauce:
- ✓ 2 tomatoes, pureed
- ✓ 1 cup chicken consommé
- ✓ 2 ½ tbsp lard, room temperature
- ✓ 1 onion, peeled and finely chopped

Directions:

- ❖ In a mixing bowl, combine all ingredients for the meatballs. Roll the mixture into bite-sized balls.
- ❖ Melt 1 tbsp of lard in a skillet over a moderately high heat. Sear the meatballs for about 3 minutes or until they are thoroughly cooked; reserve.
- ❖ Melt the remaining lard and cook the onions until tender and translucent. Add in pureed tomatoes and chicken consommé and continue to cook for 4 minutes longer.
- ❖ Add in the reserved meatballs, turn the heat to simmer and continue to cook for 6 to 7 minutes.
- ❖ Storing
- ❖ Place the meatballs in airtight containers or Ziploc bags; keep in your refrigerator for up to 3 to 4 days.
- ❖ Freeze the meatballs in airtight containers or heavy-duty freezer bags. Freeze up to 3 to 4 months. To defrost, slowly reheat in a saucepan. Bon appétit!

Nutrition: 252 Calories; 9.7g Fat; 5.3g Carbs; 34.2g Protein; 1.4g Fiber

309) Typical Mediterranean-style Cheesy Pork Loin

Cooking Time: 25 Minutes   **Servings: 4**

Ingredients:

- ✓ 1 pound pork loin, cut into 1-inch-thick pieces
- ✓ 1 tsp Mediterranean seasoning mix
- ✓ Salt and pepper, to taste
- ✓ 1 onion, sliced
- ✓ 1 tsp fresh garlic, smashed
- ✓ 2 tbsp balsamic vinegar
- ✓ 1/2 cup Romano cheese, grated
- ✓ 2 tbsp butter, room temperature
- ✓ 1 tbsp curry paste
- ✓ 1 cup roasted vegetable broth
- ✓ 1 tbsp oyster sauce

Directions:

- ❖ In a frying pan, melt the butter over a moderately high heat. Once hot, cook the pork until browned on all sides; season with salt and black pepper and set aside.
- ❖ In the pan drippings, cook the onion and garlic for 4 to 5 minutes or until they've softened.
- ❖ Add in the Mediterranean seasoning mix, curry paste, and vegetable broth. Continue to cook until the sauce has thickened and reduced slightly or

- ✓ 2 tbsp black olives, pitted and sliced

about 10 minutes. Add in the remaining ingredients along with the reserved pork.

- ❖ Top with cheese and cook for 10 minutes longer or until cooked through.
- ❖ Storing
- ❖ Divide the pork loin between four airtight containers; keep in your refrigerator for 3 to 5 days.
- ❖ For freezing, place the pork loin in airtight containers or heavy-duty freezer bags. Freeze up to 4 to 6 months. Defrost in the refrigerator. Enjoy!

Nutrition: 476 Calories; 35.3g Fat; 6.2g Carbs; 31.1g Protein; 1.4g Fiber

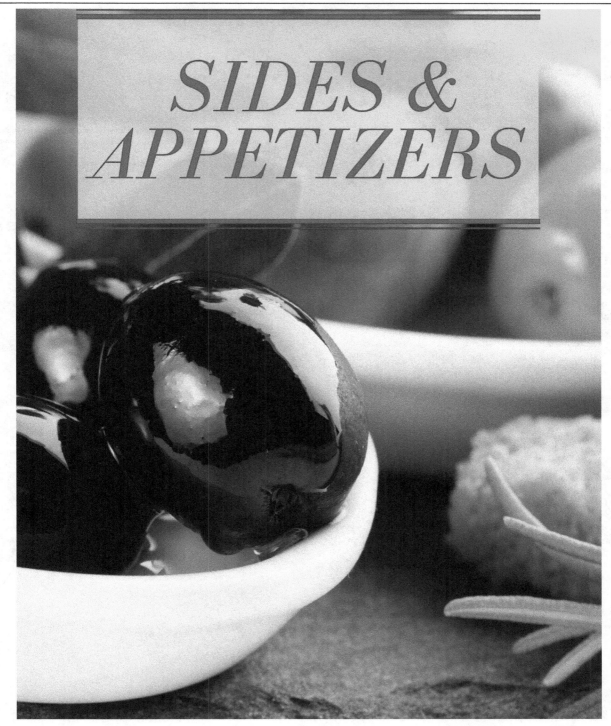

SIDES & APPETIZERS

310) MEDITERRANEAN-STYLE BAKED ZUCCHINI STICKS

Cooking Time: 20 Minutes   **Servings:** 8

Ingredients:

- ¼ cup feta cheese, crumbled
- 4 zucchini
- ¼ cup parsley, chopped
- ½ cup tomatoes, minced
- ½ cup kalamata olives, pitted and minced
- 1 cup red bell pepper, minced
- 1 tbsp oregano
- ¼ cup garlic, minced
- 1 tbsp basil
- sea salt or plain salt
- freshly ground black pepper

Directions:

- ❖ Start by cutting zucchini in half (lengthwise) and scoop out the middle.
- ❖ Then, combine garlic, black pepper, bell pepper, oregano, basil, tomatoes, and olives in a bowl.
- ❖ Now, fill in the middle of each zucchini with this mixture. Place these on a prepared baking dish and bake the dish at 0 degrees F for about 15 minutes.
- ❖ Finally, top with feta cheese and broil on high for 3 minutes or until done. Garnish with parsley.
- ❖ Serve warm.

Nutrition: 53, Total Fat: 2.2 g, Saturated Fat: 0.9 g, Cholesterol: 4 mg, Sodium: 138 mg, Total Carbohydrate: 7.5 g, Dietary Fiber: 2.1 g, Total Sugars: 3 g, Protein: 2.g, Vitamin D: 0 mcg, Calcium: 67 mg, Iron: 1 mg, Potassium: 353 mg

311) ARTICHOKE OLIVE PASTA

Cooking Time: 25 Minutes   **Servings:** 4

Ingredients:

- salt
- pepper
- 2 tbsp olive oil, divided
- 2 garlic cloves, thinly sliced
- 1 can artichoke hearts, drained, rinsed, and quartered lengthwise
- 1-pint grape tomatoes, halved lengthwise, divided
- ½ cup fresh basil leaves, torn apart
- 12 ounces whole-wheat spaghetti
- ½ medium onion, thinly sliced
- ½ cup dry white wine
- 1/3 cup pitted Kalamata olives, quartered lengthwise
- ¼ cup grated Parmesan cheese, plus extra for serving

Directions:

- ❖ Fill a large pot with salted water.
- ❖ Pour the water to a boil and cook your pasta according to package instructions until al dente.
- ❖ Drain the pasta and reserve 1 cup of the cooking water.
- ❖ Return the pasta to the pot and set aside.
- ❖ Heat 1 tbsp of olive oil in a large skillet over medium-high heat.
- ❖ Add onion and garlic, season with pepper and salt, and cook well for about 3-4 minutes until nicely browned.
- ❖ Add wine and cook for 2 minutes until evaporated.
- ❖ Stir in artichokes and keep cooking 2-3 minutes until brown.
- ❖ Add olives and half of your tomatoes.
- ❖ Cook well for 1-2 minutes until the tomatoes start to break down.
- ❖ Add pasta to the skillet.
- ❖ Stir in the rest of the tomatoes, cheese, basil, and remaining oil.
- ❖ Thin the mixture with the reserved pasta water if needed.
- ❖ Place in containers and sprinkle with extra cheese.
- ❖ Enjoy!

Nutrition: 340, Total Fat: 11.9 g, Saturated Fat: 3.3 g, Cholesterol: 10 mg, Sodium: 278 mg, Total Carbohydrate: 35.8 g, Dietary Fiber: 7.8 g, Total Sugars: 4.8 g, Protein: 11.6 g, Vitamin D: 0 mcg, Calcium: 193 mg, Iron: 3 mg, Potassium: 524 mg

312) ITALIAN CHICKEN BACON PASTA

Cooking Time: 35 Minutes   **Servings: 4**

Ingredients:

- ✓ 8 ounces linguine pasta
- ✓ 3 slices of bacon
- ✓ 1 pound boneless chicken breast, cooked and diced
- ✓ Salt
- ✓ 1 6-ounce can artichoke hearts
- ✓ 2 ounce can diced tomatoes, undrained
- ✓ ¼ tsp dried rosemary
- ✓ 1/3 cup crumbled feta cheese, plus extra for topping
- ✓ 2/3 cup pitted black olives

Directions:

- ❖ Fill a large pot with salted water and bring to a boil.
- ❖ Add linguine and cook for 8-10 minutes until al dente.
- ❖ Cook bacon until brown, and then crumble.
- ❖ Season chicken with salt.
- ❖ Place chicken and bacon into a large skillet.
- ❖ Add tomatoes and rosemary and simmer the mixture for about 20 minutes.
- ❖ Stir in feta cheese, artichoke hearts, and olives, and cook until thoroughly heated.
- ❖ Toss the freshly cooked pasta with chicken mixture and cool.
- ❖ Spread over the containers.
- ❖ Before eating, garnish with extra feta if your heart desires!

Nutrition: 755, Total Fat: 22.5 g, Saturated Fat: 6.5 g, Cholesterol: 128 mg, Sodium: 852 mg, Total Carbohydrate: 75.4 g, Dietary Fiber: 7.3 g, Total Sugars: 3.4 g,

Protein: 55.6 g, Vitamin D: 0 mcg, Calcium: 162 mg, Iron: 7 mg, Potassium: 524 mg

313) LOVELY CREAMY GARLIC SHRIMP PASTA

Cooking Time: 15 Minutes   **Servings: 4**

Ingredients:

- ✓ 6 ounces whole-wheat spaghetti, your favorite
- ✓ 12 ounces raw shrimp, peeled, deveined, and cut into 1-inch pieces
- ✓ 1 bunch asparagus, trimmed and thinly sliced
- ✓ 1 large bell pepper, thinly sliced
- ✓ 3 cloves garlic, chopped
- ✓ 1¼ tsp kosher salt
- ✓ 1½ cups non-fat plain yogurt
- ✓ ¼ cup flat-leaf parsley, chopped
- ✓ 3 tbsp lemon juice
- ✓ 1 tbsp extra virgin olive oil
- ✓ ½ tsp fresh ground black pepper
- ✓ ¼ cup toasted pine nuts

Directions:

- ❖ Bring water to a boil in a large pot.
- ❖ Add spaghetti and cook for about minutes less than called for by the package instructions.
- ❖ Add shrimp, bell pepper, asparagus and cook for about 2-4 minutes until the shrimp are tender.
- ❖ Drain the pasta.
- ❖ In a large bowl, mash the garlic until paste forms.
- ❖ Whisk yogurt, parsley, oil, pepper, and lemon juice into the garlic paste.
- ❖ Add pasta mixture and toss well.
- ❖ Cool and spread over the containers.
- ❖ Sprinkle with pine nuts.
- ❖ Enjoy!

Nutrition: 504, Total Fat: 15.4 g, Saturated Fat: 4.9 g, Cholesterol: 199 mg, Sodium: 2052 mg, Total Carbohydrate: 42.2 g, Dietary Fiber: 3.5 g, Total Sugars: 26.6 g, Protein: 43.2 g, Vitamin D: 0 mcg, Calcium: 723 mg, Iron: 3 mg, Potassium: 3 mg

314) SPECIAL MUSHROOM FETTUCCINE

Cooking Time: 15 Minutes   **Servings: 5**

Ingredients:

- ✓ 12 ounces whole-wheat fettuccine (or any other)
- ✓ 1 tbsp extra virgin olive oil
- ✓ 4 cups mixed mushrooms, such as oyster, cremini, etc., sliced
- ✓ 4 cups broccoli, divided
- ✓ 1 tbsp minced garlic
- ✓ ½ cup dry sherry
- ✓ 2 cups low-fat milk
- ✓ 2 tbsp all-purpose flour
- ✓ ½ tsp salt
- ✓ ½ tsp freshly ground pepper
- ✓ 1 cup finely shredded Asiago cheese, plus some for topping

Directions:

- ❖ Cook pasta in a large pot of boiling water for about 8- minutes.
- ❖ Drain pasta and set it to the side. Add oil to large skillet and heat over medium heat.
- ❖ Add mushrooms and broccoli, and cook for about 8-10 minutes until the mushrooms have released the liquid.
- ❖ Add garlic and cook for about 1 minute until fragrant. Add sherry, making sure to scrape up any brown bits.
- ❖ Bring the mix to a boil and cook for about 1 minute until evaporated.
- ❖ In a separate bowl, whisk flour and milk. Add the mix to your skillet, and season with salt and pepper.
- ❖ Cook well for about 2 minutes until the sauce begins to bubble and is thickened. Stir in Asiago cheese until it has fully melted.
- ❖ Add the sauce to your pasta and give it a gentle toss. Spread over the containers. Serve with extra cheese.

Nutrition: 503, Total Fat: 19.6 g, Saturated Fat: 6.3 g, Cholesterol: 25 mg, Sodium: 1136 mg, Total Carbohydrate: 57.5 g, Dietary Fiber: 12.4 g, Total Sugars: 6.4 g, Protein: 24.5 g, Vitamin D: 51 mcg, Calcium: 419 mg, Iron: 5 mg, Potassium: 390 mg

315) ORIGINAL LEMON GARLIC SARDINE FETTUCCINE

Cooking Time: 15 Minutes   **Servings: 4**

Ingredients:

- ✓ 8 ounces whole-wheat fettuccine
- ✓ 4 tbsp extra-virgin olive oil, divided
- ✓ 4 cloves garlic, minced
- ✓ 1 cup fresh breadcrumbs
- ✓ ¼ cup lemon juice
- ✓ 1 tsp freshly ground pepper
- ✓ ½ tsp of salt
- ✓ 2 4-ounce cans boneless and skinless sardines, dipped in tomato sauce
- ✓ ½ cup fresh parsley, chopped
- ✓ ¼ cup finely shredded parmesan cheese

Directions:

- ❖ Fill a large pot with water and bring to a boil.
- ❖ Cook pasta according to package instructions until tender (about 10 minutes).
- ❖ In a small skillet, heat 2 tbsp of oil over medium heat.
- ❖ Add garlic and cook for about 20 seconds, until sizzling and fragrant.
- ❖ Transfer the garlic to a large bowl.
- ❖ Add the remaining 2 tbsp of oil to skillet and heat over medium heat.
- ❖ Add breadcrumbs and cook for 5-6 minutes until golden and crispy.
- ❖ Whisk lemon juice, salt, and pepper into the garlic bowl.
- ❖ Add pasta to the garlic bowl, along with garlic, sardines, parmesan, and parsley; give it a gentle stir.
- ❖ Cool and spread over the containers.
- ❖ Before eating, sprinkle with breadcrumbs.
- ❖ Enjoy!

Nutrition: 633, Total Fat: 27.7 g, Saturated Fat: 6.4 g, Cholesterol: 40 mg, Sodium: 771 mg, Total Carbohydrate: 55.9 g, Dietary Fiber: 7.7 g, Total Sugars: 2.1 g, Protein: 38.6 g, Vitamin D: 0 mcg, Calcium: 274 mg, Iron: 7 mg, Potassium: mg

316) DELICIOUS SPINACH ALMOND STIR-FRY

Cooking Time: 10 Minutes   **Servings: 2**

Ingredients:

- ✓ 2 ounces spinach
- ✓ 1 tbsp coconut oil
- ✓ 3 tbsp almond, slices
- ✓ sea salt or plain salt
- ✓ freshly ground black pepper

Directions:

- ❖ Start by heating a skillet with coconut oil; add spinach and let it cook.
- ❖ Then, add salt and pepper as the spinach is cooking.
- ❖ Finally, add in the almond slices.
- ❖ Serve warm.

Nutrition: 117, Total Fat: 11.4 g, Saturated Fat: 6.2 g, Cholesterol: 0 mg, Sodium: 23 mg, Total Carbohydrate: 2.9 g, Dietary Fiber: 1.7 g, Total Sugars: 0.g, Protein: 2.7 g, Vitamin D: 0 mcg, Calcium: 52 mg, Iron: 1 mg, Potassium: 224 mg

317)   ITALIAN BBQ CARROTS

Cooking Time: 30 Minutes   **Servings: 8**

Ingredients:

- ✓ 2 pounds baby carrots (organic)
- ✓ 1 tbsp olive oil
- ✓ 1 tbsp garlic powder
- ✓ 1 tbsp onion powder
- ✓ sea salt or plain salt
- ✓ freshly ground black pepper

Directions:

- ❖ Mix all the Ingredients: in a plastic bag so that the carrots are well coated with the mixture.
- ❖ Then, on the BBQ grill place a piece of aluminum foil and spread the carrots in a single layer.
- ❖ Finally, grill for 30 minutes or until tender.
- ❖ Serve warm.

Nutrition: 388, Total Fat: 1.9 g, Saturated Fat: 0.3 g, Cholesterol: 0 mg, Sodium: 89 mg, Total Carbohydrate: 10.8 g, Dietary Fiber: 3.4 g, Total Sugars: 6 g, Protein: 1 g, Vitamin D: 0 mcg, Calcium: 40 mg, Iron: 1 mg, Potassium: 288 mg

318)   ORIGINAL RED ONION KALE PASTA

Cooking Time: 25 Minutes   **Servings: 4**

Ingredients:

- ✓ 2½ cups vegetable broth
- ✓ ¾ cup dry lentils
- ✓ ½ tsp of salt
- ✓ 1 bay leaf
- ✓ ¼ cup olive oil
- ✓ 1 large red onion, chopped
- ✓ 1 tsp fresh thyme, chopped
- ✓ ½ tsp fresh oregano, chopped

- ✓ 1 tsp salt, divided
- ✓ ½ tsp black pepper
- ✓ 8 ounces vegan sausage, sliced into ¼-inch slices
- ✓ 1 bunch kale, stems removed and coarsely chopped
- ✓ 1 pack rotini

Directions:

- ❖ Add vegetable broth, ½ tsp of salt, bay leaf, and lentils to a saucepan over high heat and bring to a boil.
- ❖ Reduce the heat to medium-low and allow to cook for about minutes until tender.
- ❖ Discard the bay leaf.
- ❖ Take another skillet and heat olive oil over medium-high heat.
- ❖ Stir in thyme, onions, oregano, ½ a tsp of salt, and pepper; cook for 1 minute.
- ❖ Add sausage and reduce heat to medium-low.
- ❖ Cook for 10 minutes until the onions are tender.
- ❖ Bring water to a boil in a large pot, and then add rotini pasta and kale.
- ❖ Cook for about 8 minutes until al dente.
- ❖ Remove a bit of the cooking water and put it to the side.
- ❖ Drain the pasta and kale and return to the pot.
- ❖ Stir in both the lentils mixture and the onions mixture.
- ❖ Add the reserved cooking liquid to add just a bit of moistness.
- ❖ Spread over containers.

Nutrition: Calories: 508, Total Fat: 17 g, Saturated Fat: 3 g, Cholesterol: 0 mg, Sodium: 2431 mg, Total Carbohydrate: 59.3 g, Dietary Fiber: 6 g, Total Sugars: 4.8 g, Protein: 30.9 g, Vitamin D: 0 mcg, Calcium: 256 mg, Iron: 8 mg, Potassium: 1686 mg

319)   ITALIAN SCALLOPS PEA FETTUCCINE

Cooking Time: 15 Minutes   **Servings: 5**

Ingredients:

- ✓ 8 ounces whole-wheat fettuccine (pasta, macaroni)
- ✓ 1 pound large sea scallops
- ✓ ¼ tsp salt, divided
- ✓ 1 tbsp extra virgin olive oil
- ✓ 1 8-ounce bottle of clam juice
- ✓ 1 cup low-fat milk

- ✓ ¼ tsp ground white pepper
- ✓ 3 cups frozen peas, thawed
- ✓ ¾ cup finely shredded Romano cheese, divided
- ✓ 1/3 cup fresh chives, chopped
- ✓ ½ tsp freshly grated lemon zest
- ✓ 1 tsp lemon juice

Directions:

- ❖ Boil water in a large pot and cook fettuccine according to package instructions.
- ❖ Drain well and put it to the side.
- ❖ Heat oil in a large, non-stick skillet over medium-high heat.
- ❖ Pat the scallops dry and sprinkle them with 1/8 tsp of salt.
- ❖ Add the scallops to the skillet and cook for about 2-3 minutes per side until golden brown. Remove scallops from pan.
- ❖ Add clam juice to the pan you removed the scallops from.
- ❖ In another bowl, whisk in milk, white pepper, flour, and remaining 1/8 tsp of salt.
- ❖ Once the mixture is smooth, whisk into the pan with the clam juice.
- ❖ Bring the entire mix to a simmer and keep stirring for about 1-2 minutes until the sauce is thick.
- ❖ Return the scallops to the pan and add peas. Bring it to a simmer.
- ❖ Stir in fettuccine, chives, ½ a cup of Romano cheese, lemon zest, and lemon juice.
- ❖ Mix well until thoroughly combined.
- ❖ Cool and spread over containers.
- ❖ Before eating, serve with remaining cheese sprinkled on top.
- ❖ Enjoy!

Nutrition: Calories: 388, Total Fat: 9.2 g, Saturated Fat: 3.7 g, Cholesterol: 33 mg, Sodium: 645 mg, Total Carbohydrate: 50.1 g, Dietary Fiber: 10.4 g, Total Sugars: 8.7 g, Protein: 24.9 g, Vitamin D: 25 mcg, Calcium: 293 mg, Iron: 4 mg, Potassium: 247 mg

320) MEDITERRANEAN OLIVE TUNA PASTA

Cooking Time: 20 Minutes   **Servings: 4**

Ingredients:

- ✓ 8 ounces of tuna steak, cut into 3 pieces
- ✓ ¼ cup green olives, chopped
- ✓ 3 cloves garlic, minced
- ✓ 2 cups grape tomatoes, halved
- ✓ ½ cup white wine
- ✓ 2 tbsp lemon juice
- ✓ 6 ounces pasta - whole wheat gobetti, rotini, or penne
- ✓ 1 10-ounce package frozen artichoke hearts, thawed and squeezed dry
- ✓ 4 tbsp extra-virgin olive oil, divided
- ✓ 2 tsp fresh grated lemon zest
- ✓ 2 tsp fresh rosemary, chopped, divided
- ✓ ½ tsp salt, divided
- ✓ ¼ tsp fresh ground pepper
- ✓ ¼ cup fresh basil, chopped

Directions:

- ❖ Preheat grill to medium-high heat.
- ❖ Take a large pot of water and put it on to boil.
- ❖ Place the tuna pieces in a bowl and add 1 tbsp of oil, 1 tsp of rosemary, lemon zest, a ¼ tsp of salt, and pepper.
- ❖ Grill the tuna for about 3 minutes per side.
- ❖ Transfer tuna to a plate and allow it to cool.
- ❖ Place the pasta in boiling water and cook according to package instructions.
- ❖ Drain the pasta.
- ❖ Flake the tuna into bite-sized pieces.
- ❖ In a large skillet, heat remaining oil over medium heat.
- ❖ Add artichoke hearts, garlic, olives, and remaining rosemary.
- ❖ Cook for about 3-4 minutes until slightly browned.
- ❖ Add tomatoes, wine, and bring the mixture to a boil.
- ❖ Cook for about 3 minutes until the tomatoes are broken down.
- ❖ Stir in pasta, lemon juice, tuna, and remaining salt.
- ❖ Cook for 1-2 minutes until nicely heated.
- ❖ Spread over the containers.
- ❖ Before eating, garnish with some basil and enjoy!

Nutrition: 455, Total Fat: 21.2 g, Saturated Fat: 3.5 g, Cholesterol: 59 mg, Sodium: 685 mg, Total Carbohydrate: 38.4 g, Dietary Fiber: 6.1 g, Total Sugars: 3.5 g,

Protein: 25.5 g, Vitamin D: 0 mcg, Calcium: 100 mg, Iron: 5 mg, Potassium: 800 mg

321) SPECIAL BRAISED ARTICHOKES

Cooking Time: 30 Minutes   **Servings: 6**

Ingredients:

- ✓ 6 tbsp olive oil
- ✓ 2 pounds baby artichokes, trimmed
- ✓ ½ cup lemon juice
- ✓ 4 garlic cloves, thinly sliced
- ✓ ½ tsp salt
- ✓ 1½ pounds tomatoes, seeded and diced
- ✓ ½ cup almonds, toasted and sliced

Directions:

- ❖ Heat oil in a skillet over medium heat.
- ❖ Add artichokes, garlic, and lemon juice, and allow the garlic to sizzle.
- ❖ Season with salt.
- ❖ Reduce heat to medium-low, cover, and simmer for about 15 minutes.
- ❖ Uncover, add tomatoes, and simmer for another 10 minutes until the tomato liquid has mostly evaporated.
- ❖ Season with more salt and pepper.
- ❖ Sprinkle with toasted almonds.
- ❖ Enjoy!

Nutrition: Calories: 265, Total Fat: 1g, Saturated Fat: 2.6 g, Cholesterol: 0 mg, Sodium: 265 mg, Total Carbohydrate: 23 g, Dietary Fiber: 8.1 g, Total Sugars: 12.4 g, Protein: 7 g, Vitamin D: 0 mcg, Calcium: 81 mg, Iron: 2 mg, Potassium: 1077 mg

322) DELICIOUS FRIED GREEN BEANS

Cooking Time: 15 Minutes   **Servings: 2**

Ingredients:

- ✓ ½ pound green beans, trimmed
- ✓ 1 egg
- ✓ 2 tbsp olive oil
- ✓ 1¼ tbsp almond flour
- ✓ 2 tbsp parmesan cheese
- ✓ ½ tsp garlic powder
- ✓ sea salt or plain salt
- ✓ freshly ground black pepper

Directions:

- ❖ Start by beating the egg and olive oil in a bowl.
- ❖ Then, mix the remaining Ingredients: in a separate bowl and set aside.
- ❖ Now, dip the green beans in the egg mixture and then coat with the dry mix.
- ❖ Finally, grease a baking pan, then transfer the beans to the pan and bake at 5 degrees F for about 12-15 minutes or until crisp.

❖ Serve warm.

Nutrition: Calories: 334, Total Fat: 23 g, Saturated Fat: 8.3 g, Cholesterol: 109 mg, Sodium: 397 mg, Total Carbohydrate: 10.9 g, Dietary Fiber: 4.3 g, Total Sugars: 1.9 g, Protein: 18.1 g, Vitamin D: 8 mcg, Calcium: 398 mg, Iron: 2 mg, Potassium: 274 mg

323) VEGGIE MEDITERRANEAN-STYLE PASTA

Cooking Time: 2 Hours   **Servings: 4**

Ingredients:

- ✓ ½ tsp salt
- ✓ ½ tsp brown sugar
- ✓ freshly ground black pepper
- ✓ 1 piece aubergine
- ✓ 2 pieces courgettes
- ✓ 2 pieces red peppers, de-seeded
- ✓ 2 garlic cloves, peeled
- ✓ 2-3 tbsp olive oil
- ✓ 12 small vine-ripened tomatoes
- ✓ 16 ounces of pasta of your preferred shape, such as Gigli, conchiglie, etc.
- ✓ 3½ ounces parmesan cheese

- ✓ 1 tbsp olive oil
- ✓ 1 small onion, finely chopped
- ✓ 2 small garlic cloves, finely chopped
- ✓ 2 14-ounce cans diced tomatoes
- ✓ 1 tbsp sun-dried tomato paste
- ✓ 1 bay leaf
- ✓ 1 tsp dried thyme
- ✓ 1 tsp dried basil
- ✓ 1 tsp oregano
- ✓ 1 tsp dried parsley
- ✓ bread of your choice

Directions:

- ❖ Heat oil in a pan over medium heat.
- ❖ Add onions and fry them until tender.
- ❖ Add garlic and stir-fry for 1 minute.
- ❖ Add the remaining Ingredients: listed under the sauce and bring to a boil.
- ❖ Reduce the heat, cover, and simmer for 60 minutes.
- ❖ Season with black pepper and salt as needed. Set aside.
- ❖ Preheat oven to 350 degrees F.
- ❖ Chop up courgettes, aubergine and red peppers into 1-inch pieces.
- ❖ Place them on a roasting pan along with whole garlic cloves.
- ❖ Drizzle with olive oil and season with salt and black pepper.
- ❖ Mix the veggies well and roast in the oven for 45 minutes until they are tender.
- ❖ Add tomatoes just before 20 minutes to end time.
- ❖ Cook your pasta according to package instructions.
- ❖ Drain well and stir into the sauce.
- ❖ Divide the pasta sauce between 4 containers and top with vegetables.
- ❖ Grate some parmesan cheese on top and serve with bread.
- ❖ Enjoy!

Nutrition: Calories: 211, Total Fat: 14.9 g, Saturated Fat: 2.1 g, Cholesterol: 0 mg, Sodium: 317 mg, Total Carbohydrate: 20.1 g, Dietary Fiber: 5.7 g, Total Sugars: 11.7 g, Protein: 4.2 g, Vitamin D: 0 mcg, Calcium: 66 mg, Iron: 2 mg, Potassium: 955 mg

324) CLASSIC BASIL PASTA

Cooking Time: 40 Minutes   **Servings: 4**

Ingredients:

- 2 red peppers, de-seeded and cut into chunks
- 2 red onions cut into wedges
- 2 mild red chilies, de-seeded and diced
- 3 garlic cloves, coarsely chopped
- 1 tsp golden caster sugar
- 2 tbsp olive oil, plus extra for serving
- 2 pounds small ripe tomatoes, quartered
- 12 ounces pasta
- a handful of basil leaves, torn
- 2 tbsp grated parmesan
- salt
- pepper

Directions:

- Preheat oven to 390 degrees F.
- On a large roasting pan, spread peppers, red onion, garlic, and chilies.
- Sprinkle sugar on top.
- Drizzle olive oil and season with salt and pepper.
- Roast the veggies for 1minutes.
- Add tomatoes and roast for another 15 minutes.
- In a large pot, cook your pasta in salted boiling water according to instructions.
- Once ready, drain pasta.
- Remove the veggies from the oven and carefully add pasta.
- Toss everything well and let it cool.
- Spread over the containers.
- Before eating, place torn basil leaves on top, and sprinkle with parmesan.
- Enjoy!

Nutrition: Calories: 384, Total Fat: 10.8 g, Saturated Fat: 2.3 g, Cholesterol: 67 mg, Sodium: 133 mg, Total Carbohydrate: 59.4 g, Dietary Fiber: 2.3 g, Total

Sugars: 5.7 g, Protein: 1 g, Vitamin D: 0 mcg, Calcium: 105 mg, Iron: 4 mg, Potassium: 422 mg

325) ORIGINAL RED ONION KALE PASTA

Cooking Time: 25 Minutes   **Servings: 4**

Ingredients:

- 2½ cups vegetable broth
- ¾ cup dry lentils
- ½ tsp of salt
- 1 bay leaf
- ¼ cup olive oil
- 1 large red onion, chopped
- 1 tsp fresh thyme, chopped
- ½ tsp fresh oregano, chopped
- 1 tsp salt, divided
- ½ tsp black pepper
- 8 ounces vegan sausage, sliced into ¼-inch slices
- 1 bunch kale, stems removed and coarsely chopped
- 1 pack rotini

Directions:

- Add vegetable broth, ½ tsp of salt, bay leaf, and lentils to a saucepan over high heat and bring to a boil.
- Reduce the heat to medium-low and allow to cook for about minutes until tender.
- Discard the bay leaf.
- Take another skillet and heat olive oil over medium-high heat.
- Stir in thyme, onions, oregano, ½ a tsp of salt, and pepper; cook for 1 minute.
- Add sausage and reduce heat to medium-low.
- Cook for 10 minutes until the onions are tender.
- Bring water to a boil in a large pot, and then add rotini pasta and kale.
- Cook for about 8 minutes until al dente.
- Remove a bit of the cooking water and put it to the side.
- Drain the pasta and kale and return to the pot.
- Stir in both the lentils mixture and the onions mixture.
- Add the reserved cooking liquid to add just a bit of moistness.
- Spread over containers.

Nutrition: Calories: 508, Total Fat: 17 g, Saturated Fat: 3 g, Cholesterol: 0 mg, Sodium: 2431 mg, Total Carbohydrate: 59.3 g, Dietary Fiber: 6 g, Total Sugars: 4.8 g, Protein: 30.9 g, Vitamin D: 0 mcg, Calcium: 256 mg, Iron: 8 mg, Potassium: 1686 mg

326) ITALIAN SCALLOPS PEA FETTUCCINE

Cooking Time: 15 Minutes   **Servings: 5**

Ingredients:

- 8 ounces whole-wheat fettuccine (pasta, macaroni)
- 1 pound large sea scallops
- ¼ tsp salt, divided
- 1 tbsp extra virgin olive oil
- 1 8-ounce bottle of clam juice
- 1 cup low-fat milk
- ¼ tsp ground white pepper
- 3 cups frozen peas, thawed
- ¾ cup finely shredded Romano cheese, divided
- 1/3 cup fresh chives, chopped
- ½ tsp freshly grated lemon zest
- 1 tsp lemon juice

Directions:

- Boil water in a large pot and cook fettuccine according to package instructions.
- Drain well and put it to the side.
- Heat oil in a large, non-stick skillet over medium-high heat.
- Pat the scallops dry and sprinkle them with 1/8 tsp of salt.
- Add the scallops to the skillet and cook for about 2-3 minutes per side until golden brown. Remove scallops from pan.
- Add clam juice to the pan you removed the scallops from.
- In another bowl, whisk in milk, white pepper, flour, and remaining 1/8 tsp of salt.
- Once the mixture is smooth, whisk into the pan with the clam juice.
- Bring the entire mix to a simmer and keep stirring for about 1-2 minutes until the sauce is thick.
- Return the scallops to the pan and add peas. Bring it to a simmer.
- Stir in fettuccine, chives, ½ a cup of Romano cheese, lemon zest, and lemon juice.
- Mix well until thoroughly combined.
- Cool and spread over containers.
- Before eating, serve with remaining cheese sprinkled on top.
- Enjoy!

Nutrition: Calories: 388, Total Fat: 9.2 g, Saturated Fat: 3.7 g, Cholesterol: 33 mg, Sodium: 645 mg, Total Carbohydrate: 50.1 g, Dietary Fiber: 10.4 g, Total Sugars: 8.7 g, Protein: 24.9 g, Vitamin D: 25 mcg, Calcium: 293 mg, Iron: 4 mg, Potassium: 247 mg

PART IV: KETO MEAL PLAN

The PURPOSE OF THIS PLAN is to show you what types of keto foods can be eaten, how you can prepare your foods, what a typical keto meal looks like, and recipes.

A keto diet contains high-fat foods that reduce carbohydrate intake. Although it is possible to eat some carbohydrates, the daily information must be deficient because it is intended to allow the body to develop ketosis. When the body is in ketosis, it is more effective at burning fat since it does not have adequate carbohydrates to use for energy.

People use two key keto diet people for weight loss. The classical ketogenic diet has macronutrients divided as follows: 20% protein, 75% fat, and 5% carbohydrates. This ratio is accompanied by the high-protein ketogenic diet: 35% protein, 60% fat, and 5% carbohydrates. Both work mainly in the same way that your body switches its primary source of energy to fat.

Here is how you should use this meal plan:

Each day should be between 1,500-1,700 calories (designed for weight loss).

Ensure you know your daily macromolecules (how much fat, protein, carbs, and grains you need to reach your goal).

Each recipe has anywhere between 2-10 servings, so be sure to prepare according to your macros and personal needs. For example, if you're just cooking for yourself, you may want to make one serving and then save the rest for another meal.

This eating plan is designed for one person. If you want to use it for multiple people, simply multiply the number of ingredients by the total number of people.

Be flexible. We don't know your personal goal, budget, cooking skills, favorite dishes, or what you don't like to eat, so we can't customize the meal plan just for you. This plan is to give you ideas on what to eat for breakfast, lunch, and dinner. So feel free to customize it to make it work for you.

Feel free to replicate any of the recipes or ingredients with your personal choices and adjust them to suit your tastes and situation.

If you follow a stringent ketogenic diet, be sure to customize this eating plan (including the snack list suggestion at the end) to make it work for you.

WEEK 1

BREAKFAST

110. CHORIZO BREAKFAST

Prep Time: 10 min   **Cooking Time**: 12 min   **Servings**: 2

Ingredients

- 1 tbsp. olive oil
- ½ cup diced red pepper
- ½ cup diced yellow onion
- 4 ounces chorizo sausage
- 2 large eggs
- Salt and pepper
- 2 slices thick-cut bacon, cooked

Directions:

1. Preheat the oven to 350°F and lightly grease two ramekins.
2. Heat the oil in a skillet over medium-high heat.
3. Add the peppers and onions and cook for 4 to 5 min until browned.
4. Divide the vegetable mixture between the two ramekins.
5. Chop the chorizo and divide between the ramekins.
6. Crack an egg into each ramekin and season with salt and pepper, to taste.
7. Bake for 10 to 12 min until the egg is set to the desired level.
8. Crumble the bacon over top and serve hot.

Nutrition: Calories 450 Fat 36 g Net Carb 4.5 g Total Carbs: 5.5 g Fiber: 1 g Protein 25 g

LUNCH

111. PORK LETTUCE WRAPS

Prep Time: 10 min   **Cooking Time**: 15 min   **Servings**: 2

Ingredients

- 1 tbsp. olive oil
- ¼ cup diced yellow onion
- ¼ cup diced green pepper
- 2 tbsp. diced celery
- 6 ounces ground pork
- ¼ teaspoon onion powder
- ¼ tsp. garlic powder
- 2 tbsp. soy sauce
- 1 tsp. sesame oil
- 4 leaves butter lettuce, separated
- 1 tbsp. toasted sesame seeds

Directions:

1. Heat the oil in a skillet over medium heat.

2. Add the onions, peppers, and celery and sauté for 5 min until tender.

3. Stir in the pork and cook until just browned.

4. Add the onion powder and garlic powder, then stir in the soy sauce and sesame oil.

5. Season with salt and pepper to taste, then remove from heat.

6.   Place the lettuce leaves on a plate and spoon the pork mixture evenly into them.

7.   Sprinkle with sesame seeds to serve.

Nutrition: Calories 500 Fat 29 g Net Carb 7.5 g Total Carbs: 10.5 g Fiber: 3 g Protein 49 g

DINNER

112. AVOCADO LIME SALMON

Prep Time: 15 min   **Cooking Time**: 15 min   **Servings**: 2

Ingredients

- 100 grams chopped cauliflower
- 1 large avocado
- 1 tbsp. fresh lime juice
- 2 tbsp. diced red onion

- 2 tbsp. olive oil
- 2 (6-ounce) boneless salmon fillets
- Salt and pepper

Directions:

1. Place the cauliflower in a food processor and pulse into rice-like grains.
2. Grease a skillet with cooking spray and heat over medium heat.
3. Add the cauliflower rice and cook, covered, for 8 min until tender. Set aside.
4. Combine the avocado, lime juice, and red onion in a food processor and blend smooth.
5. Heat the oil in a large skillet over medium-high heat.
6. Season the salmon with salt and pepper, then add to the skillet skin-side down.
7. Cook for 4 to 5 min until seared, then flip and cook for another 4 to 5 min.
8. Serve the salmon over a bed of cauliflower rice topped with the avocado cream.

Nutrition: Calories 570 Fat 44 g Net Carb 4 g Total Carbs: 12 g Fiber: 8 g Protein 36 g

DAY 2

BREAKFAST

113. LOW-CARB BREAKFAST EGG MUFFINS WITH SAUSAGE GRAVY

Prep Time: 15 min   **Cooking Time**: 35 min   **Servings**: 6

Ingredients

For the muffins:

- 12 large eggs
- Sea salt
- Black pepper

- 1 pound thin shaved deli ham
- 4 ounces shredded mozzarella cheese

- 4 ounces grated parmesan cheese
- Low-carb sausage gravy

For the gravy:

- 🏳 1/2 ground pork sausage
- 🏳 8 ounces softened cream cheese
- 🏳 3/4 cups beef broth
- 🏳 Sea salt
- 🏳 Black pepper

Directions:

1. Prepare the eggs and gravy.
2. Whisk eggs together with salt and pepper to taste.
3. Cook the sausage over medium heat until thoroughly cooked through. Add in the cream cheese and the broth and stirring constantly, cook until the mixture comes to a soft simmer and thickens.

Assemble the muffins:

1. Place two pieces of ham in the bottom of each muffin cup, careful to overlap and try and cover the whole surface. Evenly divide sausage gravy between each muffin.
2. Pour eggs into each muffin, dividing the mixture evenly.

4. Then reduce the heat to medium-low, still stirring constantly and simmer for 2 more min.
5. Season to taste with salt and pepper.
6. Set mixture aside.
7. Preheat oven to 325°F.

3. Top each muffin with equal parts of the two types of cheeses.
4. Bake for approximately 30-40 min or until muffin is firm and cheese is melted.

Nutrition: Calories 607 Fat 46 g Net Carb 3 g Total Carbs: 6 g Fiber: 3 g Protein 42 g

LUNCH

114. SPICED PUMPKIN SOUP

Prep Time: 15 min   **Cooking Time**: 40 min   **Servings**: 3

Ingredients

- 🏳 2 tbsp. unsalted butter
- 🏳 1 small yellow onion, chopped
- 🏳 2 cloves minced garlic
- 🏳 1 teaspoon minced ginger
- 🏳 ½ teaspoon ground cinnamon
- 🏳 ¼ teaspoon ground nutmeg
- 🏳 Salt and pepper, to taste
- 🏳 ½ cup pumpkin puree
- 🏳 1 cup chicken broth
- 🏳 3 slices thick-cut bacon
- 🏳 ¼ cup heavy cream

Directions:

1. Melt the butter in a large saucepan over medium heat.
2. Add the onions, garlic, and ginger and cook for 3 to 4 min until the onions are translucent.
3. Stir in the spices and cook for 1 min until fragrant. Season with salt and pepper.
4. Add the pumpkin puree and chicken broth, then bring to a boil.

5. Reduce heat and simmer for 20 min, then remove from heat.
6. Puree the soup using an immersion blender, then return to heat and simmer for 20 min.
7. Cook the bacon in a skillet until crisp, then remove to paper towels to drain.
8. Add the bacon fat to the soup along with the heavy cream. Crumble the bacon over top to serve.

Nutrition: Calories 250 Fat 20 g Net Carb 6 g Total Carbs: 8 g Fiber: 2 g Protein 0 g

DINNER

115. EASY CHICKEN WITH SPINACH AND BACON

Prep Time: 10 min   **Cooking Time**: 20 min   **Servings**: 2

Ingredients

- 1 chicken breast, boiled
- 1 slice bacon, chopped
- 2 tbsp butter
- 1/2 cup spinach, chopped
- 1 tbsp onion in slices
- 2 tbsp cream cheese
- 1 tsp Italian seasoning
- 1 tsp salt
- 1/2 tsp black pepper

Directions:

1.   First, let the chicken boil in hot water. Afterwards, shred it with a fork or with your hands. Set aside.

2.   Pan fry the chopped bacon in melted butter. When the bacon starts producing fats, gently drop the shredded chicken in and cook for 2-3 min.

3.   Toss in the spinach and onion into the pan. Leave to soften the vegetables.

4.   Mix in the cream cheese and stir continuously to blend the ingredients. Add more flavor with the Italian seasoning, pepper, and salt.

5.   Transfer to a serving plate and enjoy your meal.

Nutrition: Calories 383 Fat 3.2 g Net Carb 0.9 g Total Carbs: 1.2 g Fiber: 0.3 g Protein 40.3 g

DAY 3

BREAKFAST

116. BAKED EGGS IN AVOCADO

Prep Time: 5 min   **Cooking Time**: 15 min   **Servings**: 3

Ingredients

- 1 medium avocado
- 2 tbsp. lime juice
- 2 large eggs
- Salt and pepper
- 2 tbsp. shredded cheddar cheese

Directions:

1. Preheat the oven to 450°F and cut the avocado in half. Scoop out some of the flesh from the middle of each avocado half.

2. Place the avocado halves upright in a baking dish and brush with lime juice.

3. Crack an egg into each and season with salt and pepper.

4. Bake for 10 min, then sprinkle with cheese.

5. Let the eggs bake for another 2 to 3 min until the cheese is melted. Serve hot.

Nutrition: Calories 610 Fat 54 g Net Carb 4.5 g Total Carbs: 18 g Fiber: 13.5 g Protein 20 g

LUNCH

117. EASY BEEF CURRY

Prep Time: 20 min **Cooking Time**: 40 min **Servings**: 3

Ingredients

- 1 medium yellow onion, chopped
- 1 tbsp. minced garlic
- 1 tbsp. grated ginger
- 1 ¼ cups canned coconut milk
- 1 pound beef chuck, chopped
- 2 tbsp. curry powder
- 1 tsp. salt
- ½ cup fresh chopped cilantro

Directions:

1. Combine the onion, garlic, and ginger in a food processor and blend into a paste.
2. Transfer the paste to a saucepan and cook for 3 min on medium heat.
3. Stir in the coconut milk, then simmer gently for 10 min.
4. Add the chopped beef along with the curry powder and salt. Stir well then simmer, covered, for 20 min. Remove the lid and simmer for another 20 min until the beef is cooked through.
5. Adjust seasoning to taste and garnish with fresh chopped cilantro.

Nutrition: Calories 550 Fat 34 g Net Carb 9 g Total Carbs: 14 g Fiber: 5 g Protein 50 g

DINNER

118. ROSEMARY ROASTED CHICKEN AND VEGGIES

Prep Time: 15 min **Cooking Time**: 35 min **Servings**: 2

Ingredients

- 4 deboned chicken thighs
- Salt and pepper
- 1 small zucchini, sliced
- 2 small carrots, peeled and sliced
- 1 small parsnip, peeled and sliced
- 2 cloves garlic, sliced
- 3 tbsp. olive oil
- 1 tbsp. balsamic vinegar
- 2 tsp. fresh chopped rosemary

Directions:

1. Preheat the oven to 350°F and lightly grease a small rimmed baking sheet with cooking spray.
2. Place the chicken thighs on the baking sheet and season with salt and pepper.
3. Arrange the veggies around the chicken then sprinkle with sliced garlic.
4. Whisk together the remaining ingredients then drizzle over the chicken and veggies.
5. Bake for 30 min then broil for 3 to 5 min until the skins are crisp.

Nutrition Calories 540 Fat 40.5 g Net Carb 8.5 g Total Carbs: 12 g Fiber: 3.5 g Protein 33 g

DAY 4

BREAKFAST

119. LEMON RICOTTA PANCAKES

Prep Time: 10 min   **Cooking Time:** 20 min   **Servings**: 2

Ingredients

- 1 large lemon, juiced and zested
- 6 ounces whole milk ricotta
- 3 large eggs
- 10 to 12 drops liquid stevia
- ¼ cup almond flour
- 1 scoop egg white protein powder
- 1 tbsp. poppy seeds
- ¾ teaspoons baking powder
- ¼ cup powdered erythritol
- 1 tbsp. heavy cream

Directions:

1. Combine the ricotta, eggs, and liquid stevia in a food processor with half the lemon juice and the lemon zest—blend well, then pour into a bowl.
2. Whisk in the almond flour, protein powder, poppy seeds, baking powder, and a pinch of salt.
3. Heat a large nonstick pan over medium heat.
4. Spoon the batter into the pan, using about ¼ cup per pancake.
5. Cook the pancakes until bubbles form on the surface of the batter, then flip them. Let the pancakes cook until the bottom is browned, then remove to a plate. Repeat with the remaining batter.
6. Whisk together the heavy cream, powdered erythritol, and reserved lemon juice and zest.
7. Serve the pancakes hot, drizzled with the lemon glaze.

Nutrition: Calories 370 Fat 26 g Net Carb 5.5 g Total Carbs: 6.5 g Fiber: 1 g Protein 29.5g

LUNCH

120. KETO BACON CHEESEBURGER WITH MUSHROOMS

Prep Time: 5 min   **Cooking Time**: 15 min   **Servings**: 4

Ingredients

- 1 lb ground beef
- 4 slices bacon
- 1 small egg

- 1 tbsp almond flour
- 1 tsp cumin
- 1/2 cup sliced mushrooms
- 1 tsp garlic powder
- 1 tsp onion powder
- 8 cheddar cheese thin slices
- Salt
- 1 tsp black pepper

Directions:

1. Season the ground beef with all of the condiments. Crack the egg into the beef and throw in the almond flour as well. Knead until well combined. Mold into 4 meatballs. Create the hollow shape of the meatballs with a soda can. Using your hands, shape the beef to form a cup before removing the can.
2. Fill the molded beef with mushroom. Wrap a slice of bacon around the sides of the cup.
3. Lay a slice of cheese on the surface of the hamburger to cover the mushroom. Leave in the 300°F oven for 10 min. Remove once the meat is cooked.
4. Lay another slice of cheese on top and rebake for an additional 5 min, enough to melt the cheese.
5. Serve and enjoy!

Nutrition: Calories 627 Fat 50.7 g Net Carb 2.2 g Total Carbs: 3 g Fiber: 0.8 g Protein 39.6g

DINNER

121. STUFFED CHICKEN BREASTS

Prep Time: 10 min   **Cooking Time**: 30 min   **Servings**: 3

Ingredients

- 1.5 lb chicken breast, approx. 3 pcs
- 1 cup chopped spinach fresh
- 1/2 cup cherry tomatoes
- 1 garlic clove
- 6 tbsp shredded cheese
- 2 tbsp olive oil
- 1/2 cup Rao's homemade tomato basil sauce (optional)

Directions:

1. Prepare all ingredients.
2. Add one tbsp of olive oil in a skillet, add spinach, quartet cherry tomatoes, and chopped garlic. Cook it until spinach is soft.
3. Make pockets in chicken breasts. Salt, pepper, you can add Mediterranean dry herbs (basil, oregano). I had three chicken breasts so I first stuffed each with one tbsp of cheese and then cooked greens. Close cuts with wooden toothpicks.
4. Brown chicken in the skillet on both sides (don't cook it) then transfer into a deep tray with the remaining tbsp of olive oil.
5. Distribute sauce evenly on top of the chicken. Cover with foil. Preheat oven to 375°F. Cook till it's done. As a final step sprinkle remaining cheese on top of the chicken, send it back to oven for a few min for cheese to melt.
6. Enjoy.

Nutrition: Calories 417 Fat 17.9 g Net Carb 2.6 g Total Carbs: 3.6 g Fiber: 1 g Protein 58.7g

DAY 5

BREAKFAST

122. EGG WITH BLUEBERRIES AND CINNAMON

Prep Time: 5 min   **Cooking Time**: 20 min   **Servings**: 4

Ingredients

- 6 large eggs
- 2 tbsp softened butter
- 1 tsp vanilla
- 1/2 cup blueberries (or 1/4 cup, depending upon taste)
- 1/2 tsp cinnamon (you could probably double this if you like cinnamon)
- 1 tbsp coconut oil

Directions:

1. Preheat oven to 375°F. In an 8" – 9" cast iron skillet (or any oven-proof skillet), heat coconut oil over medium heat.
2. In a medium bowl beat eggs, butter, cinnamon, and vanilla together with a hand mixer until combined and fluffy (about 1-2 min).
3. Pour egg mixture into heated pan and allow bottom to cook slightly (about 2 min). Gently drop blueberries into egg mixture and place pan in oven. Cook for 15-20 or until cooked through and browned on top (but not burned).
4. Remove from oven and allow to cool slightly.

Nutrition: Calories 188 Fat 15 g Net Carb 1 g Total Carbs: 4 g Fiber: 3 g Protein 8 g

LUNCH

123. LETTUCE ROLLS WITH GROUND BEEF

Prep Time: 10 min   **Cooking Time**: 15 min   **Servings**: 4

Ingredients

- 4 lettuce leaves
- ½ lb ground beef
- 1 tbsp olive oil
- 2 tbsp chopped onion
- 1 small tomato, chopped
- ½ tsp paprika
- 1 small avocado, chopped
- 2 tbsp sour cream
- ½ tsp salt
- ½ tsp black pepper

Directions:

1. In a hot frying pan with a tbsp of olive oil, sauté the onion and tomato. Gently plop the beef into the sautéed onion and tomato. Season with pepper, salt, paprika, and any other spice of your choice. Sear for 7-10 min over medium-high heat.
2. Lay the lettuce leaf on a flat board. Scoop out some of the cooked beef and place this on one side of the leaf. Top with avocado and sour cream. Roll the leaf firmly. Repeat until all of the ingredients are used up. Transfer to a plate and enjoy!

Nutrition: Calories 127 Fat 8.5 g Net Carb 1.4 g Total Carbs: 2.1 g Fiber: 0.7 g Protein 10.6 g

DINNER

124. HOMEMADE SAGE SAUSAGE PATTIES

Prep. Time: 25 min.   **Cooking Time**: 15 min   **Servings**: 8

Ingredients

- 1 pound ground pork
- 3/4 cup shredded cheddar cheese
- 1/4 cup buttermilk
- 1 tbsp. finely chopped onion
- 2 teaspoons rubbed sage
- 3/4 teaspoon salt
- 3/4 teaspoon pepper
- 1/8 teaspoon garlic powder
- 1/8 teaspoon dried oregano

Directions:

1. In a bowl, combine all ingredients, mixing lightly but thoroughly. Shape into eight 1/2-inch-thick patties. Refrigerate 1 hour.

2. In a large cast-iron or other heavy skillet, cook patties over medium heat until a thermometer reads 160° 6-8 min on each side.

Nutrition: Calories 162 Fat 11 g Carbohydrates: 1 g Protein 13 g

DAY 6

BREAKFAST

125.   SWEET BLUEBERRY COCONUT PORRIDGE

Prep Time: 5 min   **Cooking Time**: 15 min   **Servings**: 2

Ingredients

- 1 cup unsweetened almond milk
- ¼ cup canned coconut milk
- ¼ cup coconut flour
- ¼ cup ground flaxseed
- 1 tsp. ground cinnamon
- ¼ teaspoon ground nutmeg
- Pinch salt
- 60 grams fresh blueberries
- ¼ cup shaved coconut

Directions:

1. Warm the almond milk and coconut milk in a saucepan over low heat. Whisk in the coconut flour, flaxseed, cinnamon, nutmeg, and salt. Turn up the heat and cook until the mixture bubbles.

2. Stir in the sweetener and vanilla extract, then cook until thickened to the desired level.

3. Spoon into two bowls and top with blueberries and shaved coconut.

Nutrition: Calories 390 Fat 22 g Net Carb 15 g Total Carbs: 37 g Fiber: 22 g Protein 10 g

LUNCH

126. STUFFED JALAPENO PEPPERS WITH GROUND BEEF

Prep Time: 15 min   **Cooking Time**: 30 min   **Servings**: 6

Ingredients

- 6 large jalapeños
- 1 tbsp olive oil
- ½ lb ground beef
- 2 tbsp chopped onion
- 1 small tomato, chopped
- 2 oz grated mozzarella cheese
- ½ tsp salt

- ⚐ ½ tsp black pepper

Directions:

1. While preparing the dish, let the oven preheat at 350°F. Heat the olive oil in a frying pan. Sauté the beef in the pan together with the onion and chopped tomato. Add salt and pepper to taste. Leave to cook for approximately 15 min.
2. Slice the jalapeños into two pieces. Empty the insides of the slices by discarding the seeds and the veins.
3. Stuff about a tbsp. ful of the cooked beef in the empty jalapeño halves. Sprinkle mozzarella cheese on the surface. Arrange the filled peppers on a baking sheet and cook in the oven for 15 min. Wait till the cheese browns.
4. Serve on a plate and enjoy!

Nutrition: Calories 127 Fat 8.5 g Net Carb 1.4 g Total Carbs: 2.1 g Fiber: 0.7 g Protein 10.6 g

---

DINNER

127. SAUTEED SAUSAGE WITH GREEN BEANS

Prep Time: 15 min   **Cooking Time**: 15 min   **Servings**: 3

Ingredients

- ⚐ 300 g pork sausage
- ⚐ 1/2 cup green beans
- ⚐ 1/2 onion, sliced
- ⚐ 1/2 tbsp olive oil
- ⚐ 2 tbsp sour cream
- ⚐ Salt and pepper, to taste

Directions:

1. Chop off both tips of the green beans then slice into two. Put aside.
2. Chop the sausage links into bite-sized chunks as well. Reserve in a bowl. For easy chopping, refrigerate the sausage for around 15 min before cutting.
3. Preheat a skillet then pour the oil into heat. Sear the sausage chunks for 5 min.
4. Once brown, toss in the onion and chopped green beans. Sauté for 4-5 min more.
5. Gently pour in the cream. Season with pepper and salt. Fold the mix with a spatula to incorporate all the ingredients together. Leave for an additional 3 min before turning off the heat.
6. Serve in a dish and enjoy warm.

Nutrition: Calories 369 Fat 32.6 g Net Carb 3.6 g Total Carbs: 4.5 g Fiber: 0.9 g Protein 15 g

---

DAY 7

BREAKFAST

128. LOW-CARB BREAKFAST QUICHE

Prep Time: 15 min   **Cooking Time**: 55 min   **Servings**: 4

Ingredients

- ⚐ 1 lb ground Italian sausage
- ⚐ 1.5 cups shredded cheddar cheese
- ⚐ 8 large eggs
- ⚐ 1 tbsp ranch seasoning

- ⚑ 1 cup sour cream

Directions:

1. Preheat oven to 350°F.
2. In an oven-safe skillet, brown ground sausage and drain the grease.
3. In a large bowl, whisk together egg, sour cream, and ranch seasoning. You may want to use a hand mixer.
4. Mix in cheddar cheese.
5. Pour egg mixture into pan and stir until everything is fully blended.
6. Cover with foil and bake for 30 min.
7. Remove foil and bake for another 25 min or until golden brown.

Nutrition: Calories 551 Fat 46 g Net Carb 3 g Total Carbs: 6 g Fiber: 3 g Protein 26 g

LUNCH

129. BACON WRAPPED ASPARAGUS

Prep Time: 5 min   **Cooking Time**: 20 min   **Servings**: 2

Ingredients

- ⚑ 12 spear fresh asparagus, medium-sized
- ⚑ 2 tbsp olive oil
- ⚑ 6 slices bacon
- ⚑ Salt and black pepper, to taste

Directions:

1. Set the oven to 350°F to preheat. After rinsing the asparagus with water, chop off the tough parts of the stem.
2. Drizzle olive oil on the asparagus spears. Salt and pepper to enhance the flavor. Wrap half a strip of bacon around each asparagus. Repeat until all the ingredients are used up.
3. Arrange the wrapped asparagus on a baking sheet in a way that they don't overlap. Leave in the oven for 20 min. Wait till the vegetable is tender.
4. Transfer to a plate. Best served warm.

Nutrition: Calories 565 Fat 54.6 g Net Carb   2.8 g Total Carbs: 4.8 g Fiber: 2 g Protein 15 g

130. LAMB CHOPS WITH ROSEMARY AND GARLIC

Prep Time: 35 min   **Cooking Time**: 15 min   **Servings**: 2

Ingredients

- 1 tbsp. coconut oil, melted
- 1 tsp. fresh chopped rosemary
- 1 clove garlic, minced
- 2 bone-in lamb chops (about 6 ounces meat)
- 1 tbsp. butter
- Salt and pepper
- ¼ pound fresh asparagus, trimmed
- 1 tbsp. olive oil

Directions:

1. Combine the coconut oil, rosemary, and garlic in a shallow dish. Add the lamb chops then turn to coat – let marinate in the fridge overnight. Let the lamb rest at room temperature for 30 min.
2. Heat the butter in a large skillet over medium-high heat. Add the lamb chops and cook for 6 min, then season with salt and pepper.
3. Turn the chops and cook for another 6 min or until cooked to the desired level.
4. Let the lamb chops rest for 5 min before serving.
5. Meanwhile, toss the asparagus with olive oil, salt, and pepper then spread on a baking sheet.
6. Broil for 6 to 8 min until charred, shaking occasionally. Serve hot with the lamb chops.

Nutrition: Calories 685 Fat 52 g Net Carb 3 g Total Carbs: 6 g Fiber: 3 g Protein 50.5 g

BREAKFAST

131.   VANILLA PROTEIN SMOOTHIE

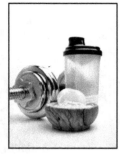

Prep Time: 5 min.   **Cooking Time**: 0 min   **Servings**: 2

Ingredients

- 1 scoop (20g) vanilla egg white protein powder
- ½ cup heavy cream
- ¼ cup vanilla almond milk
- 4 ice cubes
- 1 tbsp. coconut oil
- 1 tbsp. powdered erythritol
- ½ teaspoon vanilla extract
- ¼ cup whipped cream

Directions:

1. Combine all of the ingredients, except the whipped cream, in a blender.
2. Blend on high speed for 30 to 60 seconds until smooth. Pour into a glass and top with whipped cream.

Nutrition: Calories 540 Fat 46 g Net Carb 7.5 g Total Carbs: 8 g Fiber: 0.5 g Protein 25 g

LUNCH

132.   CHEESEBURGER SALAD

Prep Time: 10 min.   **Cooking Time**: 10   **Servings**: 2

Ingredients

- 7 ounces ground beef
- Salt and pepper
- 3 tbsp. mayonnaise
- 1 tbsp. diced pickles
- 1 tsp. mustard
- ½ teaspoon ketchup
- Pinch smoked paprika
- 3 ounces chopped romaine lettuce
- 1/3 cup diced tomatoes
- ¼ cup shredded cheddar cheese

Directions:

1. Brown the ground beef over high heat then season with salt and pepper to taste.
2. Drain the fat from the beef and remove from heat.
3. Combine the mayonnaise, pickles, mustard, ketchup, and paprika in a blender.
4. Blend the mixture until smooth and well combined.
5. Combine the lettuce, tomatoes, and cheddar cheese in a mixing bowl.
6. Toss in the ground beef and the dressing until evenly coated.

Nutrition: Calories 395 Fat 27.5 g Total Carbs: 9 g Fiber: 1 g Protein 27.5 g

DINNER

133. CHICKEN ZOODLE CLARISSA

Prep Time: 10 min.   **Cooking Time**: 25   **Servings**: 2

Ingredients

- 2 (6-ounce) chicken breasts
- 1 tbsp. olive oil
- Salt and pepper
- 2 tbsp. butter
- ¼ cup heavy cream
- ¼ cup grated Parmesan cheese
- 200 grams zucchini

Directions:

1. Heat the oil in a large skillet over medium-high heat.
2. Season the chicken with salt and pepper to taste then add to the skillet. Cook for 6 to 7 min. on each side until cooked through then slice into strips.
3. Reheat the skillet over medium-low heat and add the butter.
4. Stir in the heavy cream and Parmesan cheese then cook until thickened.
5. Spiralize the zucchini then toss it into the sauce mixture with the chicken.
6. Cook until the zucchini is tender, about 2 min., then serve hot.

Nutrition: Calories 595 Fat 40 g Net Carb 3 g Total Carbs: 4 g Fiber: 1 g Protein 55 g

DAY 2

BREAKFAST

134. HAM AND CHEESE WAFFLES

Prep Time: 15 min.   **Cooking Time:** 25   **Servings**: 2

Ingredients

- 4 large eggs, divided
- 2 scoops (40 g) egg white protein powder
- 1 teaspoon baking powder
- 1/3 cup melted butter
- ½ teaspoon salt
- 1 ounce diced ham
- ¼ cup shredded cheddar cheese

Directions:

1. Separate two of the eggs and set the other two aside.
2. Beat 2 of the egg yolks with the protein powder, baking powder, butter, and salt in a mixing bowl.
3. Fold in the chopped ham and grated cheddar cheese. Whisk the egg whites in a separate bowl with a pinch of salt until stiff peaks form.
4. Fold the beaten egg whites into the egg yolk mixture in two batches.
5. Grease a preheated waffle maker then spoon ¼ cup of the batter into it and close it. Cook until the waffle is golden brown, about 3 to 4 min., then remove.
6. Reheat the waffle iron and repeat with the remaining batter. Meanwhile, heat the oil in a skillet and fry the eggs with salt and pepper.
7. Serve the waffles hot, topped with a fried egg.

Nutrition: Calories 575 Fat 46.5 g Net Carb 5 g Total Carbs: 5 g Fiber: 0 g Protein 35 g

LUNCH

135. PAN-FRIED PEPPERONI PIZZAS

Prep Time: 10 min   **Cooking Time:** 25   **Servings**: 3

Ingredients

- 6 large eggs
- 6 tbsp. grated Parmesan cheese
- 3 tbsp. psyllium husk powder
- 1 ½ tsp. Italian seasoning
- 3 tbsp. olive oil
- 9 tbsp. low-carb tomato sauce, divided
- 4 ½ ounces shredded mozzarella, divided
- 1 ½ ounces diced pepperoni, divided
- 3 tbsp. fresh chopped basil

Directions:

1. Combine the eggs, Parmesan, and psyllium husk powder with the Italian seasoning and a pinch of salt in a blender.
2. Blend until smooth and well combined, about 30 seconds, then rest for 5 min.
3. Heat 1 tbsp. of oil in a skillet over medium-high heat.
4. Spoon 1/3 of the batter into the skillet and spread in a circle then cook until browned underneath.
5. Flip the pizza crust and cook until browned on the other side. Remove the crust to a foil-lined baking sheet and repeat with the remaining batter.
6. Spoon 3 tbsp. of low-carb tomato sauce over each crust. Top with diced pepperoni and shredded cheese then broil until the cheese is browned.
7. Sprinkle with fresh basil then slice the pizza to serve.

Nutrition: Calories 545 Fat 42 g Net Carb 4.5 g Total Carbs: 12 g Fiber: 7.5 g Protein 32 g

DINNER

136. CABBAGE AND SAUSAGE SKILLET

Prep Time: 10 min.   **Cooking Time**: 20   **Servings**: 4

Ingredients

- 6 large Italian sausage links
- ½ head green cabbage, sliced
- 2 tbsp. butter
- ¼ cup sour cream
- ¼ cup mayonnaise
- Salt and pepper

Directions:

1. Cook the sausage in a skillet over medium-high heat until evenly browned then slice them.
2. Reheat the skillet over medium-high heat then add the butter. Toss in the cabbage and cook until wilted, about 3 to 4 min.
3. Stir the sliced sausage into the cabbage then stir in the sour cream and mayonnaise.
4. Season with salt and pepper then simmer for 10 min.

Nutrition: Calories 350 Fat 24.5 g Net Carb 10 g Total Carbs: 12 g Fiber: 2 g Protein 22 g

BREAKFAST
137. JACK SAUSAGE EGG MUFFINS

Prep Time: 10 minutes   **Cooking Time**: 30   **Servings**: 3

Ingredients

- 10 ounces ground breakfast sausage
- ½ cup diced yellow onion
- ¼ teaspoon garlic powder
- Salt and pepper
- 3 large eggs, whisked
- 2 tablespoons heavy cream
- ½ cup shredded pepper jack cheese

Directions:

1. Preheat the oven to 350°F and grease three ramekins with cooking spray. Stir together the ground sausage, diced onion, garlic powder, salt, and pepper in a mixing bowl.
2. Divide the sausage mixture evenly in the ramekins, pressing it into the bottom and sides, leaving the middle open.
3. Whisk together the eggs and heavy cream with salt and pepper. Divide the egg mixture among the sausage cups and top with shredded cheese.
4. Bake for 25 to 30 minutes until the eggs are set and the cheese browned.

Nutrition: Calories 455 Fat 37 g Net Carb 3 g Total Carbs: 3.5 g Fiber: 0.5 g Protein 26 g

LUNCH

138. BACON BURGER BITES

Prep Time: 10 minutes   **Cooking Time**: 15   **Servings**: 16

Ingredients

- 1 lb ground beef
- 8 slices bacon, halved
- 1 large egg, beaten
- 1/2 cup almond flour
- 1/2 tsp garlic powder
- 6 slices mozzarella cheese
- Pickled Jalapeños (optional)
- Salt and pepper, to taste

Directions:

1. Season the meat with garlic powder, salt, and pepper. Crack the egg on the meat and mix well with the almond flour. Knead with your hands or with a spoon to flavor it entirely and create a consistent mixture.
2. Mold into 16 mini meatballs.
3. Prepare 8 strips of bacon and divide into two, making 16 bacon slices. Wrap one slice around one ball.
4. Crispy fry the bacon in two tablespoons of oil using a nonstick frying pan. Remember to cook all sides of the balls.
5. Transfer to a dish once the meatballs turn golden on every side and the bacon is crispy to your liking.
6. Slice the jalapeno into slivers and the cheese into small squares.
7. Top the hot meatballs with a piece of cheese and a slice of jalapeño. Push a toothpick through the ball to hold the tower together. Let the cheese melt on top of the meatball.
8. Enjoy warm with any dip of your choice!

Nutrition: Calories 173 Fat 14.1 g Net Carb 0.6g Total Carbs: 0.7 g Fiber: 0.1 g Protein 10.4 g

DINNER

139. CHICKEN ALFREDO WITH BROCCOLI

Prep Time: 10 minutes   **Cooking Time**: 15   **Servings**: 4

Ingredients

- 1 lb boneless chicken breast, cut in slices
- 1/2 cup spinach, cut in slices
- 1 cup broccoli florets
- 4 slices bacon (fried and cut into crisp bacon bits)
- 1 tbsp butter
- 1/2 cup heavy cream
- 1 garlic clove minced
- 2 tbsp onion, chopped
- 1/2 tsp salt
- 1/2 tsp pepper

Directions:

1. Give the broccoli the right tenderness and color by placing them in a bowl and pouring some boiling water in. Leave for 10 minutes.
2. On a hot frying pan, sauté the chicken in melted butter with the garlic and onion for 5 minutes.
3. Gently plop the spinach and broccoli into the pan. Add the bacon and cream as well. Season with salt and pepper to your liking. Leave for another 5 minutes.
4. Pour in a bowl and serve warm.

Nutrition: Calories 311ng Fat 19.5 g Net Carb 2.5g Total Carbs: 3.3 g Fiber: 0.8 g Protein 31.1 g

DAY 4

BREAKFAST

Prep Time: 10 minutes   **Cooking Time**: 15   **Servings**: 4

Ingredients

- 3 cups broccoli
- 1 large egg
- ¼ cup Parmesan cheese, freshly grated
- 1 ½ cup cheddar cheese, shredded
- 2 tsp almond flour
- ½ tsp garlic powder
- Kosher salt
- Black pepper

Directions:

1. Wash and dry your fresh broccoli bunch. Discard all of the leaves before chopping into chunks. Make sure to chop enough chunks for 3 cups.
2. Transfer the chopped broccoli pieces into a food processor. Continue pulsing until you get rice-size bits. Set the microwave to "cooking." Leave the broccoli rice in the microwave for a minute and a half. Crack the egg in a bowl. Add the garlic, cheddar cheese, and almond flour together with the riced broccoli. Beat with a spoon until combined. Season with a dash of pepper and salt.
3. Pat the mixture into a baking tray covered with waxed paper. Cover all sides of the tray evenly.
4. Sprinkle a generous amount of Parmesan cheese on top. Put in the oven for 10 minutes. The oven should be set at 300°F.
5. Take the tray out of the oven. Top with half a cup of cheddar cheese. Rebake for 5 more minutes to melt the cheese. Once ready, remove from the heat. Allow cooling for around 5 minutes then remove the paper.
6. Cut into rectangular shapes and enjoy!

Nutrition:Calories 258 Fat 18.7 g Net Carb 4.1g Total Carbs:6.2 g Fiber: 2.1 g Protein 17.4 g

140. SALMON SUSHI ROLLS

Prep Time: 30 minutes   **Cooking Time**: 20   **Servings:** 4

Ingredients

Sushi Fillings:

- 2 eggs
- 120 g fresh salmon (or smoked salmon)
- 100 g avocado (1 small)
- 100 g cucumber (1 small)

Sushi Rice:

- 3 cup cauliflower rice (shredded cauliflower)
- 150 g cream cheese, softened
- 2 tbsp rice vinegar
- 1/2 tsp salt, to taste

- 1/2 tsp So Nourished Erythritol (optional)

Other ingredients:

- 2 sheets Nori
- 2 tbsp white sesame seeds
- 1 tsp black sesame seeds (for decoration, optional)
- Sushi dip (optional)
- 1 tbsp ginger, grated
- 1 tbsp lemon juice
- 2 tbsp coconut aminos

Directions:

Making vinegared sushi rice:

1. Wash and cut the cauliflower into small pieces to prepare the cauliflower rice. You can use a knife or a food processor (better choice) to process until obtaining the rice-like pieces.
2. Place the riced cauliflower in a closed container and cook it in the microwave for three minutes. Allow them to cool down. You can also steam or cook the cauliflower in a frying pan. In a mixing bowl, add rice vinegar, sweetener, and salt. Add cauliflower rice and cream cheese in. Stir everything well with a wooden spoon until you obtain a homogeneous dough.

Prepare sushi fillings and assemble:

1. Peel off the avocado and cucumber skins. Slice into slivers. Slice the salmon into thin slivers too.

Scramble egg with a pinch of salt, fry it in a pan, then cut into thin strips.
2. Prep a sushi roller with transparent plastic on both sides to avoid sticking the mixture onto the roller.
3. Place the sushi mat roller on a flat surface. Lay a rectangular nori sheet on top.
4. Split the rice mixture into 2 parts for the 2 nori sheets. Scoop out one part and spread this mixture uniformly over the nori sheet.
5. Arrange the strips of avocado, salmon, egg, and cucumber on one short edge of the sheet. Make sure that the roller can be reeled in that direction.
6. With extra care, roll the filled side up to the other edge of the sheet. Repeat the procedure with the other sheets and remaining mixture.
7. Ideally, chill in the fridge for half an hour before cutting the roll. If desired, simply slice the roll without refrigerating. Slice all sushi rolls into bite-size pieces. This should make 4 servings.

Nutrition: Calories 310 Fat 24 g Net Carb 5.1g Total Carbs: 9.3 g Fiber: 4.2 g Protein 16.4 g

DINNER

141. BUFFALO CHICKEN WINGS

Prep Time: 10 minutes   **Cooking Time**: 15   **Servings**: 4

Ingredients

- 12 chicken wings (whole wings)
- 4 cloves garlic, peeled
- 2 tbsp coconut flour
- 50 ml hot sauce
- 1 tbsp vinegar
- 1 tbsp pepper
- 1 tbsp paprika
- ½ tbsp celery salt
- 1 pinch Stevia (optional)
- 1 lemon (optional)
- Olive oil for deep frying
- 1 tsp salt
- 1 tsp chili pepper

Directions:

1. Coat the chicken wings with lemon on all sides. Set aside for 3 minutes, then wash and dry thoroughly. For a simpler method, just wash and dry the wings without putting in the lemon. Smash together the paprika, pepper, garlic, salt, hot pepper, hot sauce, and vinegar with a mortar
2. Marinate the chicken wings with the mixed spices. Chill in the fridge for an hour while flipping the wings occasionally. Transfer the wings to a plate and coat with coconut flour all over to cover the entire sides.
3. Pour the oil in a deep fryer set at 375°F.
4. Brown the wings in the oil for around 10-15 minutes.
5. Remove from the heat once the wings turn brown on the sides. Serve on a platter.

Nutrition: Calories 300 Fat 17.8 g Net Carb 3.4 g Total Carbs: 7.1 g Fiber: 3.7 g Protein 28.6 g

---

DAY 5

BREAKFAST

142. AVOCADO SMOOTHIE WITH COCONUT MILK

Prep Time: 10 minutes   **Cooking Time**: 5   **Servings**: 1

Ingredients

- 1 cup coconut milk, unsweetened
- 1 tsp ginger, fresh and grounded
- 1/2 avocado
- 5 leaves spinach
- 1 tsp lime juice (optional)
- 1 tsp Stevia (optional)
- 1 tsp chia seeds

Directions:

1. Wash your ginger and spinach thoroughly.
2. Peel the ginger and avocado. Slice them into pieces.
3. Using a blender, mix all of the ingredients (except chia seeds and stevia) for a minute to obtain a smooth and uniform mixture. Optionally, pour some water and lime juice into the blender to produce the desired thickness. Include some ice cubes and the sweetener into the mix just to flavor it up. Transfer to a glass and garnish with a teaspoon of chia seeds on top. Serve immediately.

Nutrition: Calories 283 Fat 25.3 g Net Carb 4.5 g Total Carbs: 14.4 g Fiber: 9.9 g Protein 3.2 g

143. SPINACH STUFFED CHICKEN

Prep Time: 10 minutes   **Cooking Time**: 20   **Servings**: 2

Ingredients

- 1 chicken breast, boneless and skinless
- 1/2 cup chopped spinach
- 1 tbsp onion, chopped
- 1 tbsp butter
- Oil for frying
- 2 tbsp cream cheese
- 1 tbsp grated mozzarella cheese
- Salt and pepper, to taste

Directions:

1. Melt your butter in a hot frying pan. Sauté the spinach and onion in the butter. Set the stove to medium-high heat and leave the vegetables to cook for about 3 minutes until soft. Mix the cream cheese in the pan. Allow dissolving for around 2 minutes. Stir to combine with the onion and spinach. Set aside. Slice a pocket in the chicken breast, deep enough to be filled. Rub both sides of the chicken with salt and pepper. Season all side, including the inside of the pocket.

2. Jampack the pocket with spinach filling and some shredded cheese. Close the breast and secure with a toothpick. Heat the olive oil in a frying pan over medium heat. Gently place the chicken on the oil and cook for 7-10 minutes with the lid on. Turn the chicken over and let it fry for another 7-10 minutes. Remove from the heat once golden.

3. Cut in the middle to spill the filling. Enjoy while warm.

Nutrition: Calories 291 Fat 13.1 g Net Carb 0.9 g Total Carbs: 1.2 g Fiber: 0.3 g Protein 41.7 g

144. LOW-CARB NACHOS

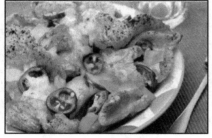

Prep Time: 20 minutes   **Cooking Time**: 25   **Servings**: 4

Ingredients

- 2 tbsp cream cheese
- 1 small egg (optional)
- 1 tsp salt
- For topping
- 1/2 lb ground beef
- 1/2 tsp dried oregano
- 1 small tomatoes, chopped
- 1 clove garlic, minced
- 1/2 tsp ground pepper
- 2 bay leaves (optional)

For guacamole

- 1 avocado medium-sized, peeled and chopped
- 1 tbsp fresh cilantro, chopped
- 1 small tomato, chopped
- 1 tbsp onion, chopped

For the chips:

- ½ cup almond flour
- 4 slices cheddar cheese (can also use grated mozzarella cheese)
- 2 tbsp butter, melted

Directions:

1. Preheat oven to 350°F.
2. Mix the almond flour, butter, oregano, cream cheese, oregano, and 1 tsp salt in a bowl. Make sure to mix until the dough looks soft so you can use a rolling pin to flatten the dough.
3. Cut small rectangles to form the crackers and place cheddar cheese on each cracker. Place them on a baking sheet and then in the oven for about 10 minutes or until they look brown. Set aside.
4. In the meantime, add oil to a preheated skillet and add the garlic clove, bay leaves, ground beef, pepper, and salt. Let it cook for 10 minutes and then add 2 chopped tomatoes. Cook for 5 more minutes and remove from heat.
5. For the guacamole, mix the avocado, 1 chopped tomato, cilantro, and onion. Add salt to taste.
6. Serve nacho crackers with meat and sour cream on top along with guacamole and enjoy!

Nutrition: Calories 507 Fat 42.1 g Net Carb 4.9 g Total Carbs: 10.5 g Fiber: 5.6 g Protein 26.1 g

DAY 6

BREAKFAST
145. COCONUT PANCAKES

Prep Time: 10 minutes   **Cooking Time**: 10   **Servings**: 2

Ingredients

Main Ingredients:

- 2 tbsp coconut flour
- 2 eggs
- ½ tbsp So Nourished Erythritol or a dash of stevia extract
- ¼ tsp baking powder
- 2 tbsp sour cream
- 2 tbsp melted butter
- ½ tsp vanilla extract

For the topping:

- 50 g strawberries
- 1 tbsp shredded coconut
- 1 tbsp almond slices
- 1 tbsp maple syrup (optional)

Directions:

1. Put the eggs, sour cream, 1 ½ tbsp. of melted butter (you'll need the rest for frying the pancakes), vanilla extract, and mix well.
2. Add the coconut flour, baking powder, erythritol to the mixture and mix again. Let the mixture sit for about 15 minutes. If the mixture is too thick, add a little bit of water (20-30 ml) and mix again until the consistency is right. In a pan on medium heat, add butter in and fry the pancakes in butter. The number of pancakes you make will depend on the size you want. We made 6 pancakes with this recipe.
3. Add the toppings and serve!

Nutrition: Calories 274 Fat 23.39 g Net Carb 4.24 g Total Carbs: 8.04 g Fiber: 3.8 g Protein 8.44 g

LUNCH
146. BROCCOLI AND CHICKEN CASSEROLE
Prep Time: 15 min   **Cooking Time**: 35 min   **Servings**: 6
Ingredients:
- 2 tbsp. butter
- ¼ cup cooked bacon, crumbled
- 2½ cups cheddar cheese, shredded and divided
- 4 oz. cream cheese, softened

- ¼ cup heavy whipping cream
- ½ pack ranch seasoning mix
- ⅔ cup homemade chicken broth

- 1½ cups small broccoli florets
- 2 cups cooked grass-fed chicken breast, shredded.

Directions:

1. Preheat your oven to 350°F.
2. Arrange a rack in the upper portion of the oven.
3. For the chicken mixture: In a large wok, melt the butter over low heat.
4. Add the bacon, 1/2 cup of cheddar cheese, cream cheese, heavy whipping cream, ranch seasoning, and broth, and with a wire whisk, beat until well combined. Cook for about 5 minutes, stirring frequently.
5. Meanwhile, in a microwave-safe dish, place the broccoli and microwave until desired tenderness is achieved.
6. In the wok, add the chicken and broccoli and mix until well combined.
7. Remove from the heat and transfer the mixture into a casserole dish. Top the chicken mixture with the remaining cheddar cheese.
8. Bake for about 25 minutes. Now, set the oven to broiler. Broil the chicken mixture for about 2–3 minutes or until cheese is bubbly.
9. Serve hot.

Nutrition: Calories: 431 Fat: 10.5g Fiber: 9.1g Carbs:4.9 g Protein: 14.1g.

DINNER

147. SALMON AND LEMON RELISH

Prep Time: 10 min   **Cooking Time:** 1 h   **Servings:** 2

Ingredients:

- 2 medium salmon fillets
- Black pepper and salt to taste
- 1 shallot, chopped

- 1 tbsp. lemon juice
- 1 big lemon
- ½ cup olive oil

- 2 tbsp. parsley, finely chopped.

Directions:

1. Grease salmon fillets with olive oil, put salt and pepper, place on a lined baking sheet, standing in the oven at 400 °F, and bake for 1 hour
2. Stir 1 tablespoon lemon juice, salt, and pepper in a bowl and leave aside for 10 minutes.
3. Cut the whole lemon in wedges and then very thinly. Put this in shallots, parsley, ¼ cup olive oil, and stir.
4. Break the salmon into medium pieces and serve with the lemon relish on the side.

Nutrition: Calories: 200 kcal Fat: 10 g Carbs: 5 g Fiber: 1 g Protein: 20 g.

DAY 7

BREAKFAST

148. PIZZA BOWL

Prep Time: 5 minutes   **Cooking Time**: 10   **Servings**: 1

Ingredients

- 1/2 green bell pepper, cut in slices
- 1 oz turkey ham, cut in small squares
- 1 tbsp red onion, cut in slices

- 2 tbsp Rao's Pizza Sauce (or tomato paste)
- 1/2 tbsp olive oil
- 1 oz grated mozzarella cheese

Directions:

1. Preheat a frying pan then pour the oil in. Fry the ham for 3 minutes. Optionally, use any meat of your choice instead of ham. Put aside.
2. Set the bell pepper on the base of a microwave-safe bowl. Layer with the onion, ham and finally, tomato paste. Then, top with mozzarella.
3. Microwave for 3 minutes and let the cheese melt. As an alternative, bake for 10 minutes in the oven preheated at 370°F. Remember to use an oven-safe pan for this.
4. Take out from the microwave (or oven) and enjoy!

Nutrition: Calories 213 Fat 15.9 g Net Carb 5.3 g Total Carbs: 7 g Fiber: 1.7 g Protein 11.7 g

LUNCH

149. CHICKEN CORDON BLEU

Prep Time: 5 minutes   **Cooking Time**: 15   **Servings**: 2

Ingredients

- 1 pc chicken breast, boneless and skinless
- 1 lemon (optional)
- 3 slices bacon
- 1 clove garlic, minced
- 1 slice smoked ham
- 1 slice cheddar cheese
- Lettuce (optional)
- Salt and pepper, to taste

Directions:

1. Spray all the sides of the chicken breast with lemon. Set aside for 3 minutes then wash and dry the chicken thoroughly. If there are no lemons available, simply wash and towel dry.
2. Season the chicken with salt, pepper, and minced garlic. Slice the cheese and ham enough to cover the chicken. Lay the ham and cheese slices on top of each chicken breast. Carefully roll the chicken, tuck the ends inside, and finally hold the pieces together with a toothpick.
3. Prepare 3 strips of bacon and wrap them around the rolled up chicken breast.
4. Set an 8-inch non-stick skillet sprayed with cooking spray over medium-high heat.
5. Sear the chicken in the pan, 5 minutes per side until there are no more pink spots on the chicken. Leave in the pan for an additional 2 minutes before removing the toothpick. Lay the chicken on top of a bed of lettuce and serve.
6. If preferred, make the breadcrumb coating for the chicken. Brush the cooked chicken with beaten egg (1 egg or less) and roll it in 2-3 tbsp of almond flour to coat entirely. Crispy fry for 3 minutes until brown.

Nutrition: Calories 56 Fat 19.3 g Net Carb 1.5 g Total Carbs: 1.7 g Fiber: 0.2 g Protein 42.5 g

DINNER

150. SCALLOPS AND FENNEL SAUCE

Prep Time: 10 min   **Cooking Time**: 10 min   **Servings**: 2

Ingredients:

- 6 scallops
- 1 fennel, trimmed, leaves chopped, and bulbs cut in wedges
- ½ lime Juice
- 1 lime zest
- 1 lime, cut in wedges
- 1 egg yolk
- tbsp. ghee, melted and heated up
- ½ tbsp. olive oil
- Black pepper and salt to taste.

Directions:

1 Season scallops with salt and pepper, put in a bowl and mix with half of the lime juice and half of the zest and toss to coat. In a bowl, mix the egg yolk with some salt and pepper, the rest of the lime juice and the rest of the lime zest and whisk well.
2 Add melted ghee and stir very well. Also, add fennel leaves and stir.
3 Brush fennel wedges with oil, place on heated grill over medium-high heat, cook for 2 minutes, flip and cook for 2 minutes more.
4 Add scallops on the grill, cook for 2 minutes, flip and cook for 2 minutes more. Divide fennel and scallops on plates, drizzle fennel and ghee mix and serve with lime wedges on the side. Enjoy!

Nutrition: Calories: 400 kcal Fat: 24 g Fiber: 4 g Carbs: 12 g Protein: 25 g.

WEEK 1

DAY 1

BREAKFAST

151. KETO COFFEE

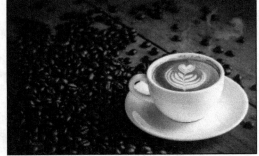

Cooking time: 60seconds

Servings: 2

Ingredient:
- 2 tbsp. organic coconut oil (or MCT oil)
- 1 tsp. vanilla extract (optional)
- 2 cups of coffee
- 2 tbsp. grass-fed of unsalted butter
- 1 tbsp. heavy whipping cream (Optional)

Prep. Time: 45 seconds

Direction:

1. Brew 2 cups of coffee with your preferred form into a big container. Try to pick something big enough (like a measuring jug) to prevent spill when we mix it.
2. If you use a pour-over process, my suggestion is the size of kosher (or somewhat smaller) salt to grind. Fill your coffee filter and wet the coffee with a little water and let it "bloom" for about 30 seconds. Then brew normally in a circular movement by pouring the sugar, carefully ensuring the coffee does not swim in sugar. Take your butter, cocoon oil and dip blender. If you like, you can mix it in a standard blender, but I feel it's more troublemaking than cleaning in a normal blender.
3. Cut 2 tbsp. Cut off of butter fed with hay. I'm shocked how few people use markings for packages – they just cut it in, they work! I like salted butter personally, but many do not. Feel free to start checking unsalted first.
4. Low the butter and add 1 tsp. Vanilla extract and 2 tbsp plunk. Coconut oil (or MCT oil if you need it) too. Finally, but not least, the 1 Tbsp. Strong cream. Heavy cream. This makes the coffee so smooth for a silky feel.
5. Mix it all with your immersion mixer. Usually, the top gets a large frothy cap between 45-60 seconds. Make sure the immersion blender is rotated up and down to emulsify all the fat in the coffee. This would also ventilate the mixture by adding extra froth. Note: You can

do it all with a regular blender bottle and mixer ball, so you don't have to shake fats every few min.

Nutrition: Calories260 Fats27.7g Net Carbs1.05g Protein1.08g.

6. Look out for the froth (it may drop down the side), but your keto proof coffee is done! Measure it and drink it in your favorite tub.

LUNCH

152. SALAD OF SESAME SALMON

Prep. Time: 5 min.   **Cooking time**: 20 min.   **Servings**: 2

Ingredient:

Salad

☞ One medium yellow pepper, chopped

☞ ¼ cup green onions, chopped

☞ One medium red pepper, chopped.

☞ One medium head lettuce, chopped

Dressing

☞ Five tbsp. coconut aminos

☞ One tsp. sesame oil

☞ Four tbsp. olive oil

☞ Two large (12-ounce each) salmon filets

☞ Two tbsp. coconut aminos

☞ One tsp. sesame oil

☞ Four tsp. olive oil

Directions:

1. Heat ¾ of the olive oil in a medium heat pot for the salad. Add sesame oil, cocoon oil and amino liquids.
2. Cut your salmon into smaller pieces if necessary. (I halved the two filets to make four parts)
3. Put your salmon in the pan and give 5-7 min. of cooking time.

4. Flip over them and cook for another 5 min. When done, they should be light rose to white on the inside. Place your salmon in a salad bowl, while your salmon is cooking.
5. Mix the dressing ingredients together in a smaller bowl.
6. After the salmon are finished, put it on top of the salad, dress up and enjoy!

Nutrition: Calories 383 Fats 27.14g Net Carbs 7.33g Protein 24.3g

DINNER

153. NACHO CHICKEN CASSEROLE

Prep. Time: 5 min.   **Cooking time**: 25 min.   **Servings**: 4

Ingredient:

☞ Salt and Pepper to Taste

☞ 1 1/2 tsp. Chili seasoning

☞ 1.75 lbs. Chicken Thighs, boneless skinless

☞ 4 oz. Cream Cheese

☞ 2 tbsp. Olive Oil

☞ 1 cup Green Chilies and Tomatoes

☞ 4 oz. Cheddar Cheese

☞ 1/4 cup Sour Cream

☞ 3 tbsp. Parmesan Cheese (~45g)

☞ One medium Jalapeño Pepper

☞ 16 oz. Frozen cauliflower, package

Directions:

1. Pre-heat 375F oven. Chop the chicken and season it, then cook in olive oil over medium to high until browned.
2. Add cream, sour cream and cheddar 3/4. Remove until melted and mixed together. Add tomatoes and chili green and mix together well. Add it all to a saucepan.

3. Frozen cauliflower microwave until cooked through. Using an immersion mixer to mix the rest of the cheese into a smooth potato. Saison to taste. Season to taste.
4. Cut jalapeño in pieces. Disseminate the cauliflower mixture over the top of the pot, then sprinkle the jalapeño pepper. Bake for fifteen-two min.

Nutrition: Calories 426 Fats 32.2g Net Carbs 4.3g Protein30.8g.

BREAKFAST

154. SAUSAGE GRAVY AND BISCUIT BAKE

Prep. Time: 10 min.   **Cooking time**: 30 min   **Servings**: 4

Ingredient:

- Two large egg whites
- One tsp. baking powder

Sausage Gravy:

- One tsp. xanthan gum
- 12 ounces ground pork breakfast sausage

- 1 cup almond flour
- Two tbsp. frozen butter

- ½ tsp. onion powder
- ½ cup half and half
- One tsp. black pepper

- ½ tsp. xanthan gum

- 1 ½ cups chicken broth
- ¼ tsp. salt, to taste

Directions:

1. Whisk the almond flour, baking powder and half a tsp. of xanthan gum together in a large cup.
2. Grate the frozen butter (or very cold). Mix with a fork in the flour mix until it appears like coarse crumbs. Set aside. Set aside.
3. The egg whites beat in a separate medium-sized bowl to steep peaks. Fold the egg whites into the flour mix until they are only mixed with a rubber spatula.
4. Chill the biscuit mixture when making the gravy in the refrigerator.
5. Brown the sausage over medium heat in a large skillet. Remove the sausage from the paper towel plate to drain the excess grate and keep in the saucepan about a tbsp. of fat.
6. Switch the heat to medium-low and sprinkle one tsp. of xanthan gum into the grease.

7. Cook the xanthan gum about a min. until it is browned lightly. Chicken, onion powder and black pepper whisk in the stock. Bring to a frying pan and let it thicken about 5 min. Sample and add salt when necessary at this time.
8. Stir in half and half and boil until thick and fluffy, about 3 min more.
9. Remove the cooked sausage and remove from the sun. Preheat the oven to a temperature of 375 ° F.
10. Pour the sausage in an 8x8 saucepan.
11. Drop the biscuit mixture in tiny spoonful's over the gravy and spread as fairly as possible. The blend is going to be dense.
12. Bake until sweet, bubbled for 18-20 min., and the biscuits are baked and browned.

Nutrition Calories374.67 Fats33.21g Net Carbs4.75g Protein14.48g.

LUNCH

155. OVEN ROASTED CAPRESE SALAD

Prep. Time: 10 min.   **Cooking time**: 30 min.   **Servings**: 6

Ingredient:

- 3 cups grape tomatoes
- 4 cloves garlic, peeled
- 4 cups baby spinach
- 1 tbsp. avocado oil

- 1 tbsp. pesto
- 10 pieces' pearl size mozzarella balls
- ¼ cup basil, fresh

- 1 tbsp. brine, reserved from cheese

Directions:

1. Heat the oven to 400 ° F and prepare a foil bakery. Spread the skinned cloves of garlic and tomatoes uniformly.

2. Drizzle the tomatoes with avocado oil and mix them to coat. Bake for about 20-30 min or until the juices are loosened, and the tops are slightly brown.

3. Drain the mozzarella sauce, set aside 1 tbsp. and mix with pesto tbsp. of salt.
4. Take the tomatoes out of the oven and place the spinach in a vast portion dish.
5. Add the spinach and roast garlic to warm tomatoes and drizzle the pesto sauce.
6. Add mozzarella balls and new ripped basil leaves.

Nutrition: Calories190.75, Fats63.49g, Net Carbs4.58g, Protein7.79g.

DINNER

156. BUFFALO CHICKEN JALAPEÑO CASSEROLE

Prep. Time: 20 min.   **Cooking time**: 55 min.   **Servings:** 6

Ingredient:

- Six slices bacon
- boneless of 2-pound chicken thighs, (6-small)
- 12 ounces' cream cheese
- Three medium jalapeños
- 4 ounces shredded cheddar cheese
- ¼ cup mayonnaise
- ¼ cup Frank's Red Hot
- 2 ounces shredded mozzarella Cheese
- Salt and pepper to taste
- De-seed if you're not a spicy fan.

Directions:

1. De-bone the chicken thighs and pre-heat oven to 400F. Season with salt and pepper, then put on a cooling rack over a cookie sheet covered in foil. Bake thighs of chicken at 400F for 40 min.
2. After 20 min of your timer, start filling. Chop 6 bacon pieces and place them in a pot over medium heat. Upon most of the bacon is crisped, add jalapeños to the pot.
3. When they are soft and fried, add cream cheese, mayo and the red-hot franks to the pot. Mix together and taste the season.
4. Remove from the oven the chicken and let it cool slightly. Remove the skins from the chicken until they are cool enough.
5. Put the chicken into a dish of casserole and spread the cream cheese mixture over it and add the cheddar and mozzarella.
6. Bake at 400F for 10-15 min. Cook for 3-5 min. to complete. Optional: Top with additional jalapeños before broiling.

Nutrition: Calories 782 Fats 66.97g Net Carbs 4.59g Protein 38.61g.

DAY 3

BREAKFAST

157. KETO COCONUT CREAM PIES

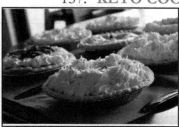

Prep. Time: 60 seconds

Cooking time: 5 min.

Servings: 2

Ingredient:

The Crust

- 4 tbsp. butter
- ¼ cup sugar substitute
- ½ cup almond flour
- ¼ cup unsweetened coconut flakes

The Custard

- 2 large egg yolks
- ¼ cup coconut flour
- 1 cup heavy whipping cream

- 🏳 1 tsp. vanilla extract
- 🏳 ½ cup water
- 🏳 ¼ cup sugar substitute

The Top

- 🏳 2 tbsp. sugar substitute
- 🏳 2-3 tbsp. unsweetened coconut flakes, toasted
- 🏳 1 cup heavy whipping cream
- 🏳 1 tsp. vanilla extract

Directions:

1. In a kettle, melt medium-low butter.
2. Stir in your sugar replacement until it dissolves in butter. Stir regularly. Mix your amber meal and coconut flakes until the mixture clumps easily together. Spoon the crust into a ramekin and flatten with a spoon.
3. Enable it to cool while making your custard
4. Heat your cream in a pot (I used the same pot as the crust). Separate the eggs and put them in a dish. It's time for the slurry!
5. Whisk your cocoa flour and the water. You should have a thick mixture of cocoa and egg.
6. Remove the vanilla from the stove to the milk.
7. Pour the slurry into the cream or spoon it.
8. Stir regularly with a whisk until the mixture thickens.
9. Let cool for about 5 min before spooning the custard on top of the crust into the ramekins.
10. Let the refrigerator set for at least one hour.
11. Heat your coconut flakes on a small pot to low. Stirring constantly. They are ready to toast when they are a perfect golden brown.
12. Remove the milk, vanilla and sugar in a big tub.
13. Beat the cream using a hand or stand mixer until it forms steep peaks.
14. Sprinkle the cream over the custard when ready to serve the custard and sprinkle the toasted coconut over it.

Nutrition: Calories 584 Net Carbs 7.25g Fats 57.33g Protein9.22g.

LUNCH

158. KETO LEMON POPPY SEED SCONES

Prep. Time: 5 seconds   **Cooking time**: 30 min.   **Servings**: 2

Ingredient:

- 🏳 1 ½ cups almond flour
- 🏳 2 tbsp. coconut flour
- 🏳 1 tbsp. psyllium husk fiber
- 🏳 1/2 tsp. baking powder
- 🏳 ¼ tsp. baking soda
- 🏳 1 tbsp. poppy seeds
- 🏳 4 tbsp. butter
- 🏳 ¼ cup erythritol
- 🏳 2 large eggs
- 🏳 ½ lemon, juice and zest
- 🏳 2 tbsp. erythritol, for sprinkling

Directions:

1. Then heat a 350F oven to a parchment paper baker. Combine almond flour, cocoa flour, psyllium husk fiber, baking powder and baking soda in a large mixing bowl. In cotton seeds, whisk until well mixed.
2. Break butter with a bell, pastry cutter or your hands into the dry ingredients to shape the dough.
3. In a separate cup, whisk eggs and sweetener together until sweetened.
4. Apply the sprinkling erythritol to the lemon on a tray. Mash sugar and zest together with a fork and set aside for dryness.
5. Break the lemon in half and squeeze the juice into the egg mixture, be careful not to get any seeds in the mixture.
6. In the dough, place the egg mixture and mix well.
7. Put the wet dough in the dome type on the prepared parchment.
8. Rate the wet dough carefully with a knife in 8 triangles and bake for 20 min.
9. Remove from an oven and cut into eight triangles. Sprinkle with lemon sugar and simmer for another 10 min.

Nutrition: Calories 206.8, Fat 18.5g Net Carbs 3.53g Protein 6.6g.

DINNER

159. LOW CARB HAMBURGER BUN

Prep. Time: 30 seconds   **Cooking time**: 2 min.   **Servings**: 1

Ingredient:

- 1 large egg
- 1 tbsp. melted butter
- 1 tbsp. chicken broth
- 1 tbsp. almond flour
- ¼ tsp. baking powder
- 1 tbsp. psyllium husk powder
- ¼ tsp. cream of tartar

Directions:

1. Crack the egg into a mug and put the melted butter into it. Remove well together until the eggs are lighter in color.
2. Apply the remaining ingredients and blend together thoroughly. You should have a slightly doughy substance.
3. Microwave for the 60-75 seconds, depending on the microwave wattage (it will buff in the mug, and reduce it greatly).
4. Cut in half and sprinkle with sugar.

Nutrition: Calories 248, Fats 19.77g, Net Carbs 3.01g, Protein 7.99g.

BREAKFAST

160. KETO AMARETTI COOKIES

Prep. Time: 5 min   **Cooking time**: 16 min   **Servings**: 10

Ingredient:

- 1 cup. Almond Flour
- 1 tbsp. Shredded Coconut
- 2 tbsp. Coconut Flour
- 1/4 tsp. Cinnamon
- 1/2 tsp. Baking Powder
- 1/2 cup Erythritol
- 1/2 tsp. Salt
- 2 large Eggs
- 1/2 tsp. Almond Extract
- 4 tbsp. Coconut Oil
- 1/2 tsp. Vanilla Extract
- 2 tbsp. Sugar-Free Jam

Directions:

1. Preheat your 350F oven. Combine all your dry ingredients and add the wet ingredients.
2. Shape your cookies on a bakery sheet lined with parchment paper. Use your finger to add an indent in the centre of each cookie.
3. Bake for about 16 min or until the cookies turn slightly golden. Let that cookie cool on a wire rack and make each indent with some sugar-free jam.
4. Sprinkle on top of each one some shredded coconut and enjoy!

Nutrition: Calories 89.38 Fats 8.11g Net Carbs 1.17g Protein 2.43g.

LUNCH

161. GRILLED SIRLOIN STEAK WITH CHIMICHURRI

Prep. Time: 10 Min   **Cooking Time**: 10 Min   **Servings**: 4

Ingredients

- 1.33 lbs. lean sirloin steak, trimmed (I recommend top sirloin)
- 1/2 tsp. black pepper
- 1 tsp. kosher salt
- 1/2 tsp. garlic powder
- 1/2 tsp. cumin
- 1 tbsp red wine vinegar
- 2 tbsp extra virgin olive oil
- 1 clove garlic, minced
- 2 tbsp parsley
- 2 tbsp cilantro
- 1 tbsp water
- 2 tbsp basil
- Salt and pepper

Directions:

1. Over medium heat preheat the grill or a grill pan.
2. In a blender or food processor, add red wine vinegar, olive oil, cilantro, basil, water, parsley, garlic, salt, and pepper. Mix until it forms a sauce, adding water if necessary. You can add red pepper flakes if you like spicy chimichurri.
3. Rub the salt, pepper, cumin, and garlic powder with the steak. Grill the steak to your desired doneness. Five min on each side for medium-rare, Get the steak removed and let it rest.
4. Thinly slice it on top of the grain and serve with chimichurri.

Nutrition Calories 280, Saturated Fat 6g, Polyunsaturated Fat 1g, Sodium 538mg, Total Carbohydrate 1g, Monounsaturated Fat 6g, Total Fat 19g, Sugars 0g, Cholesterol 87mg, Dietary Fiber 0g, Protein 25g.

DINNER

162. SOY CHICKEN AND VEGETABLES

Prep. Time: 10 Min   **Cooking Time**: 25 Min   **Servings**: 4

Ingredients

- 1/4 cup low sodium soy sauce
- 1 tbsp rice wine vinegar
- 2 tbsp oyster sauce
- 1 tbsp sesame oil

Salt and pepper

- 1 tbsp freshly grated ginger
- 1 cup carrots, sliced

- 1.33 lbs boneless skinless chicken thighs
- 2 cloves garlic, minced
- 1 cup mushrooms, halved

- 1 tsp. corn-starch
- 1 cup shelled edamame

- 2 cups broccoli florets
- 1 cup sugar snap peas

- 2 green onions, sliced

Directions:

1. To 425 degrees, heat the oven. Sprinkle with cooking spray on a large baking sheet. First, cover the baking sheet in foil for easier clean-up and then spray. In a small cup, add the soya sauce, rice vinegar, oyster sauce, corn-starch, sesame oil, garlic, and ginger and stir together.
2. On both sides, season the chicken with pepper. Place and drizzle with around half the soy mixture

on the baking sheet so that both sides are coated. Put the mixture in the oven and cook for ten min.

3. Remove it from the oven and spread the vegetables around the chicken on the baking sheet. Drizzle the remaining soy mixture with it. Return to the oven and cook for 10-15 min until the chicken is cooked and the vegetables are crisp and tender.

Nutrition: Calories 320, Sugars 4g, Monounsaturated Fat 3g, Saturated Fat 2g, Dietary Fiber 6g, Polyunsaturated Fat 3g, Total Fat 11g, Total Carbohydrate 17g, Cholesterol 131mg, Sodium 1048mg, Protein 39g.

DAY 5

BREAKFAST

163. KETO WHIPPED CREAM

Prep. Time: 60 seconds   **Cooking time**: 5 min   **Servings**: 2

Ingredient:

- 1 cup heavy cream, chilled well
- 1 tsp. vanilla extract
- 1 tbsp. erythritol, powdered

Directions:

1. Using a spice grinder or small blender to powder erythritol. Set aside the remaining ingredients.
2. Pour in a large, dry blender bowl with cold heavy cream. When washed beforehand, make sure all water is wiped from the blending bowl as only a small quantity of water can ruin whipped cream.
3. Start mixing the cream slowly with a hand mixer. Step up as the cream thickens so as not to sprinkle the cream.
4. Add powdered erythritol and vanilla extract after approximately 60 seconds of whipping.
5. Continue to whip to form medium peaks. The peaks on your beaters should be notified when they are taken out of the cream.
6. Move the cream to a bowl to serve your favourite dish. You can save 2-3 days in the fridge in an airtight jar.

Nutrition: 103 Calories, 0.9g Net Carbs, 10.8g Fats, 0.9g Protein.

LUNCH

164. KALE SOUP AND SAUSAGE

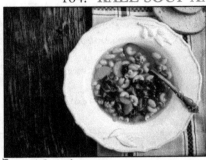

Prep. Time: 10 min

Cooking time: 25 min

Servings: 2

Ingredient:

- 1 Tbsp. butter
- 1 lb. sweet Italian sausage, ground
- One medium carrot, peeled and diced
- One medium yellow onion, chopped
- 2 tbsp. red wine vinegar
- Two cloves garlic, crushed
- 1 tsp. dried basil
- 1 tsp. dried oregano
- ¼ – ½ tsp. crushed red pepper flakes
- 1 tsp. dried rubbed sage
- 1 cup heavy whipping cream
- 4 cups low-sodium chicken broth
- 3 cups kale, chopped
- ½ medium head cauliflower, cut into small florets
- ½ tsp. freshly ground black pepper
- ½ – 1 tsp. sea salt, or to taste

Directions:

1. Heat a large casserole or Netherlands oven over medium heat. Attach ground sausage and split the beef. Cook and stir it occasionally, for 5 min, until browned and cooked.
2. Remove cooked sausage using a slotted spoon and make the drainage on a sheet covered with paper towels. Drippings discard but do not wash the pan.
3. Melt medium heat butter. Attach onion and carrot when bubbling subsides. Cook until the onion becomes brown and translucent on the outside.
4. Mix garlic into the mixture of onion and carrot. Cook one min. Cook one min. Add vinegar of red wine and cook until sip, scrap browned bits for approximately 1 min.
5. Remove the flakes of oregano, basil, wise and red pepper. Pour in heavy cream and stock. Increase medium-high sun. When the soup cooks, add colic and turn heat to medium-low. Simmer uncovered for about ten min, until cauliflower is fork-tender. Stir in the cooked sausage and kale. Cook for like 2 min, and/or till the sausage and kale wilts are restored.
6. Season with salt and pepper to taste. The amount of salt required can vary because of variations in broth marks.

Nutrition: Calories 298 Fats 24g Net Carbs 6g Protein 16g

DINNER

165. LOW CARB CORNED BEEF CABBAGE ROLLS

Prep. Time: 30 min   **Cooking time:** 6 hours 5min   **Servings:** 4

Ingredient:

- pounds corned beef
- 1 medium onion
- 15 large savoy cabbage leaves
- 1 large lemon
- ¼ cup white wine
- 1 large bay leaf
- ¼ cup coffee
- 1 tbsp. rendered bacon fat
- 1 tbsp. NOW Erythritol
- 1 tbsp. brown mustard
- 2 tsp. kosher salt
- 1 tsp. whole peppercorns
- 2 tsp. Worcestershire
- 1 tsp. mustard seeds
- ¼ tsp. cloves
- ½ tsp. red pepper flakes
- ¼ tsp. allspice

Directions:

1. Connect to the slow cooker the corned beef, liquids and spices. Let this cook on low for 6 hours.
2. Put a pot of water to a boil when it is about to be taken.
3. Add the 15 cod leaves plus 1 sliced onion for 2-3 min to the boiling water.
4. Remove the cod from the water and blanch for 3-4 min in ice water. Continue to boil in the water the onion.
5. Dry chops, cut meat, apply ointments and roll fillings into the chops.
6. Optional: Serve with a new lemon squeeze!

Nutrition: Calories481.4 Fats25.38g Net Carbs4.2g Protein34.87g

DAY 6

BREAKFAST

166. GRILLED BUFFALO CHICKEN SANDWICHES

Prep. Time: 5 Min   **Cooking Time**: 15 Min   **Servings**: 4

Ingredients

- 1 lb. boneless skinless chicken breasts
- Cooking spray
- 1 tsp. paprika
- 1/4 cup blue cheese
- 1 tsp. chili powder
- 1/4 cup buffalo sauce
- Salt and pepper
- 1/4 cup nonfat plain Greek yogurt
- 4 tsp. butter
- 4 reduced calorie hamburger buns

Directions:

1. Cut the chicken into thinner cutlets or pound it. Season with paprika, chili powder, salt, and pepper and sprinkle with cooking spray.
2. Over medium-high heat, heat a grill, grill pan, or skillet. If required, sprinkle with cooking spray. Cook the chicken on each side for 3-4 min or until it has cooked through.
3. Meanwhile, yogurt and blue cheese are mixed together to produce a burger sauce. With salt and pepper, season. The butter is melted and stirred into the buffalo sauce. Toss this mixture with the cooked chicken breasts.
4. Put the sandwiches together and add lettuce, tomatoes, onions, and any other toppings that you want.

Nutrition: Calories 285, Saturated Fat 4g, Cholesterol 72mg, Monounsaturated Fat 0g, Total Fat 8g, Total

Carbohydrate 19g, Sugars 3g, Sodium 403mg, Polyunsaturated Fat 0g, Dietary Fiber 3g, Protein 31g.

LUNCH

167. GRILLED PORK CHOPS WITH PEACH SALSA

Prep. Time: 10 Min   **Cooking Time**: 15 Min   **Servings**: 4

Ingredients

- 1.33 lbs. boneless lean center cut pork chops
- 1 tsp. chili powder (or more)
- 2 tbsp. olive oil, divided
- Salt and pepper
- 1/2 tsp. salt
- 2 peaches, chopped
- 1/2 tsp. pepper
- 2 tbsp. cilantro
- 1/4 red onion, chopped
- 1 tbsp. lime juice

Directions:

1. Preheat to medium-high heat on the grill or a grill pan. You may use the broiler as well.
2. Brush the olive oil with the pork chops and sprinkle on both sides with chili powder, salt, and pepper.
3. Grill on each side for 4-5 min (or to the desired level). Let yourself rest for 5 min. Place on a baking sheet on a wire rack to broil and broil for 4-5 min per side.
4. Toss the lime juice, peaches, cilantro, onion, and olive oil together to make the salsa: season with salt and pepper season. Over pork, serve. Grill the peaches before making the salsa for a fun twist.

Nutrition: Calories 287, Monounsaturated Fat 2g, Saturated Fat 3g, Total Carbohydrate 9g, Polyunsaturated Fat 1g, Total Fat 12g, Sodium 381mg, Cholesterol 100mg, Sugars 7g, Dietary Fiber 1g, Protein 35g.

DINNER

168. PASTA WITH FRESH TOMATO SAUCE

Prep. Time: 40 Min   **Cooking Time**: 10 Min   **Servings**: 4

Ingredients

- 1 tsp. thyme
- 2 lbs. tomatoes, diced (about ½ inch.)
- 1/2 cup fresh basil (or parsley)
- 2 tbsp. olive oil
- 8 oz. high fiber pasta
- 2 tbsp. balsamic vinegar
- Salt and pepper
- 2 garlic cloves, minced

Directions:

1. Toss together the tomatoes, olive oil, basil (or parsley), thyme, vinegar, garlic, salt, and pepper. Let it sit for 30 min at room temperature (up to 4 hours.)
2. Cook the pasta according to package instructions when ready to eat. Toss in the warm tomato pasta and eat.

Nutrition: Calories 281, Saturated Fat 1g, Polyunsaturated Fat 0g, Total Fat 13g, Cholesterol 0mg, Dietary Fiber 9g, Sodium 14mg, Total Carbohydrate 52g, Sugars 9g, Monounsaturated Fat 0g, Protein 8g.

DAY 7

BREAKFAST

169. BACON CRUSTED FRITTATA MUFFINS

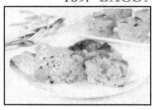

Prep. Time: 5 min

Cooking time: 30 min

Servings: 5

Ingredient:

- ½ tsp. onion powder
- 18 slices bacon
- ½ tsp. cayenne pepper
- 7 large eggs
- 1 cup cheddar cheese
- 4 tbsp. heavy whipping cream
- ½ tsp. ground black pepper
- ½ tsp. celery salt

Directions:

1. Preheat your 375F oven.
2. Break your bacon pieces in half and mold them in a cupcake bowl around the outsides and underneath of each well. You can use roughly 2 bacon slices per well, often more to fill in excess gaps.
3. Bake the bacon baskets 15 min in the oven before cooking. While the bacon is being fried, whisk some eggs, cream and spices together. Feel free to add some additional fresh herbs.
4. Put 1-2 dc. Cheddar cheese at the base of any frittata bacon. Put approximately 1/4 of an egg mixture in any bacon mold and do your best not to leave out any egg. Put them in the oven for a further 12-15 min or until they begin browning on top.
5. Take off the oven, let it cool. Serve or shop later!

Nutrition: Calories 467.57 Net Carbs 2.23g Fats 41.83g Protein 19.35g.

LUNCH

170. GRILLED CHICKEN WITH PEACH CUCUMBER SALSA

Prep. Time: 10 Min   **Cooking Time**: 10 Min   **Servings**: 4

Ingredients

- 1.33 lbs. boneless skinless chicken breast
- 1 tbsp. honey (leave out for Low Carb, Paleo, Whole30)
- 1 tbsp. olive oil
- 1 tsp. cumin
- 1 tbsp. soy sauce
- 2 peaches, diced
- 1/2 tsp. pepper
- 1/4 cup red onion, diced
- 2 Persian cucumbers, diced
- 1 tbsp. lime juice
- 1/4 cup cilantro, minced
- 1 tbsp. rice wine vinegar

Directions:

1. Put the olive oil, the honey, the soy sauce, the cumin and the pepper together. With this mixture, clean the chicken.
2. Mix the peaches, the cucumber, the red onion, the lime juice, the olive oil, and the rice vinegar. With salt and pepper, season.
3. On a medium hot grill, grill the chicken for 3-5 min on each side, depending on the thickness of your chicken. After grill marks emerge, flip it and the chicken is quickly removed from the grill.
4. With the cucumber salsa and peach on top, serve the chicken.

Nutrition: Calories 265, Saturated Fat 2g, Polyunsaturated Fat 0g, Cholesterol 243mg, Total Fat 10g, Total Carbohydrate 11g, Sodium 556mg, Dietary Fiber 2g, Sugars 8g, Monounsaturated Fat 0g, Protein 34g.

DINNER

171. BAKED SCAMPI

Prep time: 30 min   **Cook time**: 15 min   **Servings** 4

Ingredients

- 1 tbsp. fresh lemon juice
- 1 tbsp. garlic, chopped
- 1 tbsp. fresh parsley, chopped
- 2 tbsp. prepared Dijon mustard
- 2 pounds (907 g) raw shrimp, medium, shelled, deveined, with tails attached
- 1 cup butter

Directions:

1. Start by preheating the oven to 450°F (235°C).
2. Mix the lemon juice, butter, garlic, parsley and mustard in a small saucepan over moderate heat until the butter melts.
3. In a baking dish, place the shrimp, then pour over the butter mixture.
4. Arrange the dish in the preheated oven and bake for 13 min or until the shrimp are easily flaked with a fork. Remove the baking pan from the oven and serve warm.

Nutrition: Calories: 420 Total Fat: 32.9g Carbs: 1.7g Protein: 29.7g Cholesterol: 320mg Sodium: 681mg

WEEK 3

BREAKFAST

172. GRILLED HAWAIIAN BOWL

Prep Time: 10 min   **Cooking Time:** 0 min   **Servings** 1

Ingredients

- 2 slices (1/4-inch-thick) grilled fresh pineapple
- 2/3 cup cooked brown rice
- 1/4 cup thinly sliced grilled red onion

- 1/3 cup chopped red bell pepper
- 3 ounces grilled pork tenderloin
- 1/2 cup grilled sliced zucchini

Honey-Soy Sauce:

- 1 1/2 tsp. rice vinegar
- 1 tbsp. lower-sodium soy sauce
- 1 tsp. canola oil

- 1 tsp. honey
- 1/8 tsp. crushed red pepper

Directions:

1. Pineapple-cooked brown rice, red onion, red bell pepper, grilled pork and zucchini.
2. Combine the soy sauce, vinegar, sugar, canola oil, and crushed red pepper in a small bowl and blend well with a whisk. Spread over a mug.

Nutrition: Calories 393 Satfat 1.4g Fat 10.8g Polyfat 2g Monofat 4.8g Carbohydrate 56g Protein 22g Cholesterol 45mg Fiber 6g Sodium 588mg Iron 3mg Sugars 22g Calcium 41mg Est. added sugars 6g

---

LUNCH

173. PORK WRAPS

Prep Time: 15 min   **Cooking Time:** 5 min   **Servings** 4

Ingredients

- 1 tbsp. minced peeled fresh ginger
- 1 tbsp. dark sesame oil
- 1 cup matchstick-cut carrot
- 5 garlic cloves, minced
- 1 cup (1-inch) pieces green onions
- 2 (3.5-ounce) packages sliced fresh shiitake mushrooms
- 1/8 tsp. kosher salt

- 4 cups thinly sliced napa cabbage
- 12 ounces boneless pork shoulder, trimmed and very thinly sliced
- 1 tsp. sugar
- Cooking spray
- 1 tbsp. hoisin sauce
- 1 1/2 tbsp. water
- 8 (6.5-inch) whole-wheat tortilla

Directions:

1. Over medium heat, heat a large skillet. In a pan, add oil; swirl to coat. Add the ginger and garlic; cook for 30 seconds, continuously stirring. Raise the heat to medium-high heat. Add the mushrooms and carrot; cook for 2 min, stirring frequently. Add the cabbage and onions; cook for 1 to 2 min or until the cabbage

wilts. Spoon the mixture of cabbage into a large bowl; stir in the salt.

2. With paper towels, wipe the pan clean. Bring the pan back to medium-high heat. Mix the sugar and pork together, tossing well to coat. Cover pan with spray for cooking. Add the mixture of pork to the pan; cook for 3 min or until the pork is browned and done, stirring occasionally. Add 1 1/2 tbsp. of water to the pan carefully, scraping the pan to loosen the browned pieces. Incorporate the hoisin sauce. Apply the mixture of cabbage to the pan; gently toss to blend. Spoon each tortilla with about 2/3 of a cup of pork mixture, roll-up.

Nutrition: Calories 391 Satfat 4.6g Fat 14.1g Polyfat 3g Monofat 6.2g Carbohydrate 40g Protein 25g Cholesterol 57mg Fiber 20g Sodium 676mg Iron 3mg Sugars 8g Calcium 231mg Est. added sugars 2g

DINNER

174. STRAWBERRY-CHICKEN SALAD WITH PECANS

Prep Time:15 min   **Cooking Time**: 5 min   **Servings** 2

Ingredients

- 1 tbsp. white balsamic vinegar
- 4 tsp. extra-virgin olive oil, divided
- 1/2 tsp. chopped fresh thyme
- 1 tsp. honey
- 1/4 tsp. kosher salt, divided
- 3/8 tsp. freshly ground black pepper, divided
- 2 cups halved strawberries, divided
- 3/8 tsp. freshly ground black pepper, divided
- 1/4 tsp. smoked paprika

- 2 (4-ounce) skinless, boneless chicken breast cutlets
- Cooking spray
- 1/4 cup thinly sliced red onion
- 4 cups fresh baby spinach
- 1 ounce reduced-fat feta cheese, crumbled (about 1/4 cup)
- 3 tbsp. chopped pecans, toasted

Directions:

1. In a medium cup, combine vinegar, one tbsp. oil, thyme, honey, 1/4 tsp. pepper, and 1/8 tsp. salt; blend with a whisk. Attach 1 cup of strawberries and toss to cover. Let it stand for 10 min at room temperature.
2. Over medium-high heat, heat a medium skillet. Brush the chicken with one tsp. of oil remaining; sprinkle with the remaining 1/8 tsp. of pepper, salt, and paprika evenly. Cover pan with spray for cooking. Add the chicken to the pan; cook on each side or until cooked, 2 to 3 min. Take the chicken out of the pan; leave to stand for 5 min. Cut into slices across the grain.
3. Divide the spinach into two plates, the remaining 1 cup of strawberries, and the onion. Using chicken slices as well as a strawberry-balsamic mixture to top evenly. Top with 1 1/2 tbsp. of pecans and two tbsp. of cheese for each serving.

Nutrition: Calories 399 Satfat 3.9g Fat 22.2g Polyfat 4g Monofat 11.7g Carbohydrate 22g Protein 31g Cholesterol 77mg Fiber 6g Sodium 619mg Iron 3mg Sugars 12g Calcium 147mg Est. added sugars 3g

DAY 2

BREAKFAST

175. TOFU AND NOODLE BOWL WITH CARAMELIZED COCONUT

Prep Time :20 min   **Cooking Time**: 15 min   **Servings** 4

Ingredients

- 1 tsp. grated peeled fresh ginger
- 2 tsp. grated fresh jalapeño pepper
- 1 garlic clove, grated
- 1 (13.5-ounce) can light coconut milk
- 6 ounces dried brown rice noodles (such as Annie Chun's)
- 1 (14-ounce) package extra-firm water-packed tofu, drained and cut into 1/2-inch cubes
- 1/2 cup unsalted vegetable stock
- 1 1/2 cups frozen edamame
- 3/4 tsp. kosher salt
- 1 1/2 tbsp. fresh lime juice
- 1/4 cup chopped unsalted, dry-roasted peanuts
- 6 ounces baby spinach

Directions:

1. Combine a large skillet with the first 4 ingredients; bring to a boil. Tofu is applied to the pan. Cook for 12 min or until the liquid is reduced to about 1/3 cup and begins to turn golden light, stirring regularly.
2. According to package instructions, prepare rice noodles, omitting salt and fat. At the last min of cooking, add the edamame to the noodles. Set aside 1/2 of a cup of cooking liquid. Drain the noodle mixture; apply cold water to rinse, then drain.
3. Add the mixture of noodles, stock, and 1/2 cup of reserved cooking liquid into the pan; toss to cover. Stir in the juice, salt, and spinach. Remove from the sun. Sprinkle peanuts on them.

Nutrition: Calories 393 Satfat 2.8g Fat 13.6g Polyfat 5g Monofat 3.4g Carbohydrate 52g Protein 18g Cholesterol 0.0mg

Fiber 5g Sodium 469mg Iron 5mg Calcium 145mg

LUNCH

176. KOREAN SHRIMP BBQ BOWL

Prep Time :20 min   **Cooking Time**: 15 min   **Servings** 1

Ingredients

- 1 ounce shiitake mushrooms
- 2 cups fresh spinach
- 2/3 cup cooked brown rice
- 1/2 tsp. canola oil
- 1/3 cup shredded cabbage
- 1 fried egg
- 1/3 cup matchstick-cut carrot
- 3 ounces pan-seared large shrimp
- 2 tbsp. chopped green onions

Spicy Aioli:

- 1 1/2 tsp. canola mayonnaise
- 2 tsp. gochujang (Korean chile sauce)
- 1 small garlic clove, minced
- 1/4 tsp. dark sesame oil

Directions:

1. Sauté the mushrooms and spinach in canola oil. Cooked brown rice with a blend of wilted spinach, carrot, cabbage, shrimp, green onions, and egg.

2. Combine the mayonnaise, gochujang, sesame oil, and minced garlic in a small bowl. Drizzle over tub.

Nutrition: Calories 400 Satfat 2.2g Fat 14.3g Polyfat 3.2g Monofat 5.3g Est. added sugars 3g Carbohydrate 43g Protein 27g Cholesterol 311mg Fiber 6g Sodium 595mg Iron 4mg Sugars 7g Calcium 177mg

DINNER

177. STEAK TACOS

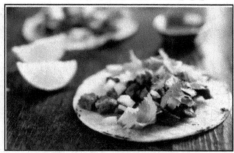

Prep. Time - 2 Hours 25 Mins

Cooking Time - 25 Mins

Servings 6

Ingredients

- 1/4 cup olive oil, divided
- 1 medium red onion, peeled and cut into 1/2-inch-thick slices
- 2 dried chiles de arbol
- 1/4 cup Mexican crema
- 5 garlic cloves, minced
- 1 (1 1/2-pound) flat iron or skirt steak
- 5 tbsp. fresh lime juice
- Cooking spray
- 3/4 tsp. kosher salt
- 3/4 cup Toasted Chile Salsa
- 12 Fresh Corn Tortillas or packaged corn tortillas, warmed

Directions:

1. Over high cook, cook a cast-iron skillet. Add onion; cook, turning once, for 5 min or until charred. Remove from pan; chop and put in a bowl.
2. Over medium heat, heat a small skillet. To the tub, apply two tbsp. of oil. Add garlic and chiles; cook two min, stirring occasionally. In a cup, apply the garlic mixture to the onion. Incorporate the juice and remaining oil. Mix half of the onion mixture (including both chiles de árbol) as well as steak in a large zip-top plastic bag; seal. Refrigerate 1 hour. Reserve the remaining mixture of onions. Remove the steak from the fridge; leave to stand for 1 hour at room temperature. Preheat the grill to a medium-high temperature.
3. Remove steak from marinade; discard marinade. Wipe off the steak with any remaining onion and garlic. Sprinkle salt with the steak. Place the steak on a spray-coated grill rack; grill over medium-high heat for 8 min or until desired, turning once. Set aside from the grill; leave to stand for 15 min.
4. Cut the steak into very thin slices around the grain. To the reserved onion mixture, add the steak and accumulated juices, toss. Put two tortillas on six plates each. Top each tortilla with the 1 1/2 ounces of steak; divide onion mixture among tacos. Place one tbsp. of Toasted Chile Salsa and one tsp. of cream each on top.

Nutrition: Calories 395 Satfat 4.6g Fat 18.3g Polyfat 1.2g Monofat 7.7g Carbohydrate 30g Protein 27g Cholesterol 81mg Fiber 3g Sodium 574mg Iron 6mg Sugars 2g Calcium 71mg Est. added sugars 0g

178. STEAK AND ROASTED SWEET POTATO BOWL

Prep Time :10 min   **Cooking Time**: 0 min   **Servings** 1

Ingredients

- 1 tbsp. salsa verde
- 1/2 cup cooked brown rice
- 2 tbsp. thinly sliced peeled avocado
- 1/3 cup black beans
- 1 1/2 ounces grilled flank steak
- 1/2 cup cubed roasted sweet potato
- 2 tbsp. fresh cilantro
- 1 tbsp. roasted pumpkin seed kernels
- 1 tsp. olive oil
- Honey-Chipotle-Lime Sauce:
- 1/2 tsp. honey
- 1 tsp. adobo sauce
- 1 tsp. fresh lime juice

Directions:

1. Mix the cooked brown rice along with the salsa verde. Black beans, avocado, sweet potato, steak, kernels of pumpkin seeds, and cilantro on top.

2. Combine the olive oil, adobo sauce, sugar, and lime juice in a small bowl and whisk in a small bowl. Sprinkle over the bowl of steak.

Nutrition: Calories 398 Satfat 2.3g Fat 12.4g Polyfat 1.2g Monofat 6.4g Carbohydrate 52g Protein 21g Cholesterol 32mg Fiber 10g Sodium 438mg Iron 3mg Sugars 7g Calcium 73mg Est. added sugars 3g

---

LUNCH

179. CHICKEN AND BLACK BEAN ENCHILADAS

Prep. Time - 1 Hour 45 Mins   **Cooking Time** - 23 Mins   **Servings** 8

Ingredients

- Cooking spray
- 1 1/2 cups chopped onion
- 1 tbsp. canola oil
- 5 garlic cloves, minced
- 1 cup chopped poblano chile
- 1 tsp. ground cumin
- 2 tsp. chili powder
- 1 cup unsalted chicken stock
- 1/2 tsp. dried oregano
- 2 (8-ounce) cans unsalted tomato sauce
- 1 tbsp. pureed canned chipotle chiles in adobo sauce
- 1 (15.5-ounce) can unsalted black beans, rinsed and drained
- 3 cups shredded cooked skinless chicken breast
- 4 ounces shredded part-skim mozzarella cheese (about 1 cup)
- 4 ounces shredded reduced-fat cheddar cheese (about 1 cup)
- 1 cup prepared salsa
- 16 (6-inch) corn tortillas
- Fresh cilantro leaves (optional)
- 1/2 cup reduced-fat sour cream

Directions:

1. Preheat the oven to 350 degrees. Using cooking spray to cover a 13 x 9-inch baking dish.

2. Heat oil over medium heat in a large skillet. Add the onion, poblano, and garlic and sauté for 4 min or

until the poblano and onion are tender. Stir in chili powder, cumin and oregano. Add stock, chipotle, and tomato sauce and simmer; cook for 5 min or until slightly thickened.

3. In a medium bowl, combine the chicken and the black beans; add half the sauce mixture. Combine the cheeses in a bowl; blend the chicken mixture with 1/2 cup cheese mixture. To combine, toss.

4. Put eight tortillas on a microwave-safe plate; cover with a paper towel that is slightly damp. Microwave for 45 seconds at HIGH or until warm. Place the tortilla on a flat work surface, operating with one tortilla at a time; spoon 1/4 cup chicken mixture on one end of the tortilla. Roll up, style jelly-roll. Repeat the process for leftover tortillas when the first batch is used up, heating up the second batch of tortillas. Arrange the enchiladas in the prepared bowl, seam side down. Sprinkle with the remaining the cheese mixture; pour the remaining sauce over the enchiladas. Bake for thirteen min or until the sauce is bubbly and the cheese is melted and golden brown, uncovered, at 350 °. When needed, serve enchiladas with salsa, sour cream, and cilantro.

Nutrition: Calories 406 Satfat 5.4g Fat 13.1g Polyfat 1.8g Monofat 2.9g Carbohydrate 42g Protein 32g Est. added sugars 1g Cholesterol 70mg Fiber 8g Sodium 531mg Iron 3mg Sugars 7g Calcium 435mg

DINNER

180. ROASTED SALMON WITH WINE COUSCOUS

Prep. Time: 45 Mins   **Cooking Time** 15 Mins   **Servings** 4

- 2 tbsp. chopped fresh chives
- 2 tbsp. 2% reduced-fat Greek yogurt
- 4 tsp. lemon juice, divided
- 2 tbsp. olive oil, divided
- 1 1/8 tsp. kosher salt, divided
- 4 (6-ounce) salmon fillets
- 2 cups finely chopped carrots
- 1/2 tsp. black pepper, divided
- 2 tsp. minced garlic
- 1/4 cup minced shallots
- 1 cup hot cooked couscous
- 1/3 cup dry white wine

Directions:

1. Preheat the oven to 450 degrees. Combine the yogurt, chives, two tsp. of oil, and one tbsp. of juice and whisk together. Sprinkle 1/2 tsp. salt and 1/4 tsp. pepper over the fish. Rub with a mixture of 2 tsp. yogurt. Over high heat, heat an ovenproof skillet. To the pan, add one tsp. of oil. Add fish, side down on the skin; cook for 2 min. Turn to the oven. Bake for 5 min at 450 °. Turn the fish over; cook for 1 min or until ready.

2. Over medium-high prepare, prepare a skillet. To the tub, apply the remaining one tbsp. of oil. Add the carrots, shallots, and garlic; cook, occasionally stirring, for 4 min. Apply the remaining one tsp. of lemon juice, the remaining 5/8 of a tsp. of salt, 1/4 of a tsp. of pepper and wine. 30 seconds to cook. Stir in couscous; toss. Serve the fish with a combination of couscous and yogurt.

Nutrition: Calories 404 Satfat 2.7g Fat 17.9g Polyfat 5.1g Monofat 8.5g Est. added sugars 0g Carbohydrate 19g Protein 37g Cholesterol 94mg Fiber 3g Sodium 667mg Iron 2mg Sugars 4g Calcium 59mg

DAY 4

BREAKFAST

181. VEGETARIAN TORTILLA SOUP

Prep. Time: 5 Min   **Cooking Time**: 25 Min   **Servings**: 4

Ingredients

- 2 tsp. olive oil
- 2 cloves garlic, minced
- 1 onion, diced
- 1 tsp. cumin
- 2 tsp. paprika
- 3/4 tsp. chili powder
- 3/4 tsp. coriander
- 14 oz. crushed tomatoes
- 1/8 tsp. cayenne pepper
- 14 oz. canned hominy, rinsed and drained
- 4 cups vegetable broth
- 2 limes
- 1 cup corn (frozen or canned)
- 1/4 cup cilantro
- 14 oz. canned black beans, rinsed and drained
- 2 corn tortillas
- 2 oz queso fresco
- 2 radishes, sliced into super thin rounds

Directions:

1. To 400 degrees, preheat the oven. Heat the olive oil over high-medium heat. Add the onion and cook for approximately 4-5 min. Garlic is added and cooked for 30 seconds. Spices are added and cook for 30 seconds.
2. Add the broth and the crushed tomatoes. Together, stir. You may want to use an immersion blender at this stage to mix the tomatoes and broth if you want a smoother soup.
3. Add the black beans and hominy. Boil for 20 min.
4. Break your tortillas into tiny strips. Use cooking spray to sprinkle and put on a baking sheet or foil. Bake until crispy for 6-8 min.
5. Crunchy strips of tortillas, cheese, cilantro, radishes, and lime juice.

Nutrition: Calories 312, Monounsaturated Fat 0g, Cholesterol 10mg, Saturated Fat 2g, Total Carbohydrate 55g, Polyunsaturated Fat 0g, Sodium 1786mg, Dietary Fiber 15g, Sugars 10g, Total Fat 8g, Protein 13g.

LUNCH

182. PARMESAN BROCCOLI PASTA

Prep. Time: 5 Min   **Cooking Time**: 20 Min   **Servings**: 4

Ingredients

- 2 tsp. olive oil
- 8 oz. high fiber pasta
- 4 cloves garlic, minced
- 1 cup skim milk (add more if needed)
- 2 cups vegetable broth
- 1/2 cup Parmesan cheese
- 3 cups broccoli florets
- Salt and pepper

Directions:

1. Heat the olive oil over high-medium heat. Add garlic and cook until fragrant, for 1-2 min. Pasta, broth, and milk should be added together. Carry to a boil and then to a simmer; turn down. Cook, sometimes stirring, for 18-20 min. After 8 min, add the broccoli. To make a creamy sauce, cook until the pasta is completely cooked, and the fluid is absorbed. Add more milk or vegetable broth if needed.
2. Stir in the cheese with Parmesan. Using salt and plenty of black pepper to season.

Nutrition: Calories 300, Saturated Fat 3g, Polyunsaturated Fat 0g, Total Carbohydrate 52g, Monounsaturated Fat 0g, Total Fat 12g, Sodium 751mg, Sugars 7g, Dietary Fiber 8g, Cholesterol 11mg, Protein 15g.

DINNER

183. CHICKEN PARMESAN ZUCCHINI BOATS

Prep. Time: 15 Min   **Cooking Time**: 35 Min   **Servings**: 5

Ingredients

- 5 zucchini
- 2 garlic clove, minced
- 1 cup part skim shredded mozzarella cheese
- 1/2 cup onion, diced
- 2 tsp olive oil
- 1/4 cup basil, chopped
- 1 lb 99% lean ground chicken (or chopped chicken breast)
- 1/2 tsp oregano
- 14 oz canned diced Italian tomatoes, drained

Directions:

1. To 400, preheat the oven.
2. To build a ship, slice the zucchini and scoop out the centers with a spatula. Finely chop the scooped-out zucchini.
3. Over medium flame heat the olive oil. Add the chicken and onion from the ground. Cook for 6-8 min until it is not pink anymore.
4. Garlic, chopped zucchini, diced tomatoes, basil, and oregano are added to the altogether. Cook until fragrant for 2-3 min.
5. Place it in a baking dish with the zucchini. Fill the mixture with chicken. With shredded cheese on top.
6. Using foil to cover and bake for 25 min. Then remove the foil and bake for another 10 min.

Nutrition Calories 267, Monounsaturated Fat 1g, Saturated Fat 4g, Sodium 359mg, Polyunsaturated Fat 0g, Dietary Fiber 4gm, Total Fat 11g, Total Carbohydrate 16g, Sugars 11g, Cholesterol 76mg, Protein 27g.

DAY 5

BREAKFAST

184. STEAK AND ROASTED SWEET POTATO BOWL

Prep. Time: 15 Min   **Cooking Time**: 0 Min   **Servings**: 1

Ingredients

- 1 tbsp. salsa verde
- 1/2 cup cooked brown rice
- 2 tbsp. thinly sliced peeled avocado
- 1/3 cup black beans
- 1 1/2 ounces grilled flank steak
- 1/2 cup cubed roasted sweet potato
- 2 tbsp. fresh cilantro
- 1 tbsp. roasted pumpkin seed kernels
- 1 tsp. olive oil
- Honey-Chipotle-Lime Sauce:
- 1/2 tsp. honey
- 1 tsp. adobo sauce
- 1 tsp. fresh lime juice

Directions:

1. Mix the cooked brown rice along with the salsa verde. Black beans, avocado, sweet potato, steak, kernels of pumpkin seeds, and cilantro on top.
2. Combine the olive oil, adobo sauce, sugar, and lime juice in a small bowl and whisk in a small bowl. Sprinkle over the bowl of steak.

Nutrition: Calories 398 Satfat 2.3g Fat 12.4g Polyfat 1.2g Monofat 6.4g Carbohydrate 52g Protein 21g Cholesterol 32mg Fiber 10g Sodium 438mg Iron 3mg Sugars 7g Calcium 73mg Est. added sugars 3g

LUNCH

185. SPICY CHICKEN WINGS

Prep Time: 20 min   **Cooking Time**: 30 min   **Servings**: 4

Ingredients:

- 2 lb. Chicken Wings
- 1 tsp. Cajun Spice
- 2 tsp. Smoked Paprika
- ½ tsp. Turmeric
- Salt - Dash
- 2 tbsp. Baking Powder
- Pepper - Dash.

Directions:

1. When you first begin the Ketogenic Diet, you may find that you won't be eating the traditional foods that may have made up a majority of your diet in the past. While this is a good thing for your health, you may feel you are missing out! The good news is that there are delicious alternatives that aren't lacking in flavor!
2. To start this recipe, you'll want to prep the stove to 400°F. As this heat up, you will want to take some time to dry your chicken wings with a paper towel. This will help remove any excess moisture and get you some nice, crispy wings!
3. When you are all set, take out a mixing bowl and place all of the seasonings along with the baking powder. If you feel like it, you can adjust the seasoning levels however you would like.
4. Once these are set, go ahead and throw the chicken wings in and coat evenly.
5. If you have one, you'll want to place the wings on a wire rack that is placed over your baking tray. If not, you can just lay them across the baking sheet.
6. Now that your chicken wings are set, you are going to pop them into the stove for 30 min.
7. By the end of this time, the tops of the wings should be crispy. If they are, take them out from the oven and flip them so that you can bake the other side.
8. You will want to cook these for an additional 30 min.
9. Finally, take the tray from the oven and allow it to cool slightly before serving up your spiced keto wings. For additional flavor, serve with any of your favorite, keto-friendly dipping sauce.

Nutrition: Calories 299 kcal Fats: 7 g Carbs: 1 g Proteins: 60 g.

DINNER

186. LEMONY ROASTED SALMON WITH WHITE WINE COUSCOUS

Prep. Time: 25 Mins   **Cooking Time**: 15 Mins   **Servings**: 4

Ingredients

- 2 tbsp. chopped fresh chives
- 2 tbsp. 2% reduced-fat Greek yogurt
- 4 tsp. lemon juice, divided
- 2 tbsp. olive oil, divided
- 1 1/8 tsp. kosher salt, divided
- 4 (6-ounce) salmon fillets
- 2 cups finely chopped carrots
- 1/2 tsp. black pepper, divided
- 2 tsp. minced garlic
- 1/4 cup minced shallots
- 1 cup hot cooked couscous

- 1/3 cup dry white wine

Directions:

1. Preheat the oven to 450 degrees. Combine the yogurt, chives, two tsp. of oil, and one tbsp. of juice and whisk together. Sprinkle 1/2 tsp. salt and 1/4 tsp. pepper over the fish. Rub with a mixture of 2 tsp. yogurt. Over high heat, heat an ovenproof skillet. To the pan, add one tsp. of oil. Add fish, side down on the skin; cook for 2 min. Turn to the oven. Bake for 5 min. at 450 °. Turn the fish over; cook for 1 min. or until ready.

2. Over medium-high prepare, prepare a skillet. To the tub, apply the remaining one tbsp. of oil. Add the carrots, shallots, and garlic; cook, occasionally stirring, for 4 min. Apply the remaining one tsp. of lemon juice, the remaining 5/8 of a tsp. of salt, 1/4 of a tsp. of pepper and wine. 30 seconds to cook. Stir in couscous; toss. Serve the fish with a combination of couscous and yogurt.

Nutrition: Calories 404 Satfat 2.7g Fat 17.9g Polyfat 5.1g Monofat 8.5g Carbohydrate 19g Protein 37g Cholesterol 94mg Fiber 3g Sodium 667mg Iron 2mg Sugars 4g Calcium 59mg Est. added sugars 0g

DAY 6

BREAKFAST

187. MEATBALLS AND PEPPERS IN GRAVY

Prep. Time: 20 Min. **Cooking Time**: 20 Min. **Servings**: 4

Ingredients

- 1 lb. 95% lean ground beef
- 2 tsp. Italian seasoning
- 1/4 cup onion, minced
- 12 oz. nonfat evaporated milk
- 1/2 tsp. pepper
- 2 tsp. olive oil
- 1/2 tsp. salt
- 1 red bell pepper, chopped
- 1 cup mushrooms, sliced
- 1 yellow bell pepper, chopped
- 3 garlic cloves, minced
- 1 summer squash, chopped
- 1.25 tbsp. whole wheat flour (substitute 1 tsp. cornstarch or arrowroot for low carb/Paleo/GF)

Directions:

1. Mix the onion, beef, salt, Italian seasoning, and pepper together. Consider adding 1⁄4-1 tsp, if you like heat—likewise, red pepper flakes.

2. Roll this mixture into 20 meatballs with a diameter of about 1 inch. Over medium flame heat the olive oil. Add the meatballs and cook until browned on all sides, for 4-5 min. Turn the heat down and continue to cook for 15 min. until it is cooked. Remove and set aside. Tent with foil to preserve the warmth.

3. Using the skillet to add the tomatoes, mushrooms, squash, and garlic. Cook until just tender, for 4-5 min.

4. Mix 1 tbsp. Of evaporated milk with the flour. Add and stir well into the pan.

5. Add the remaining evaporated milk and cook until the sauce is thick, for around 5-8 min.—season with salt and pepper. To mix everything, add the meatballs to the pan and stir.

Nutrition: Calories 280, Saturated Fat 3g, Polyunsaturated Fat 0g, Monounsaturated Fat 2g, Total Fat 8g, Sodium 472mg, Cholesterol 74mg, Dietary Fiber 2g, Sugars 13g, Total Carbohydrate 19g, Protein 33g.

LUNCH

188. HAM QUICHE WITH CHEESE

Prep Time: 10 min   **Cooking Time:** 30 min   **Servings:** 6

Ingredients:

- 8 eggs
- 1 cup Zucchini
- ½ cup Shredded heavy Cream
- 1 cup Ham, Diced
- 1 tsp. Mustard
- Salt – Dash.

Directions:

1. For this recipe, you can start off by prepping your stove to 375°F and getting out a pie plate for your quiche. Next, it is time to prep the zucchini. First, you will want to go ahead and shred it into small pieces. Once this is complete, take a paper towel and gently squeeze out the excess moisture. This will help avoid a soggy quiche.
2. When the step from above is complete, you will want to place the zucchini into your pie plate along with the cooked ham pieces and your cheese.
3. Once these items are in place, you will want to whisk the seasonings, cream, and eggs together before pouring it over the top.
4. Now that your quiche is set, you are going to pop the dish into your stove for about 40min.
5. By the end of this time, the egg should be cooked through, and you will be able to insert a knife into the center and have it come out clean.
6. If the quiche is cooked to your liking, take the dish from the oven and allow it to chill slightly before slicing and serving.

Nutrition: Calories 211 kcal Fats: 25 g Carbs: 2 g Proteins: 20 g.

DINNER

189. TANGY SHRIMP

Prep Time: 15 min   **Cooking Time**: 15 min   **Servings**: 2

Ingredients:

- 3 cloves Garlic
- ¼ cup Olive oil
- ½ lb. Jumbo shrimp
- 1 Lemon
- Cayenne pepper, to taste.

Directions:

1. Sauté the garlic and cayenne with the olive oil.
2. Peel and devein the shrimp.
3. Cook within 2 to 3 min. per side.
4. Put pepper, salt, and lemon wedges.
5. Use the rest of the garlic oil for a dipping sauce. Serve.

Nutrition: Calories: 335 kcal Carbs: 3 g Protein: 23 g Fats: 27 g.

DAY 7

BREAKFAST

190. CRUNCH BOWL WITH SALMON

Prep Time: 15 min   **Cooking Time**: 0 min   **Servings** 1

Ingredients

- 2 tbsp. matchstick-cut carrot
- 2/3 cup cooked quinoa
- 1 tsp. chopped dry-roasted peanuts
- 2 tbsp. steamed edamame
- 2 tbsp. chopped red bell pepper
- 3 ounces broiled salmon
- 1/4 cup shredded red cabbage

Sesame-Peanut Sauce:

- 1 tsp. lower-sodium soy sauce
- 1/2 tsp. fresh lime juice
- 1 tsp. creamy peanut butter
- 1/2 tsp. dark sesame oil
- 1/2 tsp. rice vinegar

Directions:

1. Top-cooked carrot quinoa, red bell pepper, edamame, salmon, and cabbage. Sprinkle peanuts on them.

2. Combine the peanut butter, soy sauce, vinegar, sesame oil, and lime juice in a small cup, stirring well. Spread over a mug.

Nutrition: Calories 397 Satfat 1.9g Fat 15.3g Polyfat 3.3g Monofat 4.3g Carbohydrate 34g Protein 31g Cholesterol 54mg Fiber 6g Sodium 302mg Iron 3mg Sugars 4g Calcium 59mg Est. Added Sugars 0g

---

LUNCH

191. CARNITAS TACOS WITH RED ONION

Prep Time: 1 Hours 30 Mins   **Cooking Time**: 25 Mins   **Servings** 6

Ingredients

- 1/2 tsp. grated orange rind
- 7 unpeeled garlic cloves
- 4 tsp. achiote paste
- 3 tbsp. fresh orange juice
- 1 3/4 tsp. kosher salt, divided
- 2 tbsp. plus 2 tsp. canola oil, divided
- 1 cup thinly sliced red onion (half-moons)

- 1 (1 1/2-pound) boneless pork shoulder, trimmed
- 1/4 cup cider vinegar
- 1/2 cup water
- 12 Fresh Corn Tortillas or packaged corn tortillas, warmed
- 2 tsp. light agave nectar or granulated sugar
- 3/4 cup Tomatillo Salsa

Directions:

1. Preheat the oven to 250 degrees.
2. Over medium heat, heat a large cast-iron skillet. Add garlic to the pan; cook 8 min. or until the skin is well charred, occasionally turning. Remove the cloves from the pan; cool and discard the skins for 5 min. In a mini chopper, combine the garlic, rind, juice, achiote paste, and two tsp. of oil; process until smooth.
3. Sprinkle the pork with one tsp. of salt. Brush the mixture of achiote evenly over the pork. In a medium Dutch oven or ovenproof saucepan, place the pork; cover and cook for 6 hours at 250 °. Take it out of the oven, and let stand for 30 min.
4. Place the onion in a medium bowl while the pork is cooking. In a saucepan over medium-high heat, mix 1/2 cup water, vinegar, agave, and the remaining 3/4 tsp. salt; bring to a boil, stirring until the salt dissolves. Pour a mixture of vinegar over the onion; stir. Cover the plastic wrap bowl; cool to room

temperature, rearranging to hold onion submerged as needed. Chill out for 1 hour, at least.

5. Put pork on a cutting board; shred with two forks. Discard any fat.
6. Over medium-high prepare, heat a large cast-iron skillet. In the pan, add two tbsp. of oil; swirl to coat. In an even layer, add 1 cup of shredded pork to the pan; cook for 3 min. or until a crust forms, turning once. Place the crispy pork on a plate. Repeat procedure with shredded pork remaining.
7. Place two warm tortillas on each of 6 plates. Add 1 1/2 ounces of crisped pork, one tbsp. of Tomatillo Salsa, and one tbsp. of pickled red onion to each tortilla.

Nutrition: Calories 390 Satfat 3.3g Fat 16.1g Polyfat 2.8g Monofat 7.7g Carbohydrate 35g Protein 27g Cholesterol 76mg Fiber 4g Sodium 593mg Iron 4mg Sugars 4g Calcium 88mg Est. added sugars 1g

DINNER

192. ASPARAGUS, HERB, AND PEA PASTA

Prep Time: 25 Mins   **Cooking Time**: 15 Mins   **Servings** 4

Ingredients

- 1 large garlic clove, thinly sliced
- 2 thin pancetta slices (about 5/8 ounce)
- 3 ounces 1/3-less-fat cream cheese (about 1/3 cup)
- 2/3 cup unsalted chicken stock
- 8 ounces uncooked pappardelle (wide ribbon pasta)
- 3 tbsp. mascarpone cheese
- 1/2 cup frozen green peas
- 1 1/2 cups (1-inch) asparagus pieces
- 1/4 tsp. freshly ground black pepper
- 1/2 tsp. kosher salt
- 1 tbsp. thinly sliced fresh chives
- 1 tbsp. chopped fresh flat-leaf parsley

Directions:

1. Place the pancetta over medium heat in a large skillet; cook for 6 min. or until the pancetta becomes crisp, stirring occasionally. Add the garlic; cook for 30 seconds, continuously stirring. Stock add; bring to a boil.
2. Lower the heat; simmer for 4 min. Add the cream cheese and mascarpone, stirring until smooth with a whisk. Strain sauce over a large bowl through a fine sieve. Solids to discard.
3. Cook pasta according to package instructions; salt and fat are omitted. For the last 2 min. of cooking, add the asparagus and peas; cook for 2 min. Then, drain. In a cup, apply the pasta mixture, salt, and black pepper to the sauce, toss to combine well. Using parsley and chives to sprinkle.

Nutrition: Calories 388 Satfat 5.8g Fat 12.3g Calcium 118mg Polyfat 1.3g Monofat 3g Carbohydrate 53g Protein 17g Cholesterol 61mg Fiber 7g Sodium 407mg Iron 7mg

CONCLUSIONS

The Mediterranean diet, often called the Mediterranean lifestyle, has been getting a lot of hype lately. More and more people are trying to eat healthier or simply starting to think about what they eat. Mediterranean diets, sometimes called the traditional Mediterranean diet or traditional lifestyle was initially designed for those who worked on farms. As surprising as it may be, there is not much difference between the Mediterranean diet and the Atkins diet. All three focus on eating healthy foods. The Mediterranean diet is based on the fact that food often contains more than one nutrient. Most fruits and vegetables have some fat: or sugar in them. The idea is to eat various foods from all parts of the world, which includes different types of meats, cheeses, grains, legumes, nuts, and other foods. In addition to being a great way to eat well naturally, the Mediterranean diet is good for your health. It has been shown to help with weight loss and cardiovascular disease prevention. It also promotes weight maintenance after weight loss. Studies have shown that it can reduce cholesterol levels in obese people and reduce blood pressure in people with hypertension. People with high cholesterol can have their grades lowered by following a Mediterranean diet. Studies have also shown that it can help fight cancer naturally, causing tumors to shrink faster than other dietary regimens.

The ketogenic diet is a diet that believes that by minimizing carbohydrates while maximizing the good fat in your system and making sure that you are getting the protein you need, that you will be happier and healthier. This book gives you the information to know what this diet is and describe its different types and areas. Most people assume that there is only one way to do it, and while there is one thing that the additional options share, there are four different options that you can choose. Each one has its unique benefits, and you should be familiar with each type to know what would be best for your body, which is why we've outlined them in the book so that you have the best possible information when starting this diet for yourself.

As many people are using this diet to their benefit, learning about food is one of the most significant parts of this, and it becomes easier once you start using this in your daily life. One of the best things you can do is pay attention to the food you are eating and how it affects your body and mind.

The Keto diet has been tried and tested for decades. It originated from a medical background to help patients with epilepsy. Many successful studies align with the knowledge that Keto works. Whether you are trying to diet for a month or a year, both are equally healthy for you. Keto is an adjustment, but it's an adjustment that will continue to benefit you for as long as you can maintain it.

This book has given you all the information you need to do this diet correctly and do it right. Use the knowledge in this book to get amazing recipes and learn directions for excellent meals for yourself.

Alexander Sandler, Elizabeth Roberts & Kristen Potter

CPSIA information can be obtained
at www.ICGtesting.com
Printed in the USA
BVHW051926270421
605944BV00008B/1915